Bayer-Symposium I

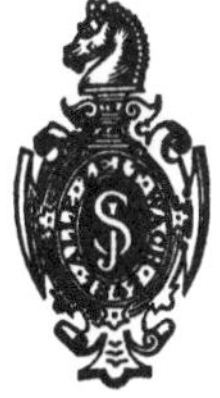

Current Problems in Immunology

Edited by

O. Westphal · H.-E. Bock · E. Grundmann

With 135 Figures

Springer-Verlag Berlin Heidelberg GmbH 1969

Professor Dr. Otto Westphal, Direktor des Max-Planck-Instituts für Immunbiologie,
7800 Freiburg-Zähringen
Professor Dr. Dr. h. c. Hans-Erhard Bock, Direktor der Medizinischen Klinik
der Universität, 7400 Tübingen
Professor Dr. Ekkehard Grundmann, Vorstand des Instituts für experimentelle Pathologie
der Farbenfabriken Bayer AG, 5600 Wuppertal-Elberfeld

Bayer-Symposium I
held at Grosse Ledder near Cologne, Germany
October 11th—13th, 1968

ISBN 978-3-662-27746-1   ISBN 978-3-662-29237-2 (eBook)
DOI 10.1007/978-3-662-29237-2

Contents

B. Clinical Part
(Moderator H.-E. BOCK, Tübingen)

List of Participants

Priv.-Doz. Dr. F.-W. Aly, Medizinische Universitätsklinik, 74 Tübingen, Olfried-Müller-Straße

Prof. Dr. E. Auhagen, Biochemisches Labor der Farbenfabriken Bayer AG, 56 Wuppertal-Elberfeld

Dr. K. Bauer, Biochemisches Labor der Farbenfabriken Bayer AG, 56 Wuppertal-Elberfeld

Prof. Dr. H. Begemann, I. Medizinische Abteilung des Städtischen Krankenhauses München-Schwabing, 8 München 23, Kölner Platz 1

Prof. Dr. Dr. h. c. H.-E. Bock, Medizinische Klinik der Universität, 74 Tübingen, Olfried-Müller-Straße

Priv.-Doz. Dr. H. Deicher, Medizinische Klinik der Medizinischen Hochschule Hannover im Krankenhaus Oststadt, 3 Hannover, Podbielskistraße 380

Prof. Dr. R. Drzeniek, Institut für Virologie der Veterinärmedizinischen Fakultät der Universität, 63 Gießen, Frankfurter Straße 87

Prof. Dr. H. Fischer, Max-Planck-Institut für Immunbiologie, 78 Freiburg-Zähringen, Stübeweg 51

Prof. Dr. K. Fischer, Abteilung für Klinische Immunpathologie, Universitäts-Kinderklinik und -Poliklinik, Universitäts-Krankenhaus Eppendorf, 2 Hamburg 20, Martinistraße 52

Dr. A. Freis, Abteilung Klinische Forschung, Farbenfabriken Bayer AG, 56 Wuppertal-Elberfeld

Dr. H. Götze, Springer-Verlag, 69 Heidelberg 1, Neuenheimer Landstraße 28—30

Prof. Dr. E. Grundmann, Institut für experimentelle Pathologie der Farbenfabriken Bayer AG, 56 Wuppertal-Elberfeld

Priv.-Doz. Dr. D. Hammer, Max-Planck-Institut für Immunbiologie, 78 Freiburg-Zähringen, Stübeweg 51

Priv.-Doz. Dr. W. Hartl, Medizinische Universitätsklinik, 74 Tübingen, Olfried-Müller-Straße

Prof. Dr. F. Hartmann, Medizinische Klinik der Medizinischen Hochschule Hannover im Krankenhaus Oststadt, 3 Hannover, Podbielskistraße 380

Prof. Dr. M. Hasek, Institut für experimentelle Biologie und Genetik, Tschechoslowakische Akademie der Wissenschaften, Prag, ČSSR

Prof. Dr. F. Haurowitz, Indiana University, Department of Chemistry, Chemistry Building, Bloomington, Indiana 47401, USA

Dr. N. Hilschmann, Max-Planck-Institut für experimentelle Medizin, Abteilung Chemie, Arbeitsgruppe Immunchemie, 34 Göttingen, Hermann-Rein-Straße 3

Dr. H. P. Hobik, Institut für experimentelle Pathologie der Farbenfabriken Bayer AG, 56 Wuppertal-Elberfeld

Prof. Dr. P. Klein, Institut für Medizinische Mikrobiologie der Universität, 65 Mainz, Langenbeckstraße 1

Dr. K. Lauenstein, Institut für experimentelle Pathologie der Farbenfabriken Bayer AG, 56 Wuppertal-Elberfeld

Prof. Dr. E. Macher, Hautklinik der Universität, 78 Freiburg i. Br., Hauptstraße 7

Prof. Dr. H. J. Müller-Eberhard, Department of Experimental Pathology, Scripps Clinic and Research Foundation, 476 Prospect Street, La Jolla, California 92307, USA

Prof. Dr. J. Oehme, Kinderklinik des Krankenhauses Holwedestraße, 33 Braunschweig, Holwedestraße 16

Prof. Dr. H. F. Oettgen, Sloan-Kettering Institute for Cancer Research, 410 East 68th Street, New York, N.Y. 10021, USA

Prof. Dr. H. Popper, Mount Sinai School of Medicine of the City University of New York, Fifth Avenue and 100th Street, New York, N.Y. 10029, USA

Prof. Dr. K. Rajewsky, Institut für Genetik der Universität, 5 Köln-Lindenthal, Weyertal 121

Priv.-Doz. Dr. D. Ricken, Medizinische Universitätsklinik für Innere- und Nervenkrankheiten, 53 Bonn, Venusberg

Dr. G. Riethmüller, Medizinische Klinik der Universität, 74 Tübingen, Olfried-Müller-Straße

Prof. Dr. I. M. Roitt, Department of Immunology, Arthur Stanley House, The Middlesex Hospital Medical School, London, W. 1, England

Prof. Dr. K. O. Rother, Max-Planck-Institut für Immunbiologie, 78 Freiburg-Zähringen, Stübeweg 51

Prof. Dr. H. Schubothe, Abteilung für klinische Immunpathologie der Medizinischen Universitätsklinik, 78 Freiburg i. Br., Hugstetter-Straße 55

Dr. H. G. Schwick, Behringwerke AG, 355 Marburg/Lahn

Dr. C. P. Sodomann, Pathologisches Institut der Universität, 53 Bonn, Venusberg

Prof. Dr. G. F. Springer, Department of Immunochemistry Research, Evanston Hospital, Northwestern University, 2650 Ridge Avenue, Evanston, Illinois 60201, USA

Prof. Dr. K. O. Vorlaender, Innere Abteilung des Luisenhospitals, 51 Aachen, Boxgraben 99

Prof. Dr. R. L. Walford, University of California, Department of Pathology, School of Medicine, The Center for the Health Sciences, Los Angeles, California 90024, USA

Priv.-Doz. Dr. H. Warnatz, Abteilung für klinische Immunologie des Universitäts-Krankenhauses Erlangen-Nürnberg, 852 Erlangen, Krankenhausstraße 12

Priv.-Doz. Dr. A. L. de Weck, Dermatologische Universitäts-Klinik, Abteilung für Allergie und klinische Immunologie, 3008 Bern, Schweiz, Inselspital

Priv.-Doz. Dr. H. J. Wellensiek, Institut für Medizinische Mikrobiologie der Universität, 65 Mainz, Langenbeckstraße 1

Prof. Dr. O. Westphal, Max-Planck-Institut für Immunbiologie, 78 Freiburg-Zähringen, Stübeweg 51

Opening Remarks

E. Grundmann

Gentlemen:

May I welcome you to our Symposium. During the next 3 days we shall have ample opportunity to discuss questions of mutual interest. I thank you all for coming, and am particularly grateful to those who have made a long journey from neighbouring countries or even from overseas.

I would like to pay special tribute to Professor Westphal with whom I share an affection for Freiburg, and to Professor Bock my clinical tutor. Both gentlemen have contributed in considerable measure to the preparation of this symposium and furthermore have agreed to act as moderators.

First of all, allow me to say a few words about our surroundings. Until 1908 Große Ledder was a typical village of the Bergische Land with about 100 inhabitants, a farm house and a manor house. Both are still in good repair and we will be dining in the former.

"Ledder" means roughly a "Ladder" in the sense of a slope or steep pathway. The house in which we are at present is also situated on a slope — which is as it should be since the area here has the reputation of being "buckliges Land" as the Cologne people would say. Here one must count on an uphill grind, which is typical of scientific work. Today Große Ledder is a convalescent and holiday home of Farbenfabriken Bayer and we are grateful to the management for putting almost the entire area at our disposal for these 3 days.

In contrast to the other guests, we are not here on holiday but to discuss some problems of immunology. This title is rather comprehensive and yet at the same time compact in that we have excluded anything related to tumor immunology and transplant rejection, even though these two fields are topical. We wish to concentrate entirely on so-called immune diseases. Under the concept of 'immune diseases' we understand here all those diseases in which immunological mechanisms are either in the foreground or play a decisive role. Even here discrimination is necessary. We intend to restrict ourselves to the immunological diseases of the blood and the immunology of chronic hepatitis, glomerulonephritis, some thyroid diseases, rheumatism and cardiovascular diseases. Naturally, with a choice of this kind, drug allergy cannot be excluded.

A prerequisite for any discussion on these clinical questions is a knowledge of immunological processes as such. The simple rule that an antigen evokes the formation of an antibody and is therewith neutralized belongs to the past.

The more we deal with the subject, the more complicated become the relationships and processes involved.

The definition of an antigen is complex enough but even more so the question of structure and mode of formation of antibodies. The distinction between humoral and cell-bound antibodies has now been accepted as a working hypothesis. Both types are being related to different cell systems — with plasma cells and with lymphocytes. The lymphatic reactions associated with the responses of the "delayed type" are proving more and more important for an understanding of clinical pictures, which in the past we have been unable to classify. The so-called autoimmune diseases are only one form. Among the humoral factors, the complement system is playing an ever increasing role, and for this reason we have placed discussions on this topic at the beginning of the symposium.

Everywhere we are gaining new knowledge and meeting new problems. We are all agreed that there is still much to learn, both from our own experiments and observations, and from those of others who already know more in their own field. Therefore, clinicians are learning from the basic findings of the theorists, and the latter from the experience and findings of the clinicians at the bedside. The main purpose of this symposium is to bring together these two groups, and if we are sitting somewhat close together here in this room then this can be taken as a paradigma.

And now: let's beginn!

A. Theoretical Part

Moderator: O. Westphal, Freiburg

Bayer-Symposium I, 5—15 (1969)

Destruction of Complement-Target Cell Complexes by Mononuclear Leukocytes[1,2]

HANS J. MÜLLER-EBERHARD, PETER PERLMANN, HEDVIG PERLMANN, and JORGE A. MANNI[3]

With 6 Figures

There are two primary mechanisms by which biological membranes may sustain irreversible damage in the course of immune reactions, one involving lymphocytes, the other humoral factors. Damage of membranes by sensitized mononuclear cells usually does not require participation of serum factors such as complement; and membrane damage by antibody and complement occurs without participation of cells. In the following, preliminary experiments will be reported which point out the existence of an additional mode of membrane damage in

Table 1. *In vitro models of mononuclear leukocyte-induced cell damage*

1. Sensitized Lymphocyte (a) + Target Cell (a).
2. Sensitized Lymphocyte (b) + Antigen (b) + Target Cell (a).
3. Normal Lymphocyte + Antibody (a) + Target Cell (a).
4. Normal Lymphocyte + PHA + Target Cell.
5. Monocyte + Antibody (a) + Target Cell (a).

which non-sensitized mononuclear leukocytes and complement appear to cooperate. The early part of this work has been presented previously [1].

The known *in vitro* models of cell damage induced by mononuclear leukocytes are listed in Table 1. The classical system consists of lymphocytes sensitized to an antigen (a) and target cells which carry (a) as a natural constituent on their surface [2]. Lymphocytes sensitized to an antigen (b), not naturally occurring on the surface of target cells, also produce damage if the antigen is coupled *in vitro* to the target cell [3]. Normal lymphocytes are able to kill target cells, provided an antibody directed to a target cell surface antigen is added to the system [3]. In this situation, the antibody combines with the target cell and apparently links it to a lymphocyte through sites in the Fc portion which have an affinity for lymphocyte

[1] This is publication number 324 from the Department of Experimental Pathology, Scripps Clinic and Research Foundation, La Jolla, California.

[2] This work was supported by United States Public Health Service Grant AI-07007, American Heart Association, Inc. Grant 68-666 and United States Atomic Energy Commission Contract AT (04-3)-730.

[3] Dr. Manni is supported by United States Public Health Service Training Grant No. 5TIGM683.

6   H. J. Müller-Eberhard, P. Perlmann, H. Perlmann, and J. A. Manni

receptors. A similar mechanism is operative in the attack of target cells by monocytes, which is mediated through γG type antibody to target cell surface antigens
[4, 5]. Finally, an apparently non-immunologic system has been described in
which normal lymphocytes are induced to kill non-sensitized target cells through
the action of phytohemagglutinin [6]. All of these systems are believed to function
independently of serum complement and by a non-phagocytic mechanism. The
precise nature of the mode of cytotoxic action of mononuclear leukocytes is unknown. Some investigators postulate that damage is produced by intimate contact
between aggressor and target cell. Others have cited evidence for the production
of cytotoxic factors by the aggressor cells [7, 8].

Membrane damage by antidody and complement is a complex process [9] which
is schematically summarized in Fig. 1. In brief, following attachment of specific
antibody to an antigen on the surface of a target cell, the cytolytic complement
reaction is triggered by activation of the first component, C1[4]. This component
consists of a calcium dependent complex of three proteins called C1q, C1r and C1s.
Through its C1q subunit, the complex is enabled to bind reversibly to antibody on
the target cell surface. Binding leads to activation of the C1s subunit. Activated
C1 exhibits esterase activity and represents the activating enzyme for C2 and C4.
The latter two components constitute the precursors for the complex enzyme C3
convertase which is assembled on the cell surface in two steps. First, C4 is cleaved
into two fragments, C4a and C4b, and the latter, which is the larger fragment, is
enabled to bind to membrane receptors. Second, C2 is cleaved into the fragments
C2a and C2b. Again, the larger of the two pieces (C2a) is bound to the cell surface,
the acceptor being C4b and thus the complex $\overline{\text{C4b, 2a}}$ is formed. Through its
enzymatic activity (C3 convertase) the complex cleaves C3 into C3a and C3b, and
C3b is then bound to the target cell. Whereas C3a possesses anaphylatoxin and chemotactic activity, binding of C3b to the $\overline{\text{C4b, 2a}}$ sites gives rise to C3 dependent
peptidase activity. It is through the action of this enzyme that C5, 6, 7 are activated and enabled to interact with membrane receptors. In the course of this reaction,
C5 is cleaved into the fragments C5a and C5b and anaphylatoxin and chemotactic
activity are generated which reside in the small C5a fragment. Unbound, cytoly-
tically inactive C5, 6, 7 remaining in the fluid phase and forming a reversible
complex constitute the third chemotactic factor derived from the complement
system. Following binding of C8 to the target cell, membrane damage becomes
evident through slow, low grade lysis of the cells. Lysis is accelerated through the
action of the terminal component C9.

In view of the apparent distinctness of the two known mechanisms of immunologic membrane damage, the question was asked whether there might be an additional type of cell damage in which mononuclear leukocytes and complement
participate in a cooperative manner. In this connection, phagocytosis was not
considered a form of direct cell damage. Chicken erythrocytes which were freshly
obtained by cardiac puncture were used as target cells. The cells were sensitized
with four hemolysin units of 19S antibody to boiled stromata of sheep erythrocytes
[10]. Complexes of target cells (E), antibody (A) and complement (C) were prepared as decribed previously using chemically and functionally purified human

---

[4] Symbols and terms are those recommended by the W.H.O. Committee on Complement
Nomenclature, Boston, 1968.

complement components [11—15]. The following intermediate complexes were utilized in this study: EA; EAC1, 4; EAC1, 4, 2; EAC1, 4, 2, 3; and EAC1, 4, 2, 3, 5, 6, 7. The complement complexes will be referred to as C4-cells, C2-cells, C3-cells and C7-cells, according to the component with which the cells have

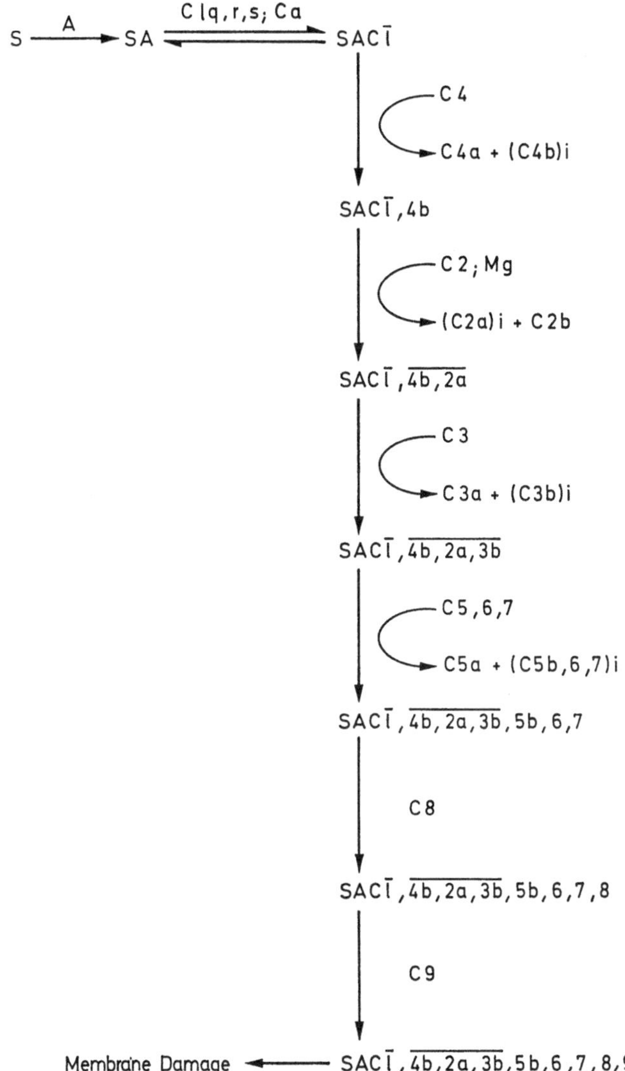

Fig. 1. Schematic description of membrane damage by complement triggered by anti membrane antibody, showing the intermediate reaction products and by-products [9]. S denotes an antigenic site on membrane surface; A, a molecule of 19 S antibody directed to S; the bars designate enzymes which are indigenous to the complement system: $\overline{\text{C1}}$, C1-esterase; $\overline{\text{C4b, 2a}}$, C3 convertase; $\overline{\text{C4b, 2a, 3b}}$, C3-dependent peptidase. Physical attachment of complement components to the cell surface has been demonstrated for all except C6 and C7. Binding of components is quite strong, except that of C1 which is readily reversible. Membrane damage becomes demonstrable following uptake of C8. Manifestation of damage is greatly accelerated by C9

Table 2. *Lysis of complement-chicken erythrocyte complexes by complement components and by two different fetal calf serum preparations*

	C2—9	C3—9	C5—9	C8, 9	FCS[a] (56°, 90′)	FCS Fraction
EAC1, 4	100[b]	—	—	—	0	0
EAC1, 4, 2[c]	—	100	—	—	0	0
EAC1, 4, 2, 3	—	—	100	—	0	0
EAC1, 4, 2, 3, 5, 6, 7	—	—	—	95	35	0

[a] Fetal calf serum (5%, v/v).

[b] Numbers indicate per cent lysis of 3×10^7 cells in 30 min at 32°.

[c] C2 was used exclusively in oxidized form.

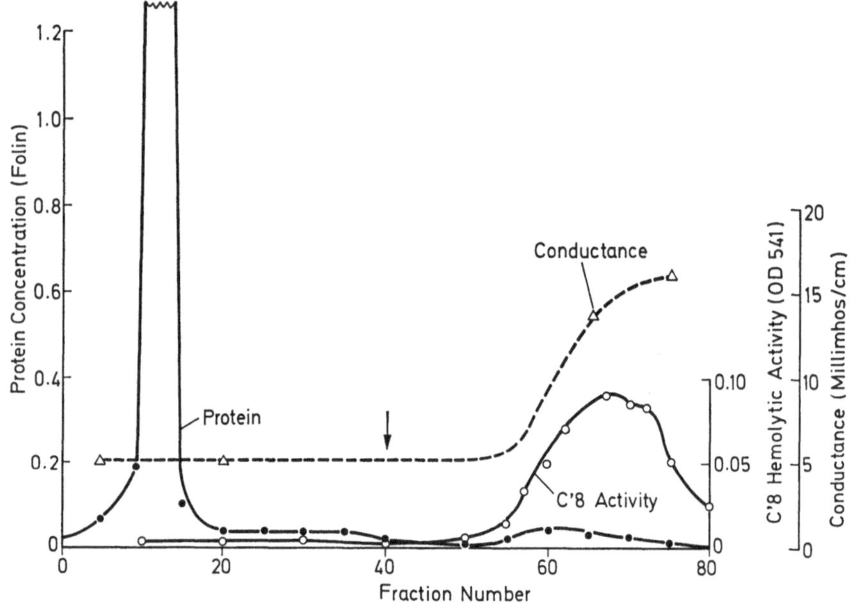

Fig. 2. Preparation of C8- and C9-depleted fetal calf serum (FCS) by chromatography for supplementation of culture medium. Twenty-five ml of FCS was dialyzed against starting buffer and applied to a 45×9.5 cm column of carboxymethyl cellulose equilibrated with phosphate buffer, pH 6.0, $\mu = 0.1$. The flow rate was 1 ml per minute and fractions of 15 ml were collected. More than 95% of the protein was eluted in the first 18 fractions. After passage through the column of 600 ml buffer, residual protein and C8 and C9 were eluted by a sodium chloride solution in starting buffer having a conductance of 28 millimhos per cm. C9 activity (not shown) had a similar distribution as C8 activity. The first 20 fractions were pooled, concentrated to 25 ml, dialyzed against 0.15 M NaCl, sterilized and heated for 90 min at 56°

reacted last[5]. The cells were labeled with [51]Chromium (^{51}Cr) by incubation of 0.1 ml of 1.5×10^8 cells/ml in Tris buffered (pH 7.8) Hank's balanced salt solution with an equal volume of 50 to 100 μc of ^{51}Cr-sodium chromate for 30 min at 37°.

---

[5] C4-cells contained 6000 to 8000 C4 molecules per cell on their surface, C2-cells contained, in addition, an equal number of oxyC2. C3-cells were prepared from C2-cells and carried 5000 to 25000 bound C3 molecules per cell.

They were washed and suspended in Parker's medium 199. Mononuclear leukocytes were obtained by sedimentation of defibrinated human blood through gelatin [16]. They were washed and suspended in Parker's medium 199 supplemented with a fetal calf serum fraction. The leukocyte preparations obtained by this method consisted of approximately 75% lymphocytes, the rest being large monocytes and polymorphonuclear leukocytes. Monocyte-rich preparations of leukocytes were obtained by flotation in 30% albumin according to the method of Bennett and

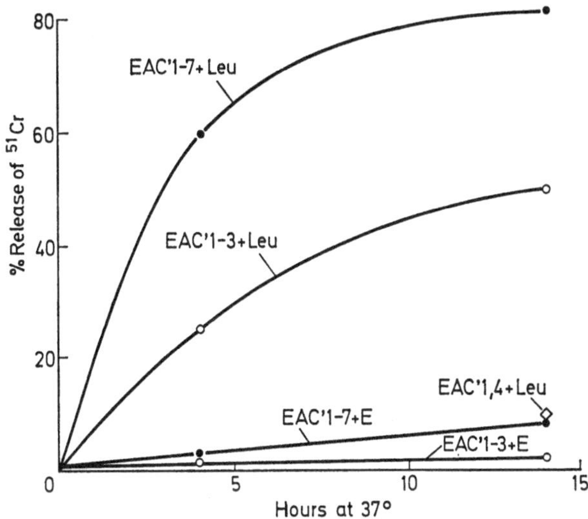

Fig. 3. Damage of complement-target cell complexes by a lymphocyte-enriched preparation of leukocytes from peripheral human blood. Target cells consisted of chicken erythrocytes which were treated with rabbit 19S antibody to boiled sheep erythrocyte stromata and with purified human complement components to obtain the indicated intermediate complexes. They were labeled with ^{51}Cr and cell damage was quantitated by measuring the proportion of radioactivity released into the medium. Thirty-eight % of the leukocyte preparation consisted of polymorphonuclear leukocytes and monocytes, the rest of small lymphocytes. The reaction mixtures contained 1×10^5 target cells, 4×10^6 leukocytes (Leu) or 1×10^7 unlabeled and untreated chicken erythrocytes (E). The reaction volume was 1.5 ml and Parker's medium 199 was used supplemented with 5% heated fetal calf serum previously depleted of C8 and C9 by chromatography. All tests were performed in duplicates, each value representing the mean of two determinations

Cohn [17]. These preparations consisted of 80% monocytes and approximately 20% small lymphocytes and they were virtually free of polymorphonuclear leukocytes. Purified lymphocytes were prepared according to Rabinowitz [18] by passage of lymphocyte-enriched leukocytes through a column of small glass beads. 0.5 ml of the various leukocyte preparations containing 2 to 4×10^6 viable cells and 0.5 ml of ^{51}Cr-labeled erythrocyte-complement complexes (1×10^5 cells) were mixed and incubated in duplicates under sterile conditions. In controls, the leukocytes were replaced by 10^6 untreated and unlabeled chicken erythrocytes. Target cell damage was detected and quantitated by measuring the release of ^{51}Cr into the fluid phase. Since some of the label was bound to cell membranes and nuclei, release of 80% of the radioactivity corresponded to 100% cell lysis.

Initially, the tissue culture medium was supplemented by 5% heat inactivated fetal calf serum. As shown in Table 2, column 5, this concentration of fetal calf serum caused lysis of C7-cells, even after heating at 56° for 90 min. This observation indicated that heating did not completely abolish the activities of C8 and C9. By a simple chromatographic technique, C8 and C9 were therefore eliminated from fetal calf serum, as shown in Fig. 2. Twenty-five ml of serum was applied to a 45×9.5 cm column of carboxymethyl cellulose, which was equilibrated with phosphate buffer, pH 6.0, $\mu = 0.1$. Under these conditions C8 and C9 were adsorbed to the cellulose, while 98% of the serum protein was eluted with the starting buffer. The eluted protein was concentrated by pressure dialysis to 25 ml, dialyzed against 0.15 M sodium chloride, passed through a bacterial filter and heated for

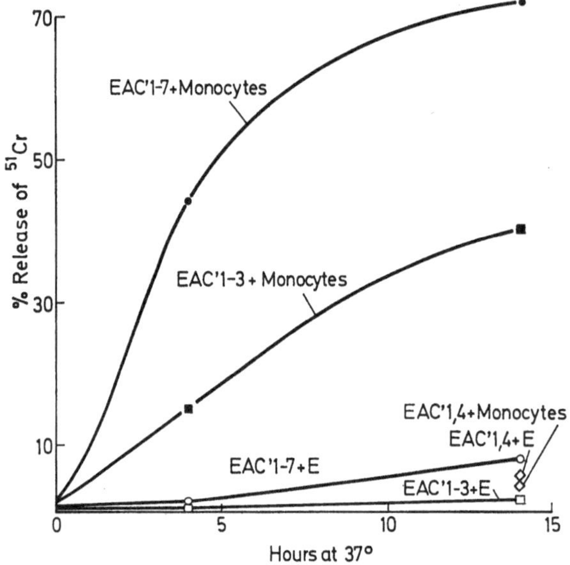

Fig. 4. Damage of complement-target cell complexes by a preparation of monocytes obtained from peripheral human blood. The isolated monocytes were essentially free of polymorphonuclear leukocytes, however, contained approximately 15% small lymphocytes. Experimental details were as described in the legend to Fig. 3, except that the number of monocytes per reaction mixture was 3×10^6

90 min at 56°. As seen in Table 2, column 6, this material did not cause detectable lysis of any of the target cell complexes used. The C8 and C9 depleted fetal calf serum was used in a final concentration of 5% (v/v) in all experiments to supplement the tissue culture medium.

Incubation of target cells with an excess of lymphocyte-enriched leukocytes led to release of ^{51}Cr from C3-cells and C7-cells but not from antibody coated cells, C2-cells and C4-cells. It is emphasized that in none of these experiments positive reactions were observed with the 19S antibody coated cells. The kinetic analysis of this reaction is shown in Fig. 3. C7-cells released the radioactive label with a greater velocity and to a greater extent than C3-cells, the reaction with C7-cells approaching completion after 5 h. Similar results were obtained in eight analogous experiments. Since these preparations of leukocytes contained varying numbers of polymorphonuclear leukocytes (20 to 35%), participation of this type of cell in the observed target cell destruction could not be ruled out. In the following, leukocyte preparations were utilized which were essentially free of polymorphs.

Fig. 4 shows the results of a kinetic experiment in which a monocyte-rich white cell preparation was used which contained approximately 25% small lymphocytes and less than 1% polymorphonuclear leukocytes. Again, a rapid release of ^{51}Cr from C7-cells was observed and a less rapid and extensive release from C3-cells. In contrast, C4-cells were unaffected by the monocytes. Three analogous experiments gave comparable results.

The effect of purified small lymphocytes on complement target cell complexes is shown in Fig. 5, which depicts the results of one of eight similar experiments.

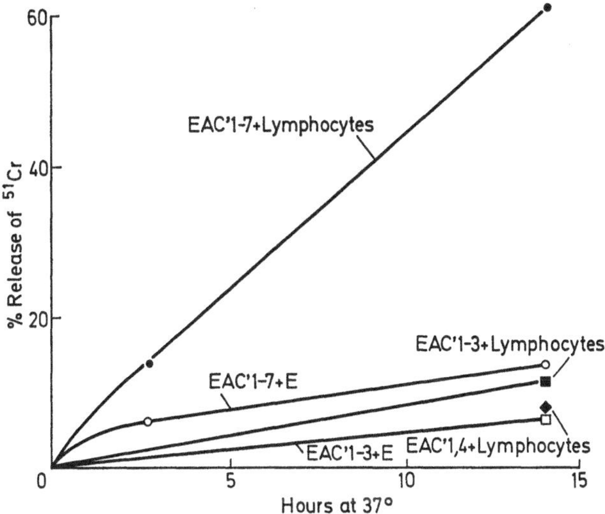

Fig. 5. Damage of complement-target cell complexes by purified lymphocytes isolated from peripheral human blood. The lymphocyte preparation was contaminated with human erythrocytes but was essentially devoid of polymorphs and monocytes. Experimental details were as described in the legend to Fig. 3, except that the number of lymphocytes per reaction mixture was 8×10^6

Unlike the previously used two types of white cell preparations, purified lymphocytes had very little, if any, effect on C3-cells. However, they caused extensive release of ^{51}Cr from C7-cells. With respect to velocity and specificity, the action of purified lymphocytes on C7-cells resembled that of C8 from human serum. Since the lymphocytes were contaminated with human erythrocytes, the possibility existed that the red cells carried on their surface small amounts of C8 which were released during incubation with target cells. This possibility, however, was ruled out by showing that a large excess of human erythrocytes, which were free of white cells, did not cause lysis of C7-cells (Table 3).

An attempt was made to assess the extent to which phagocytosis might contribute to the observed target cell damage. If phagocytosis occurred, it was expected that the radioactive label of the target cells would be found inside the phagocytic cells, at least in the early periods of incubation. Therefore, after 3 h of incubation with purified lymphocytes and with lymphocyte-enriched leukocytes, respectively, the cell mixtures were centrifuged and the cell free medium was removed. The cells were then treated for 30 sec with distilled water, following which isotonicity was re-established. In another experiment the sedimented cells were resuspended and incubated in a dilution of serum obtained from the human blood donor from whom the white cells were derived. Both treatments were expected to affect the target cells outside white cells but not those inside phagocytic cells at the time of treatment. The unlysed cells were separated from the medium by centrifugation and the distribution of radioactivity was determined. As shown in Table 4, the amount of ^{51}Cr which could not be released from the cells by these measures was small. It was therefore concluded that the proportion of target cells found inside phagocytic

Table 3. *Comparison of effect of erythrocytes (E) and lymphocytes on complement-target cell complexes*

^{51}Cr-Target cells	Per cent release of ^{51}Cr		
	Human E	Chicken E	Lymphocytes
EAC1—3	4	4	8
EAC1—7	8	7	43

Number of target cells: 1×10^5
Human E: 2×10^8
Chicken E: 3×10^7
Lymphocytes: 4×10^6

Table 4. *Role of phagocytosis in leukocyte-dependent damage of complement-target cell complexes*

	% ^{51}Cr released in 3 h incubation with		% residual ^{51}Cr released by H$_2$O	
	Leu.	Ly.	Leu.	Ly.
EAC1, 4	1	0.5	104	104
EAC1—3	18	3	95	97
EAC1—7	56	25	100	104

E: Labeled with ^{51}Cr   Leu.: 20% PMN   Ly.: 0.5% PMN

cells after 3 h of incubation was minimal and that therefore phagocytosis did not play a major role in the mechanism of target cell destruction.

In order to ascertain whether the cytolytic effect required metabolically active aggressor cells, the effect of anti-metabolites on damage of C7-cells by purified lymphocytes was investigated. As shown in Table 5, pretreatment of lymphocytes with actinomycin D or antimycin A caused definite inhibition of the cytolytic capacity of these cells. In contrast, puromycin in the concentration tested had no effect in this particular experiment. It was concluded that the cells had to be intact with respect to their energy generating mechanism.

If target cell damage was dependent on direct contact with the aggressor cells, sonicated white cells should not exhibit cytolytic activity. It was found, however, that following disintegration of purified lymphocytes and removal of cellular debris by ultracentrifugation (50,000 r.p.m., 45 min) an active principle was present in free solution. As shown in Fig. 6, approximately 35% of the cytolytic activity of intact lymphocytes was liberated by sonication of an identical number of cells. The activity was destroyed by heating at 56° for 30 min. The soluble factor acted only on C7-cells and not on C3-cells or untreated chicken erythrocytes. It is thus not a general cytotoxic factor but a factor of limited and specific function which resembles C8. Preliminary exploration of the molecular size of this material

Table 5. *Effect of anti-metabolites on damage of EAC1—7 by lymphocytes*

Inhibitor	Concentration	% inhibition after 4 h incubation
Puromycin[a]	20 µg/ml	0
Actinomycin D[b]	10 µg/ml	40
Antimycin A3[b]	10^{-5} M	100

[a] Present during reaction.
[b] Lymphocytes pretreated for 45 min at 37°.

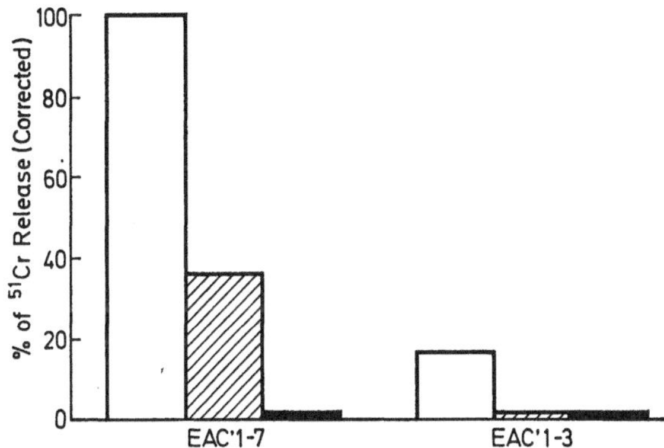

Fig. 6. Damage of EAC1—7 cells by intact and sonically disintegrated, purified lymphocytes. For comparison, the effect on EAC1—3 cells is also shown. 1×10^5 target cells were incubated at 37° for 15 h in a total reaction volume of 1.5 ml containing 5×10^6 intact lymphocytes (white bars) or the soluble material from the same number of lymphocytes (gray bars) obtained by sonication (30 sec at 0°) and subsequent removal of cellular debris (50,000 r.p.m., 30 min). The soluble lymphocyte constituents were also tested following heating at 56° for 30 min (black bars). Target cell damage was expressed in per cent release of ^{51}Cr by intact lymphocytes. ☐ intact; ▨ sonicated; ■ sonicated and heated

by Sephadex filtration suggests that it is intermediate to that of albumin and of γG-globulin.

The underlying mechanism of the observed cytolytic phenomena is not readily explained. Obviously, monocytes and lymphocytes exert their cell damaging effects in different ways, as indicated by the differential susceptibility of target cell complexes to their action. Monocytes are known to contain on their surface sites through which they can interact with the third component of complement bound to other cells [19, 20]. The ability of monocytes to attack C3-cells may well depend on this C3 specific receptor. Although monocytes are capable of phagocytosis, the manner in which they impaired C3-cells under the conditions employed in this study does not seem to be primarily phagocytic. Others have previously reported a cell damaging capacity of monocytes which is non-phagocytic [4, 5] and which depended on the presence of γG type antibody directed to target cell antigens. The reactions described in this paper are different in that they do not involve γG type antibody. Although a certain percentage of lymphocytes also have been found to possess sites capable of interacting with bound C3 [20], purified lymphocytes lacked the ability to attack C3-cells. Their marked effect on C7-cells may well be a function of the soluble factor which could be liberated by sonication, although this remains to be demonstrated. One possible explanation of the nature of the soluble lymphocyte factor is that it is identical with C8 of the complement system. If this hypothesis were correct, C8 would either be synthesized by mononuclear leukocytes or specifically carried on their surface. The lymphocyte factor resembled C8 purified from human serum [21] in thermolability, behavior on Sephadex filtration and specificity of action. Alternatively, the cytolytic factor is chemically distinct from C8, sharing with it only functional characteristics. Further work is needed to distinguish between these two alternatives and to cast light on the molecular processes through which monocytes and lymphocytes damage complement coated target cells.

Acknowledgment

The authors wish to express their gratitude to Miss Susan Muench for dedicated and skillful technical assistance.

References

1. Perlmann, P., H. Perlmann, H. J. Müller-Eberhard, and J. A. Manni: Cytotoxic effects of leukocytes triggered by complement bound to target cells. Science (1969) (in press).
2. Wilson, D. B., and R. E. Billingham: Lymphocytes and transplantation immunity. Advanc. Immunol. 7, 189 (1967).
3. Perlmann, P., and G. Holm: Studies on the mechanism of lymphocyte cytotoxicity. In: Mechanism of inflammation induced by immune reactions, p. 325, Miescher, P. A., and P. Grabar, Eds. Basel: Schwabe and Co. 1968.
4. LoBuglio, L., R. S. Cotran, and J. H. Jandl: Red cells coated with immunoglobulin G: Binding and sphering by mononuclear cells in man. Science 158, 1582 (1967).
5. Granger, G. A., and R. S. Weiser: Homograft target cells: Contact destruction *in vitro* by immune macrophages. Science 151, 97 (1966).
6. Holm, G., and P. Perlmann: Cytotoxic potential of stimulated human lymphocytes. J. exp. Med. 125, 721 (1967).
7. Ruddle, N. H., and B. H. Waksman: Cytotoxicity mediated by soluble antigen and lymphocytes in delayed hypersensitivity. III. Analysis of mechanism. J. exp. Med. 128, 1267 (1968).
8. Kolb, W. P., and G. A. Granger: A cell free cytotoxic factor produced by lymphoid cells during mutual *in vitro* aggressor lymphoid cell-target cell destruction. Fed. Proc. 27, 687 (1968).
9. Müller-Eberhard, H. J.: Complement. Ann. Rev. Biochem. Vol. 38 (1969) (in press).
10. Mayer, M. M.: Complement and complement fixation. In: Experimental immunochemistry, p. 133. Kabat, E. A., and M. M. Mayer, Eds. Springfield (Illinois): Charles C. Thomas 1961.
11. Cooper, N. R., and H. J. Müller-Eberhard: A comparison of methods for the molecular quantitation of the fourth component of human complement. Immunochemistry 5, 155 (1968).

12. Polley, M. J., and H. J. Müller-Eberhard: The second component of human complement: Its isolation, fragmentation by C1 esterase, and incorporation into C3 convertase. J. exp. Med. **128**, 533 (1968).
13. Müller-Eberhard, H. J., A. P. Dalmasso, and M. A. Calcott: The reaction mechanism of β_{1C}-globulin (C'3) in immune hemolysis. J. exp. Med. **123**, 33 (1966).
14. Nilsson, U. R., and H. J. Müller-Eberhard: Isolation of β_{1F}-globulin from human serum and its characterization as the fifth component of complement. J. exp. Med. **122**, 277 (1965).
15. — — Studies on the mode of action of the fifth, sixth and seventh component of human complement in immune haemolysis. Immunology **13**, 101 (1967).
16. Holm, G., and P. Perlmann: Quantitative studies on phytohemagglutinin-induced cytotoxicity by human lymphocytes against homologous cells in tissue culture. Immunology **12**, 525 (1967).
17. Bennett, W. E., and Z. A. Cohn: The isolation and selected properties of blood monocytes. J. exp. Med. **123**, 145 (1966).
18. Rabinowitz, Y.: Separation of lymphocytes, polymorphonuclear leukocytes and monocytes on glass columns, including tissue culture observations. Blood **23**, 811 (1964).
19. Huber, H., M. J. Polley, W. D. Linscott, H. H. Fudenberg, and H. J. Müller-Eberhard: Human monocytes: Distinct receptor sites for the third component of complement and for immunoglobulin G. Science **162**, 1281 (1968).
20. Lay, W. H., and V. Nussenzweig: Receptors for complement on leukocytes. J. exp. Med. **128**, 991 (1968).
21. Manni, J. A., and H. J. Müller-Eberhard: Purification of human C'8 and inhibition of its activity by specific antibody. Fed. Proc. **27**, 479 (1968).

Prof. Dr. H. J. Müller-Eberhard
Department of Experimental Pathology,
Scripps Clinic and Research Foundation,
476 Prospect Street, La Jolla,
California 92037, U.S.A.

Discussion

FISCHER (Freiburg): I would like to ask Dr. Müller-Eberhard whether he thinks that also in vivo target cell destruction has to be preceded by the formation of the C-1-7 complex on the target cell?

We can demonstrate cytotoxicity in systems for which we can exclude the presence of such complexes. Under these conditions lysis might be effected solely by what you call C8 of lymphocyte origin.

But would it be justified to consider this lysis as mediated by the complement system?

In our laboratory Otto Götze has demonstrated that C8 causes irreversible membrane damage which is merely drastically enhanced by addition of C9. We favour the idea that C8 may be an encyme which affects the phospholipid metabolism of the targe cell membrane. [O. Götze, J. Haupt, and H. Fischer: Nature (Lond.) **217**, 1165 (1968)].

MÜLLER-EBERHARD (La Jolla): 1. Regarding the time-course of events: Damage of C7-cells by C8 is also a slow process. Kinetically, both systems might well be very similiar; only after addition of C9 does the reaction proceed more rapidly.

2. If it is now in fact C8 that is liberated by the lymphocytes, what are the implications for classical, lymphocyte mediated cytotoxicity? At this juncture

we do not propose that C8 is operative in the classical mechanism although this possibility should be considered and should be further explored.

KLEIN (Mainz): The course of lysis concerning the C3 cells is different from that of C7 cells. If one assumes that the C3 cells are damaged by a substance which comes from lymphocytes and which is apparently not identical with C8, one would imply a double function of these lymphocytes.

MÜLLER-EBERHARD (La Jolla): We know that at least two mechanisms are involved. A cell free extract of monocytes cannot attack C3 cells although intact monocytes can. In contrast extracts of monocytes are quite able to damage C7 cells.

KLEIN (Mainz): Have you tried to find out whether extracts of monocytes are able to convert C3 cells into C7 cells?

MÜLLER-EBERHARD (La Jolla): Yes, this is apparently not possible.

RAJEWSKY (Cologne): Is the cytotoxic principle, which is synthesized by lymphocytes only specific for 1 to 7 loaded erythrocytes or does it also attack normal erythrocytes?

MÜLLER-EBERHARD (La Jolla): In our experiments it had no effect on untreated cells.

HAMMER (Freiburg): How stable is your C7 erythrocyte-complex in vitro in comparison with your C3 complex? Is C8 specific with regard to Gamma G or Gamma A globulin?

MÜLLER-EBERHARD (La Jolla): Both complexes are stable for many hours. C8 has nothing to do with Gamma globulin, in any case it shows no cross-reaction with Gamma A or Gamma G.

ROTHER (Freiburg): You have worked with chicken erythrocytes. They are 100 to 1000 times more sensitive to the post-C3 complement reaction steps when compared with sheep erythrocytes. Chicken erythrocytes may thus pick up minute amounts of C8 and C9 activity that escape detection in the sheep erythrocyte system.

MÜLLER-EBERHARD (La Jolla): The reaction also works with sheep erythrocytes.

FISCHER (Freiburg): In our system the target cells are incubated in a medium which contains serum, and this serum of course contains C8 and C9. Would you agree that in your system lysis might occur even without lymphocytes?

MÜLLER-EBERHARD (La Jolla): In all our experiments we used a chromatographic fraction of fetal calf serum, which had been depleted of C8 and C9.

WESTPHAL (Freiburg): Is there another method, other than the liberation of C^{51} or the liberation of haemoglobin, or any other more sensitive method?

MÜLLER-EBERHARD (La Jolla): We intend using radioactive iron instead of chromium.

WESTPHAL (Freiburg): Some investigators feed the cells first with radioactive phosphate and then determine the excretion of labelled phosphate.

ROITT (London): A very sensitive test for antibodies directed against antigens on the surface of lymphocytes is opsonic adherence to macrophages. C8 might be demonstrable in this way. It would interest me to know whether one of the antigens which play a role in the immunosuppressive action of antilymphocyte serum might be C8.

MÜLLER-EBERHARD (La Jolla): We have looked into this question using a potent antilymphocytic serum. This single serum contained no anti-C8 activity.

OETTGEN (New York): Have you found natural antibodies against chicken cells in the serum of any of your lymphocyte donors?

MÜLLER-EBERHARD (La Jolla): So far we have found no differences in lymphocyte reactivity amongst 30 different donors. I do not know whether there were any antibodies against chicken erythrocytes in their serum, but this is of no consequence in our system.

Bayer-Symposium I, 18—24 (1969)

Anticomplementary Activity of Guinea Pig Serum Euglobulin: Its Relation to C 1 and to TAMe Esterase[1]

P. Klein

With 7 Figures

The interaction of complement with a suitable antigen-antibody aggregate triggers a chain of chemical reactions involving consecutively the nine factors of complement (C1 to C9). The triggering reaction is identical with the material fixation of C1 to the immune complex; this leads to the formation of Ag-Ab-C1. By its fixation C1 is converted from its chemically inert form to a highly reactive state ("fixed" or "activated" C1). The reactivity of fixed C1 is directed first against C4. Consequently C4 rapidly disappears from the fluid phase in the presence of fixed C1. A strikingly similar process occurs spontaneously in a fraction of guinea pig serum [5, 6].

If freshly precipitated guinea pig serum euglobulin is redissolved in a suitable buffer (pH 7, 6; ionic strength 0.15) it turns anticomplementary. This process of "conversion" occurs spontaneously; it is favored by incubating the euglobulin solution at 37 °C. During the conversion the preparation acquires not only a marked anticomplementary potency but also a demonstrable enzymatic activity. The anticomplementary activity is directed against guinea pig C4 and causes its rapid destruction. The enzymatic activity is directed against p-Toluene-L-argininmethyl-ester (TAMe) and is responsible for its hydrolytic degradation.

The observation that guinea pig euglobulin turns anticomplementary was first made in 1907 [1]; however no attention was paid to this phenomenon until Lepow and associates discovered an analogous process in human euglobulin [8]. They found that during the incubation of human euglobulin the C1 activity gradually disappears; in the same time a new factor was found to be generated. This factor was not active in hemolysis but it inactivated human C4 and C2 and exhibited a marked capacity to hydrolyse N-acetyl-L-tyrosine-ethyl-ester (ATEe). These three activities could not be dissociated by chemical fractionation of the human euglobulin. The authors concluded that one and the same factor is responsible for esterolysis and for the inactivation of C4 and C2. This factor was regarded as a derivative of C1 and consequently termed "C1-esterase". According to this concept C1 is a proenzyme; during the euglobulin conversion this proenzyme is "activated" i.e. it is transformed into the C1-esterase. The natural substrates of

---

[1] This work was done at the Institute of Medical Microbiology, Johannes Gutenberg-Universität, Mainz. The work was supported by the Deutsche Forschungsgemeinschaft (Grant Kl 124/10) and by the Landesversicherungsanstalt Rheinland-Pfalz. The members of the working group are the following: Dr. W. Opferkuch, Dr. R. Ringelmann, M. Loos and the speaker.

C1-esterase are C4 and C2. The enzymatic digestion of these complement factors by C1-esterase renders them reactive with respect to certain sites of the immune complex. The synthetic ester ATEe is merely regarded as a artificial substrate of the C1-esterase.

The above outlined hypothesis is based on a rich material of indirect evidence [7, 9]. Some of its implications can be summarized in four points:

1. The activation of C1 can be induced by two ways: Either by its fixation to an immune complex or in the absence of the latter by physico-chemical factors.

2. The activation of C1 is irreversible, i.e. an activated C1 cannot be reconverted to its non-activated state.

3. The generation of the anticomplementary activity of euglobulin in the absence of immune complexes is identical with a spontaneously occuring activation of C1. The destruction of C4, of C2 and of ATEe by converted euglobulin is not

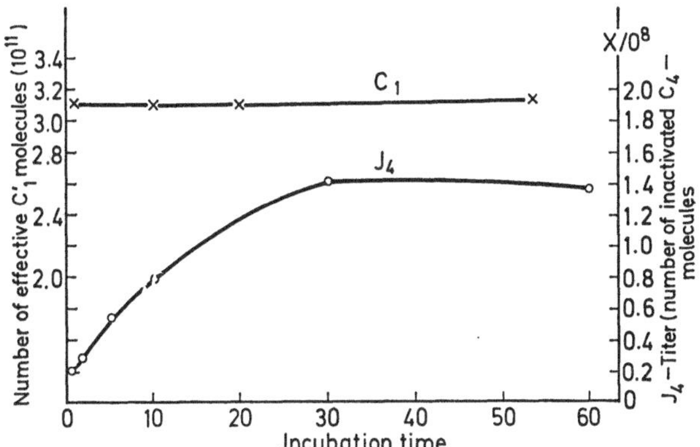

Fig. 1. Conversion of g. p. euglobulin: Course of lytic C_1-activity and of J_4-potency

only due to one and the same species of molecule but to one and the same type of molecular site. Fixed C1 exhibits the same functional and material properties as the C1-esterase from spontaneously converted euglobulin.

4. The kinetics of the destruction of C4 and of C2 by converted euglobulin are in essence the same as the kinetics of ATEe hydrolysis induced by the same factor.

Since the experimental evidence for the C1-esterase concept rests almost exclusively on investigations made with human serum an attempt was made to examine the validity of these postulates for guinea pig serum [3, 4, 10]. The following measurements refer to three activities. The activity of free nonbound C1 will be referred to as "C1-titer"; the C4-inactivating potency will be designated "I_4-activity," finally the esterolytic activity against TAMe will be represented as "enzymatic activity." Fig. 1 shows the course of the spontaneous conversion of guinea pig euglobulin.

During the incubation of the euglobulin, samples were taken at intervals and subjected to two measurements: First the C1-titer was estimated in terms of effective C1-molecules per ml euglobulin. Second the capacity of the euglobulin to inactivate purified guinea pig C4 was determined and formulated as C4-destruction rate ("I_4-titer"); the results were referred to 1 ml of euglobulin and given in terms of inactivated C4-molecules per 15 min incubation. It can be seen in Fig. 1 that during the whole conversion process the C1-titer shows no change at all. On the other hand the C4-inactivating capacity (I_4-activity) after a short lag period increases gradually until it reaches its maximum value. This observation is at variance with the data given for human complement.

We may assume that the material bearer of the I_4-activity is identical with the C1-molecule; this implies that during the conversion process some or all of the C1-molecules acquire a second activity namely the capacity to destroy C4. If this assumption is correct one must expect that the activities of C1 and I_4 cannot be separated by subjecting converted euglobulin to any chemical or physico-chemical fractionation procedure. An attempt was made to verify this postulate.

Converted euglobulin was subjected to ultracentrifugation in a sucrose gradient. It was found that the C1-activity can be recovered to about 80% from those fractions, the sedimentation rate of which corresponds to about S 19 whereas the

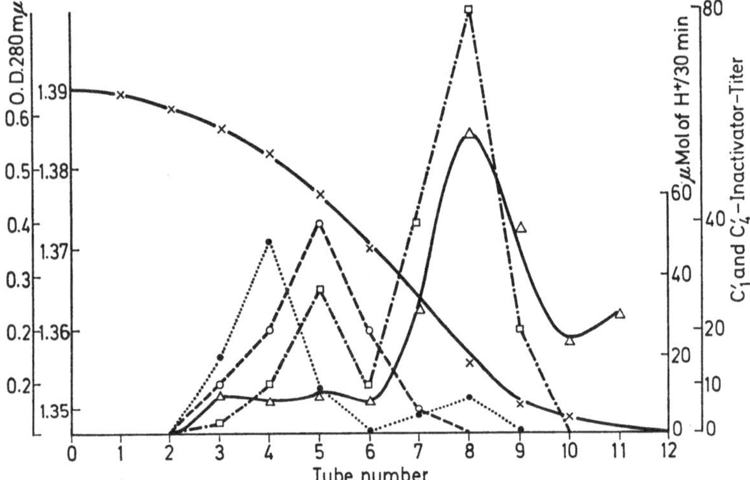

Fig. 2. Euglobulin in sucrose-gradient centrifugation (40—10%) Δ———Δ protein, O···O C_1activity, □—·—□ C_4inactivator, ●········● TAMe-esterase, × — × — × refraction index

I_4-activity was found in the 7S-fractions. Fig. 2 shows the separation of C1 and of I_4 by the first run of ultracentrifugation. The low I_4-activity shown by some of the C1-fractions, is a contamination; increasing separation can be obtained by a second ultracentrifugation of these fractions.

The results shown in Fig. 1 and Fig. 2 do not support the assumption that in converted euglobulin the activities of C1 and of I_4 are located on one and the same molecule. It seems more consistent to conclude at this point that the generation of I_4 during the euglobulin conversion does not involve C1. This would mean that the precursor of I_4 is a factor distinct from C1. To test this hypothesis an attempt was made to characterize C1 and I_4 from converted guinea pig euglobulin in terms of its serological specifity.

The purification of hemolytically active C1 is performed by its precipitation from serum according to Nelson's method. Afterwards the preparation is repeatedly precipitated and redissolved by exposing it alternatively to an ionic strength of

0.065 (precipitation) and of 0.15 (re-dissolution). The following ultracentrifugation yields a preparation of about 10^{13} effective molecules per mg protein. — Another way to purify C1 consists on adsorbing it specifically to immune aggregates. The resulting AgAbC1 complex releases C1 if it is exposed to an ionic strength of $\mu = 1.2$. — The purification procedure of I_4 is shown in Fig. 3. Fig. 4 shows the activity range of I_4 with respect to complement components and intermediate cells.

Rabbit immune sera were made against C1 and against I_4. These immune sera were examined with reference to their capacity to block the hemolytic function of C1 and the C4-destroying function of I_4. Fig. 5 shows that the blocking effect of the immune sera against C'1 and against I_4 is strictly limited to their homologous antigen; in other words, C1 and I_4 are serologically distinct.

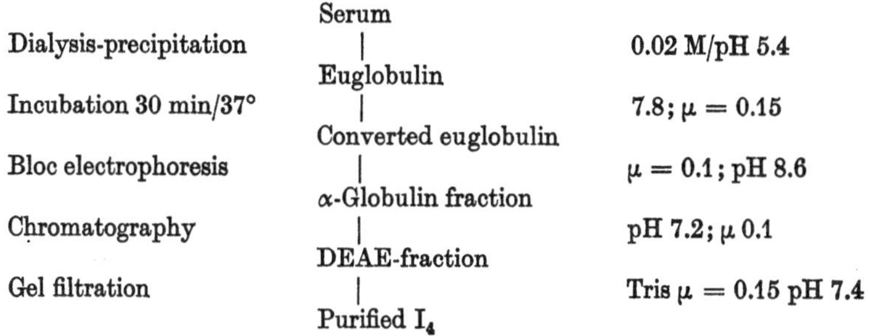

Fig. 3. Purification of C_4 inactivator

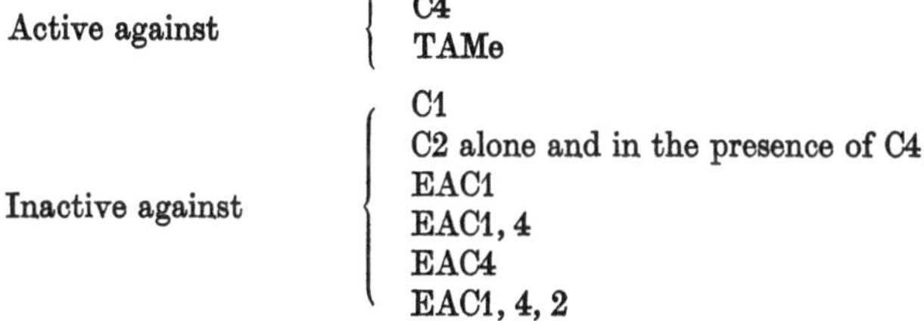

Fig. 4. Activity range of purified I_4

The TAMe hydrolizing activity of the converted euglobulin is located in those fractions that contain I_4. Accordingly the purified I_4 preparation inactivates C4 and hydrolyses TAMe. On the other hand the highly purified preparations of C1 did not exhibit any detectable TAMe hydrolizing activity. These findings show that the generation process of the esterolytic activity in converted euglobulin does not involve C1. However the possibility must be taken into consideration that the TAMe hydrolysis and C4 inactivation are both mediated by one and the same molecular site. If this is the case one would expect that the C4-destruction and the TAMe hydrolysis show similarities as far as their kinetics are concerned. An attempt was made to examine the influence of temperature upon the rate of both processes.

Fig. 6 shows that the rate of TAMe hydrolysis is sharply raised by higher temperatures of incubation. On the other hand it can be seen that the C4 inactivation is very little influenced by changing the reaction temperature. This

                                    P. Klein

finding indicates that the I_4-activity and the esterolytic activity are basically distinct processes. In other experiments it was found that the rate of TAMe hydrolysis is not influenced by the presence of C4.

Finally an experiment was made to see whether in the system EAC1 + C4 the generation of SAC1, 4 sites is influenced by the reaction temperature. Consequently EAC1 cells were incubated with a limited amount of purified C4 and the resulting SAC1, 4 were estimated by adding consecutively C2 and afterwards chelated complement. Fig. 7 shows that the reaction temperature has little in-

Immune sera	Blocking titre of the immune serum when tested against…	
	EAC1	C4-inactivator
Anti-AgAbC1	320	∅
Anti-C4-inactivator	∅	80

Fig. 5. Blocking effect of homologous immune sera upon EAC1 and upon C_4inactivator

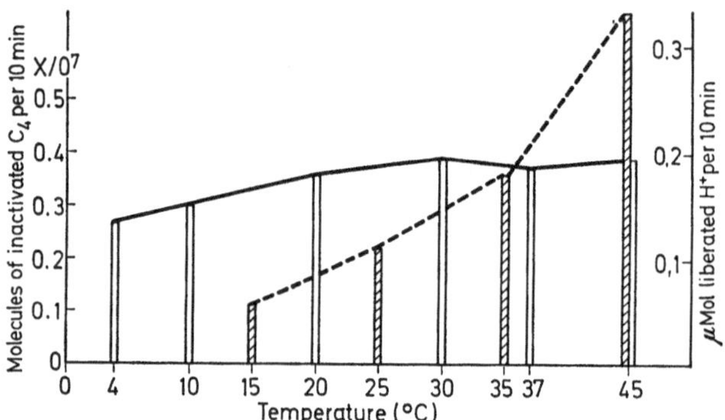

Fig. 6. Influence of temperature upon the rate of C_4inactivation and TAMe hydrolysis both induced by I4. ——— C_4inactivation rate, - - - - TAMe hydrolysis

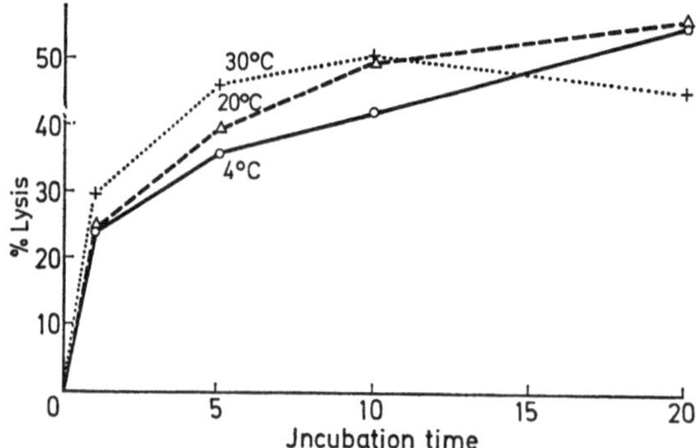

Fig. 7. Influence of temperature upon the fixation of C_4 to EAC_1. System: $[EAC_1 + C_4$ (limited)]; incubation at 4°, 20°, and 30 °C. Exposure to C2 and to C_{EDTA}

fluence upon the outcome of the reaction. This result does not support the assumption that fixed C1 acts upon C4 as an enzyme.

Conclusions — Discussion

The data presented in this paper indicate that the concept of C1-esterase as developed on the basis of experiments with human serum cannot easily be applied to explain the outcome of our experiments with guinea pig serum. According to these experiments the following conclusions can be made: The conversion of euglobulin results in the generation of an anticomplementary factor and of an esterolytic principle. The anticomplementary factor is directed against C4; the esterolytic principle is active against TAMe. The C4-inactivating factor (I_4) is generated from a precurser which seems to be distinct from C1. The kinetics of the interaction of I_4 with C4 do not indicate that I_4 is an enzyme. On the other hand the TAMe hydrolysis shows the kinetic characteristics of an enzymatic reaction. This leads to the interpretation that two distinct factors are responsible for the C4-inactivation and for the TAMe hydrolysis. Finally the possibility should be taken into consideration that the interaction of EAC1 with C4 is not an enzymatic process; this is suggested by the observation that the generation rate of SAC1, 4 sites is not markedly influenced by changes of the reaction temperature.

Earlier experiments have shown that fixed C1 is strongly active with respect to C4, whereas native, i.e. non-fixed C1 is inert [2]. Later it was shown, that from an AgAbC1-complex which was highly active against C4 a C1-preparation could be dissociated which in the absence of an immune complex proved to be inert against C4. Yet the same preparation again could be rendered highly active against C4 when it was fixed to an immune aggregate [3, 11]. This indicates that the activation of C1 might be a reversible process; it could be imagined that the activity against C4 depends upon a certain conformational state of the C1 molecule. This conformational state may be reversibly acquired and lost by the fixation of C1 to the immune complex and by its dissociation from the latter. This hypothesis would imply that there are two distinct pathways for the inactivation of C4 in the fluid phase: The first pathway is identical with the fixation of C4 to the complex AgAbC1; the second pathway is identical with the interaction of I_4 with C4. In the light of this speculation one could theorize of whether the I_4-factor can be regarded as a regulation factor outside of the very complement system.

Summary

The spontaneous conversion of guinea pig euglobulin results in the generation of a factor that inactivates C4; besides, an enzymatic activity appears which is directed against TAMe. The generation process of both activities is independent from C1. A serological analysis of the C4-inactivating euglobulin factor (I_4) and of C1 suggests that both factors are distinct. The inactivation rate of C4 by I_4 is not markedly influenced by changes in temperature whereas the TAMe hydrolysis exhibits a pronounced temperature dependence. Finally the generation rate of SAC1, 4 sites in the system EAC1 + C4 is largely independent from the reaction temperature. The implications of these findings are discussed with reference to the C1-esterase concept.

References

1. Brand. E.: Über das Verhalten der Komplemente bei der Dialyse. Berl. klin. Wschr. 1907, 1075.
2. Colli, A., W. Opferkuch und P. Klein: Studien über den Mechanismus der Immunhämolyse: Der Bindungsmodus der vierten Komplementkomponente. Z. ges. Hyg. 147, 213 (1961).
3. Klein, P.: Inactivation of C'4 by guinea pig euglobulin. Proc. Sympos. Protides of the biological fluids, Brügge 15, 433 (1967).
4. — Communication, Complement workshop June 1968, Boston Mass.
5. —, and H. J. Wellensiek: Complement: Hemolytic function and chemical properties. Int. Rev. exp. Path. 4, 246—332 (1965).
6. Müller-Eberhard, H. J.: Chemistry and reaction mechanisms of complement. Advanc. Immunol. 8, 1—69 (1968).
7. —, U. F. Nilsson, A. P. Dalmasso, Margaret J. Polley, and Mary A. Calcott: A molecular concept of immune cytolysis. Arch. Path. 82, 205 (1966).
8. Lepow, J. H., A. D. Ratnoff, and R. L. Levy: Studies on the activation of a proesterase associated with partially purified first component of human complement. J. exp. Med. 107, 451 (1958).
9. — Complement: A review (including esterase activity). In: Mechanisms of hypersensitivity, p. 267 (J. H. Shaffer, Ed.). Boston/Mass.: Little and Brown 1959.
10. Ringelmann, R.: Esterolytic activity of guinea pig euglobulins. Proc. Sympos. Protides of the biological fluids, Brügge 15, 463 (1967).
11. Steinbrecher, A.: Die Beziehung der ersten Komplement-Komponente zur esterolytischen und antikomplementären Aktivität: Vergleichende Untersuchungen bei verschiedenen Säugetieren. Doctoral Thesis, Naturwiss. Fakultät, Johannes Gutenberg-Universität, Mainz 1966.

Prof. Dr. P. Klein
Institut für Medizinische Mikrobiologie der
Universität, 65 Mainz, Langenbeckstraße 1

Discussion

SCHWICK (Marburg): I quite believe that C-1-esterase — if it is present at all — or simply C1 might well possess different properties in guinea pigs than in humans. I am thinking of plasminogen which in man is certainly a different molecule from that of cattle. [Bergström, K.: Arkiv Kemi 21, 517 (1961). — Hoepfinger, L. M., I. Y. S. Cham, and E. T. Mertz: Fifteenth Annual Symposium on Blood. Detroit, January 20, 1967].

MÜLLER-EBERHARD (La Jolla): Is your purified guinea pig-C1 able to inactivate C4 ? Can your purified C4-inactivator (I_4) attach free C4 to EA cells ?

KLEIN (Mainz): Our purified C1 component has no C4 inactivating potency. Our yield of C1 in highly purified preparations lies between 3 and 10% in terms of effective molecules per protein molecules (19S). If under defined conditions C1 is fixed to cells it can be removed. We repeated this experiment many times and found that by dissociation of AgAbC1, a C1-preparation can be obtained which is unable to inactivate C4 but which is nevertheless haemolytically active. If this finding is confirmed at a larger scale it means that guinea pig C1 is reversibly activated by being attached to the AgAb-complex. Once it is removed from the complex it turns again to its previous state being inert against C4.

MÜLLER-EBERHARD (La Jolla): Is the C4 inactivator also able to inactivate C2 as it is known of C1 esterase ?

KLEIN (Mainz): No; in this respect our C4-inactivator is substantial different from that which in human complement is named C1 esterase.

Bayer-Symposium I, 25—30 (1969)

Experimental Inhibition of Complement

K. LAUENSTEIN

With 3 Figures

Four methods are available to elucidate the biological significance of the serum-complement system:

1. The demonstration of complement components at the site of the immunological event.

2. Investigation with animals possessing a genetic C defect.

3. Experiments with anticomplement substances and

4. Turnover studies with individual C-components.

We have been interested for some years now in our institute in the inhibition of serum-complement in animal experiments. The motive for these investigations came from experiments designed to study the mechanism of action of heparin. We had found that in animal experiments heparin possessed marked anti-inflammatory properties (1962). It was found, however, that the long established complement inhibiting component of heparin is without significance in the usual chemically induced inflammation models. Also, a fall in serum complement occurs in vivo only at doses at which blood coagulation is already inhibited. The duration of action is very short. Two hours after intraperitoneal injection the complement is again within the normal range. In all these experiments the total complement i.e. the total haemolytic activity of the serum was determined by applying the usual immune-haemolytic methods to the sera obtained by cardiac-puncture using sheep cells and rabbit antiserum.

At one time, working together with H. Fischer and H. G. Siedentopf (1965) we determined the site of action of heparin and also other heparinoids within the complement chain. We found that heparin inhibits the first component of serum complement. At the same time, Borsos, Rapp and Crisler (1965) found that carrageenin, also a heparinoid, inhibits the first complement component by forming heparinoid precipitates with C1. Also they found in vivo an inhibition of complement only at doses at which bleeding time was already considerably prolonged. One must, therefore, conclude that heparin and the heparinoids are not suitable as inhibitors for studies on the biological action of total complement.

We have tested nearly all known in vitro active complement inhibitors in animal experiments, either on the rat or on the guinea pig. These substances were either too toxic for animal tests, or they showed no action.

The action of aggregated human γ-globulin on the serum complement level was of too short duration to carry out animal experiments. Also copper-chlorophyllin which, according to the literature, is active in vivo proved to be too weak in action.

We were not able to examine the C3 inactivating factor which Nelson isolated from cobra venom. In the search for an anticomplement substance which is also active in vivo and non-toxic, we then tested a whole series of new substances both in vitro and in vivo. Some high molecular components made available from our Leverkusen Chemical Laboratories by Dr. Pieper proved to be of particular interest.

Among these the sulphated high-polymers all possessed anticoagulant properties. This type of compound was not investigated further. It was finally found that the poly-N-oxide of the nicotinic acid ester of polyvinyl alcohol was the most active.

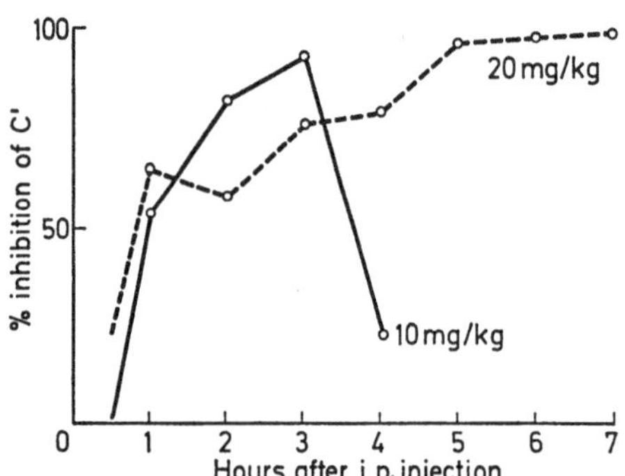

This substance which was only just soluble in water was highly active in the rat at doses of 10 to 20 mg/kg. A fall in total haemolytic activity of serum complement occurred barely 1 h after i.p. injection, being optimal between 2 to 3 h. After about 6 h the complement level was again normal. This effect can be repeated any number of time by renewed administration; we treated animals up to 3 weeks with one or two daily injections.

Fig. 1. Complement inhibition in rats. Male Wistar I rats (breeder Winkelmann, Paderborn) weighting 120 to 140 g, were injected 10 resp. 20 mg/kg Poly-N-oxide of the nicotinic acid ester of polyvinylalcohol (PVA-NA). Each point represents the C-activity of the pooled sera of 10 animals. Estimation of whole C according to Kabat and Mayer

To some extent it is possible in this way to achieve 100% inhibition of serum complement, i.e. the residual activity lies within the deviation of our method. Such a marked inhibition can, however, only be obtained with the rat. With the guinea-pig we achieved at the most a 50% reduction of serum complement. Increasing the dose further was without effect. We were unable to influence complement levels in the rabbit, dog, and in man — as we discovered later.

The substance which we first used still consisted of a mixture of fractions with a very variable molecular weight. After further separation and purification, it was found that only those fractions with a molecular weight of about 50,000 to 90,000 possessed notable activity.

In in vitro experiments the substance showed the following properties: If high serum dilutions were used i.e. with about two haemolytic units of complement in the usual immune-haemolytic arrangement and the substance added only in vitro, then no inhibition was demonstrable. Not until large quantities of serum were used did an almost complete inhibition of complement occur. This applies to rats and guinea pigs. Also under these conditions, no inhibition of dog, rabbit, and human serum was observed.

By incubation tests using E- and EA-cells respectively with the inhibitor and then washing out the inhibitor on the centrifuge, could it be shown that the complement lysis of both cell types was not changed. Also the substance does not excert an unspecific sensitising action as described by Cowan (1954) and Dalmasso and Müller-Eberhard (1964) for polyethylene glycol.

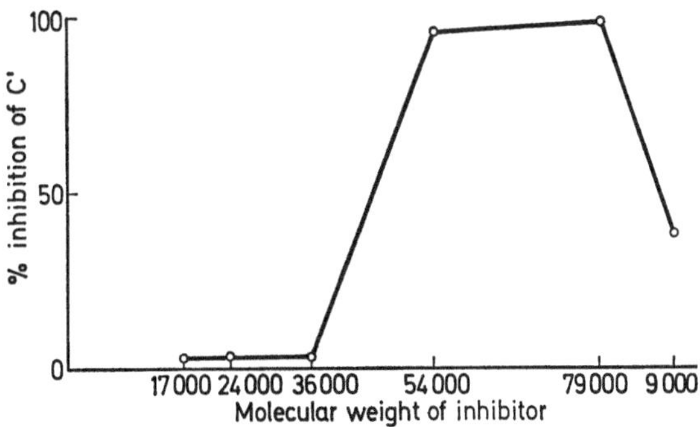

Fig. 2. Complement inhibition by PVA-NA of different molecular weight

Investitations to determine the site of action of the inhibitor within the complement system using C defective rat serum produced in vivo, have so far shown that all complement components are reduced in their concentration. We tested the defect serum with EAC1-, EAC14-, EAC142-, EAC1423-, and EAC1423567-cells. With the aid of such a defective serum, we were only able to make EAC14-cells i.e. only up to the limiting component.

Taking into consideration both the in vivo blood level investigations and the in vitro tests, then we have the following picture: We have an inhibitor which in vivo in the rat leads to a marked inhibition of serum complement and in the guinea pig to a less marked inhibition. The inhibitor is without effect in the dog, rabbit, and in man.

In a modified in vitro-test in the presence of excess serum proteins, the same species distribution is found, that is, activity in the rat and guinea pig, no activity in the dog, rabbit, and guinea pig. No single complement component is inhibited but rather all components — at least as far as we have tested, so that we are probably concerned here with a consumption of complement. It is apt to assume that similar to polyethyleneglycol a decomplementation by aggregated γ-globulin or an inhibitor-protein-complex is involved.

However, so far we have no experimental proof for such a hypothesis. We only know that the substance is excreted very slowly and incompletely and that considerable stores are found in the cells of the reticulo-endothelial system.

There is a certain parallel to the anticomplement action of aggregated γ-globulin in that γ-globulins of different species behave quite differently.

What effect then does administration of the inhibitor have on different immune-models? Since the inhibitor was only effective in the rat and in the guinea pig, we used only these two species.

Skin transplants on Wistar rats were rejected as usual in spite of daily or twice daily administration of the inhibitor. The in-bred mouse behaved the same, we transplanted from the C3H- onto the CPBN-mouse and vice versa. We have been unable to show that the graft-versus-host reaction with the in-bred baby mouse is influenced. Furthermore, we found no influence of the PCA reaction in the guinea pig. However, there was a marked influence of a reaction of the Arthus type in the guinea pig. As a model we used the local Forssman reaction with

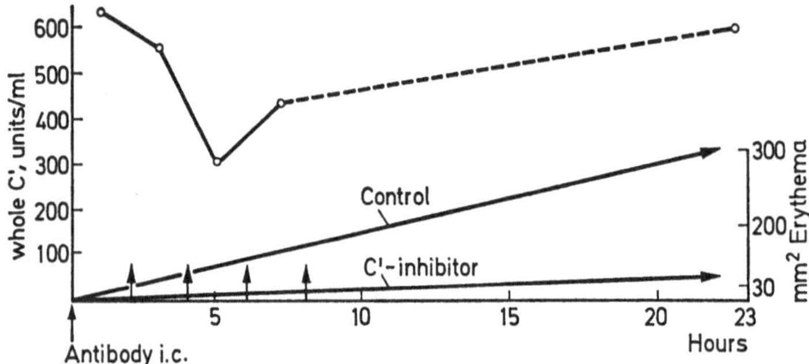

Fig. 3. Inhibition of the local Forssman reaction by PVA-NA. Pirbright white guinea pigs (male, 250 to 300 g, breeder Winkelmann, Paderborn) were injected 0.05 ml Ambozeptor 1:3000 (rabbit, Behringwerke AG, Marburg) intracutanously. Each point represents the mean value of 10 animals. Treatment with 4 injections of 25 mg/kg PVA-NA

rabbit serum. Parallel with a marked fall of serum complement the treated animals showed a definite influence of the skin reaction measured by the area of inflammation. It is essential that the reduction in complement is carried out immediately before or after the injection of the antibody. If treatment is delayed for several hours, then the reaction is not influenced. From this it is also improbable that the inhibitor possesses an unspecific anti-inflammatory action. If in the same test we give a substance which is very similar chemically, has the same molecular weight, the same basic chain, but with another side-chain which we know does not inhibit complement, then the local Forssman reaction is not influenced.

The substance is also effective in the Forssman-shock of the guinea pig. As is known the situation here is quite different from that prevailing with reactions of the anaphylactic system and where, in contrast to other anaphylactic reactions, involvement of complement was demonstrated (Witebsky and Neter, 1935).

If one examines the complement level of the surviving guinea pigs, it would appear that a 30 to 50% reduction of serum complement is sufficient for survival or lengthening of the survival time.

In recapitulation of our in vivo-tests, we have not, therefore, in spite of effective reduction of the complement level, been able to influence immune-models in which the cellular immune response is prominent and where γ-globulins do not play an essential role (skin transplantations, graft-versus-host reactions, and the Tbc-reactions of the guinea pig). Also the PCA-reaction of the guinea pig, which is not dependent on complement, was not influenced. Our results with these reactions are a further indication that serum complement is not essentially involved here.

In Forssman-shock and with the local Forssman reaction in which the involvement of complement has been demonstrated, we were able to achieve a definite influence.

Table 1. *Forssman-shock of the guinea pig. Guinea pigs were injected 0,3 ml Ambozeptor 1:8000 (Behringwerke AG, Marburg) intravenously. Complement estimation in the pooled sera. PVA-NA treatment 2 h before injection of Ambozeptor*

Animal	Pretreated with	Forssman antiserum	Death min after antiserum	Whole C units/ml
1	Saline	none	none	500
2				
3	Saline	+	2	360
4		+	1	
5		+	3	
6		+	2	
7		+	2	
8	25 mg/kg i.p.	none	none	370
9	C-Inhibitor			
10	25 mg/kg i.p.	+	15	90
11	C-Inhibitor	+	20	
12		+	3	
13		+	20	
14		+	16	

We have investigations underway with substances which are also able to inhibit human serum complement in vitro. We hope that one day we shall find substances which are not stored but consist of chains capable of degradation. There is, we believe, a justifiable hope that substances of this type might be able to favourably influence at least those autoaggression-diseases in which antibodies against membrane antigens are of importance, for example acquired haemolytic anaemia and thrombocytopenia.

References

Borsos, T., H. J. Rapp, and C. Crisler: J. Immunol. **94**, 662 (1965).

Complement. Ciba Foundation Symposium. London: Churchill 1965.

Cowan, K. M.: Dissertation submitted to the School of Hygiene and Public Health, The Johns Hopkins University 1954.

Dalmasso, A. P., and H. J. Müller-Eberhard: Proc. Soc. exp. Biol. (N. Y.) **117**, 643 (1964).

Lauenstein, K., H. Friedrich, and G. L. Haberland: Med. exp. (Basel) **6**, 200 (1962).
—, H. G. Siedentopf und H. Fischer: Z. Naturforsch. **20 b**, 575 (1965).
Rapp, H. J., and T. Borsos: J. Amer. med. Ass. **198**, 1347 (1966).
Witebsky, E., and E. Neter: J. exp. Med. **61**, 489 (1935).

Dr. K. Lauenstein
Institut für experimentelle Pathologie
der Farbenfabriken Bayer AG,
56 Wuppertal-Elberfeld

Discussion

ROTHER (Freiburg): We have had similar experiences. When studying heparinoids and polystyrenes, complement inhibiting properties regularly went along with inhibition of the coagulation process.

DE WECK (Berne): Also with different polymers species differences are to be found e.g. polylysines and polyamines have an action on the leucocyte aggregation of the guinea pig but not of the rabbit.

SPRINGER (Evanston): With which serum do you carry out the Forssman-shock?

LAUENSTEIN (Wuppertal): We use rabbit serum immunised with sheep erythrocytes.

MÜLLER-EBERHARD (La Jolla): Together with Dr. Fjellström we carried out tests in Ja Jolla with dialdehyde-dextran. It was found that this substance reacts with all serum proteins. My question is, have you carried out electrophoretic investigations on the effect in your inhibitor on serum proteins?

LAUENSTEIN (Wuppertal): We have carried out such investigations. In spite of specific staining of our inhibitor we were not successful in demonstrating aggregates with serum proteins.

KLEIN (Mainz): You did not mention earlier investigations some of which I believe were carried out in Wuppertal; in these investigations an anticomplementary action was found in vitro for Aspirin, Germanin and Resochin.

LAUENSTEIN (Wuppertal): All these substances only have an action in vitro and only at very high doses.

KLEIN (Mainz): Have you any indication that when using various inhibitors an activation of the complement inhibitors takes place?

LAUENSTEIN (Wuppertal): No.

WESTPHAL (Freiburg): Can one in fact inhibit complement also by highly purified antibodies against individual complement components.

MÜLLER-EBERHARD (La Jolla): As far as I know such investigations have been carried out using highly purified antibodies to C3 and this component completely disappears. I should like to say something else regarding the cobra factor. It is a glycoprotein having a molecular weight of approximately 140,000. This substance itself has no effect whatsoever on purified C3. However, if one adds this factor in highly purified form to serum then it is bound in the presence of bivalent cations to a previously unknown protein of the β globulin fraction. This β globulin has a molecular weight of approximately 90,000 and we call it the C3 serum protinactivator and its complex with cobra factor the C3 inactivator complex. The complex inactivates C3 by cleaving the C3 molecule enzymatically. When cobra factor is injected into an animal (1 to 2 mg/kg body weight) the C3 inactivator complex forms in the animals circulation and eliminates C3, so that it can no longer be detected in serum either by hemolytic or immunochemical assay. The action of cobra factor in vivo lasts about 4 days. During this time one may carry out investigations of the role of complement in immune reactions.

FISCHER (Freiburg): The inhibiting action of the cobra factor resembles to some extent the action of polyvinylpyridine-N-oxide (PPNO) which prevents cell damage in silicosis. PPNO protects macrophages against damage by quartz-crystals. Has anybody tried to protect macrophages by the cobra factor ?

LAUENSTEIN (Wuppertal): Our complement inhibitor is not effective against silicosis, whereas on the other hand polyvinylpyridine-N-oxide does not inhibit the serum complement.

HAMMER (Freiburg): I have a question to ask Dr. Müller-Eberhardt: Might it be possible to prolong the decomplementation by cobra factor by making these animals on which one wishes to test immunopathological effects tolerant to this factor ?

MÜLLER-EBERHARD (La Jolla): Together with Dr. Weigle we have tried this with rabbits and with guinea pigs. We have not, however, succeeded in making these animals tolerant.

Bayer-Symposium I, 32—46 (1969)

Molecular and Stereochemical Properties Required of Antigens for the Elicitation of Allergic Reactions[1]

A. L. DE WECK, and C. H. SCHNEIDER

With 6 Figures

Antigens are molecules possessing several different immunological functions. At the present time, a more precise definition of these various functions under the terms of immunogenicity, antigenicity, allergenicity, and tolerogenicity may appear useful (Table 1). Whereas natural macromolecular antigens are usually able to perform simultaneously all possible functions of an antigen, the chemical manipulations of antigenic determinants and of carrier molecules and the preparation of synthetic antigens has permitted us in recent years to analyze somewhat better the molecular characteristics required for the one or the other function of antigens. Beside its theoretical interest, such an analysis has also permitted to obtain more insight in the molecular mechanism of various types of allergic reactions. Furthermore, the practical implications of this work lie at hand: according to circumstances, it could be most desirable in human medicine to prepare and administer antigens possessing solely one or the other of the possible functions.

Molecular analysis of the antigens' functions may be considered to have started with Landsteiner and his first immunochemical experiments with hapten-protein conjugates (Landsteiner, 1945). The precipitation of antibody by plurivalent hapten-protein conjugates, i.e. proteins carrying several antigenic determinants per molecule and the specific inhibition of precipitation by univalent haptens became the basis of immunochemistry for more than 30 years before it was realized that the question of uni- or plurivalent antigens is also most relevant for the allergenic function *in vivo*, although some phenomena of hapten inhibition of allergic reactions *in vivo* had been reported before (Campbell and McCasland, 1944; Klopstock and Selter, 1929; Tillet *et al.*, 1929). It is only in 1960 that Ovary and Karush reported a quantitative analysis of the inhibition of anaphylactic reactions in guinea pigs by monovalent haptens (Ovary and Karush, 1960). At the same time, in Eisen's laboratory, experiments were initiated with mono-, bi- and plurivalent antigens and with antibody fragments in order to assess the molecular aspects of antigen-antibody complex formation required for the elicitation of cutaneous anaphylaxis in animals and in man (Farah *et al.*, 1960; Parker *et al.*, 1962a). The preparation of a plurivalent non immunogenic conjugate of penicillin with a homopolymer of lysine (penicillolyl-polylysine) enabled for the first time to put to practical use the separation of the immunogenic and antigenic functions and to obtain an antigen suitable for skin testing but unable to sensitize

---

[1] This work has been supported in part by the Swiss National Foundation for Scientific Research and by the Emil Barell Foundation of F. Hoffmann — La Roche, Inc., Basle.

normal individuals (Parker *et al.*, 1962b). Studies on the immunological functions of hapten-substituted polylysines have been then considerably extended by Levine (Levine, 1965a; Levine, 1965b).

Although studies with artificial polypeptide antigens have also contributed considerably to increase our knowledge on the molecular requirements for the immunogenic, antigenic and tolerogenic functions of antigens, this presentation will be restricted to the allergenic function i.e. the ability of eliciting allergic inflammatory reactions in already sensitized individuals. The choice of the penicilloyl (BPO) structure as antigenic determinant permitted to compare allergic reactions in rabbits and guinea pigs with those of a large population of sensitized human beings. Although some data on the allergenic function of pluri-, tri-, bi- or monovalent antigens carrying other antigenic determinants [such as the dini-

Table 1. *Functions of an "antigen"*

Immunogenicity: capacity to induce antibody formation and/or delayed-type hypersensitivity.

Antigenicity (sensu stricto): capacity to react specifically with antibody.

Allergenicity: capacity to elicit allergic inflammatory reactions (anaphylaxis, Arthus, delayed) in sensitized individuals.

Tolerogenicity: capacity to induce specific immunological tolerance.

---

trophenyl (DNP) or the p-azobenzenearsonate group] are available, it is with penicilloyl antigens that the largest experimental evidence has been collected for the time being.

1. Elicitation of the Anaphylactic Reaction

The term of anaphylactic reaction is used here in a rather restricted sense to define the molecular processes occuring on the surface of a histamine-containing cell (e.g. mast cell, blood leucocyte) and leading to the release of histamine. As models of such reactions were studied the active and passive systemic or cutaneous anaphylaxis in guinea pigs, the Schulz-Dale reaction of sensitized guinea pig ileum and the wheal-and-erythema skin reaction of penicilloyl specificity in patients allergic to penicillin.

Plurivalent antigens (i.e. carrying several antigenic determinants per molecule) are most probably the rule among natural allergens. More than 15 antigenic determinants have been identified on an albumin molecule (Kaminski, 1965). It may be important to know whether a natural antigen molecule carries several antigenic determinants which are all different and non cross-reacting with each other (e.g. a, b, c, d etc.) or whether identical antigenic determinants are present on the same molecule (e.g. a_3, b_4). In the first case, lattice formation and antibody precipitation will only occur if antibodies specific for several determinants (e. g. anti-a, anti-b, anti-c etc.) are present at the same time, enabling the formation of a mixed lattice constituted by antibodies of different specificities (Fig. 1). With natural antigen molecules of relatively low molecular weight such as insulin, we are probably faced with a peculiar situation where a given antigenic determinant is not repeated on the same molecule (Fig. 1). The precipitability of such a molecule will therefore depend on the extent to which antibodies of varying specificities have been formed against that antigen or on the extent to which the antigen may form aggregates. This may explain the paradoxical behaviour and the variable precipitability of anti-insulin antisera, when compared with binding data obtained with radioactive insulin (Johner, 1968).

On the other hand, artificial plurivalent hapten-protein conjugates carry by definition several identical antigenic determinants on the same carrier molecule. These determinants are identical as far as the hapten only is considered. However, when using protein carriers, structural differences in the points of attachement of haptenic groups may be responsible for a microheterogeneity of the antigen which may be reflected in heterogeneity of the antibodies formed (Eisen and Siskind,

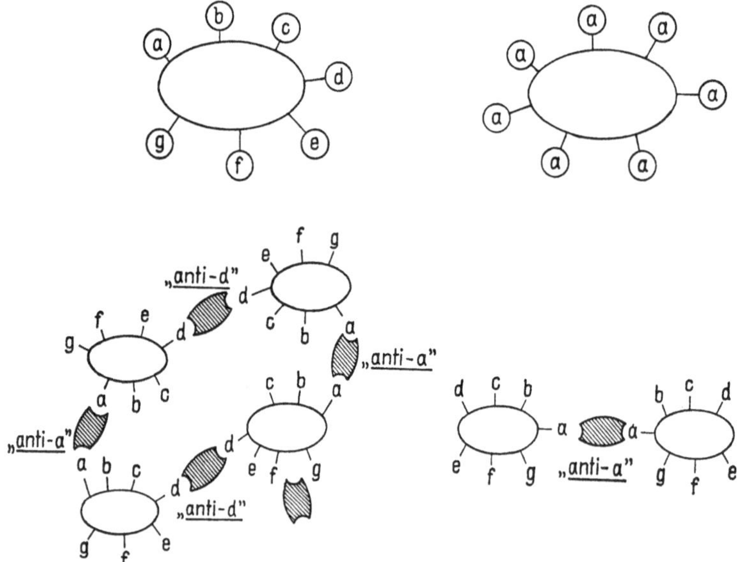

Fig. 1. Precipitation by antibodies of mixed specificity

1964). By the use of well defined homopolymer peptide carriers (such as polylysines) this type of heterogeneity appears to be reduced to a minimum.

It is apparent from Table 2 that anaphylactic reactions are initiated by a passive phenomenon, namely the linking of antibody molecules by a plurivalent antigen. Apart from its possible involvement in the antibody's specificity (specificity for part of the carrier adjacent to the haptenic group or "carrier specificity"), the carrier molecule plays no other role than that of a passive link. The immunogenic property of the carrier itself play no role at all in the elicitation phenomenon.

By varying the degree of substitution by antigenic determinants and the size of the polylysine carrier, Levine (1965a and 1965b) has been able to demonstrate that only a few of the available antigenic determinants are effectively occupied by antibody in the anaphylactic reaction (Fig. 2 and 3). Provided there are at least two antigenic determinants per molecule, the degree of substitution or the size of the carrier do not markedly influence the efficiency of the system. An

Table 2

Antigen	Immunogenicity Induction of anti-BPO Ab	Elicitation of anaphylactic reactions					
		in vitro			*in vivo*		
		Ab ppt.	C′ fix.	S-Dale	PCA	SA	WER
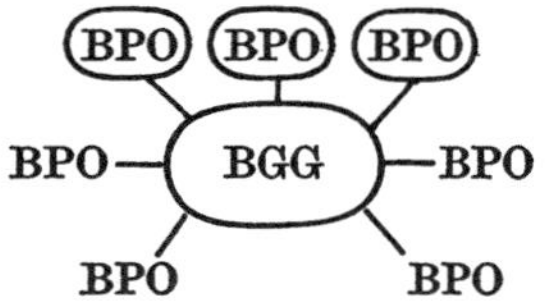 *Plurivalent* immunogenic: BPO-BGG	+++	+++	+++	+++	+++	+++	+++
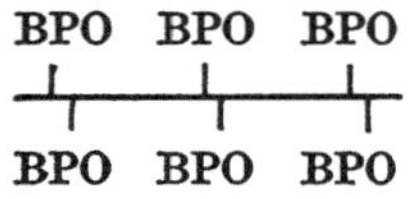 non immunogenic: BPO$_6$-PLL$_{12}$	—	+++	+++	+++	+++	+++	+++
Bivalent non immunogenic: BPO$_2$-HEX	—	—	—	++	++	++	++
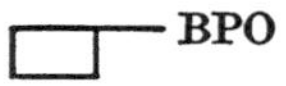 *Truly monovalent* immunogenic: BPO$_1$-BAC	+++	— inh	—	—	—	—	—
non immunogenic: BPO-EACA	— inh	— inh	—	inh	inh	inh	inh
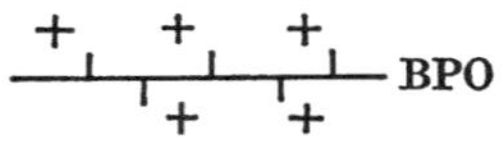 *Pseudo monovalent* immunogenic: BPO$_1$-PLL$_{12}$	++	— inh	+++	+++	+++	+++	+++

SA: Systemic anaphylactic shock in guinea pigs.
WER: Wheal- and -erythema reaction in human penicillin allergics.
inh: Specific inhibition.

optimal eliciting antigen appears to carry 4 to 5 antigenic determinants within a relatively short distance. This suggests very strongly that the reaction between antigen and antibody does not occur in free solution, but consists in the linking of antibody molecules which are restricted in their mobility e.g. by fixation on the surface of a cell membrane. The observations of Levine, which we have been able to confirm as well in guinea pigs as in man (de Weck, 1968) are a powerful argument in favour of the bridging theory of anaphylaxis formulated by Ovary and Taranta (1963).

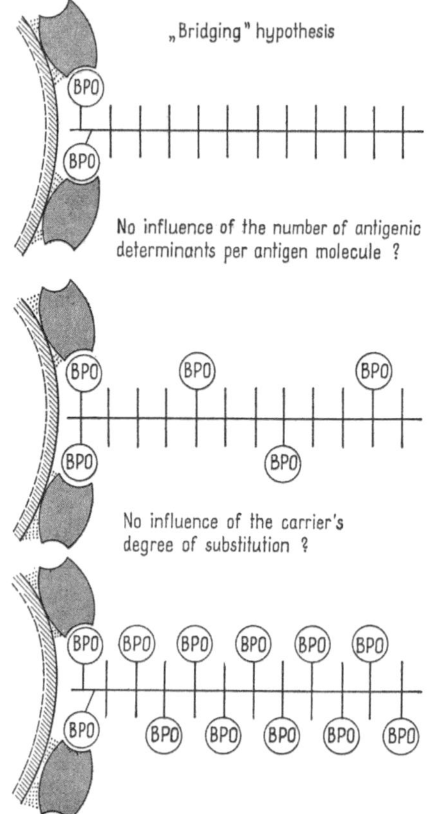

Fig. 2. Elicitation of anaphylactic reaction

More compelling even for the bridging theory is the fact established first by Parker *et al.* (1962a), confirmed by Ovary (1963), Levine (1965a) and ourselves (de Weck, 1968), that bivalent antigens which are unable to precipitate antibody, which do not yield complement-fixing complexes and which do not cause Arthus reactions, are nevertheless capable of eliciting all types of anaphylactic reactions, as well *in vitro* as *in vivo*, in experimental animals and in man. We have recently been investigating in the penicilloyl system some of the stereochemical factors involved in the bridging of two antibody combining sites by a bivalent antigen. As shown in Fig. 4, there appears to be an optimal distance between antigenic determinants in order to achieve bridging. Assuming the penicil-

loyl determinant to be completely engulfed in the antibody combining site, the
bridging distance between two combining sites would be about 10 Angström.
Another argument in favour of the bridging hypothesis is the phenomenon of
anaphylaxis inhibition in excess of bivalent antigen (Fig. 5). Whereas it appears
almost impossible to cause hapten inhibition with a plurivalent antigen, marked
inhibition in excess of bivalent antigen is readily obtained, as well in systemic
(de Weck and Schneider, 1969), as in local anaphylaxis. Bivalent antigens are by
no means the most efficient in eliciting anaphylactic reactions and antigens carry-

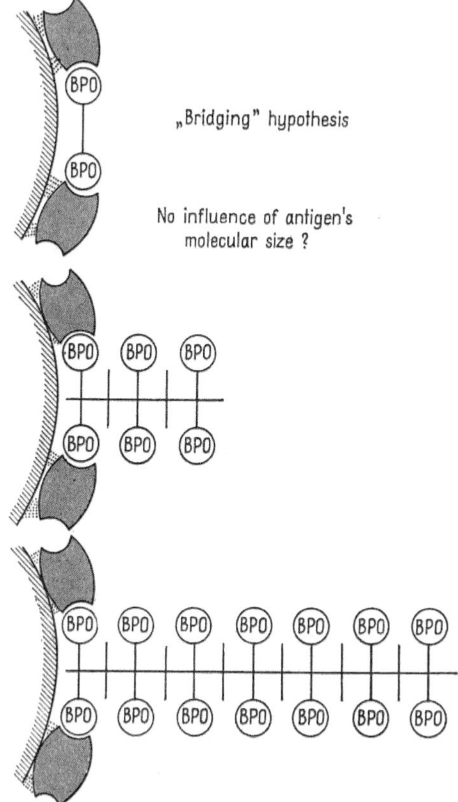

Fig. 3. Elicitation of anaphylactic reaction

ing 3 to 6 antigenic determinants are certainly more efficient. As antibodies
responsible for anaphylactic reactions appear to be cytotropic and bound to the
cell surface by their F_c fragment, a visual expression of the bridging reaction on
the surface of the mast cell may be represented as in Fig. 6. Whereas early re-
presentations of the antibody molecule and the Edelman model still considered
the antibody molecule as an ovoid possessing one combining site at each end
(as shown schematically in Figs. 1 to 5), recent investigations confirmed by
direct observations with the electron microscope (Valentine and Green, 1967)
rather ascribe to the IgG immunoglobulin molecule the shape of a fork (as in
Fig. 6).

The role of monovalent antigens in anaphylaxis, which for a while appeared quite clear to most investigators, has now become somewhat controversial. It had almost become classical that monovalent haptens and especially monovalent conjugates (e.g. a hapten-amino acid compound where the reactive hapten has no longer the capacity to form eventual plurivalent conjugates *in vivo*) are incapable of eliciting anaphylactic reactions *in vitro* or *in vivo*. Moreover, such compounds have repeatedly been demonstrated as able to inhibit specifically such reactions when given in sufficient excess together with or prior to the eliciting plurivalent antigen. However, several authors have reported in recent years that some appar-

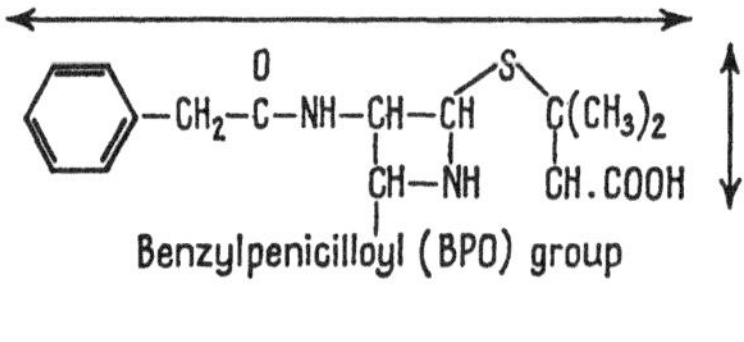

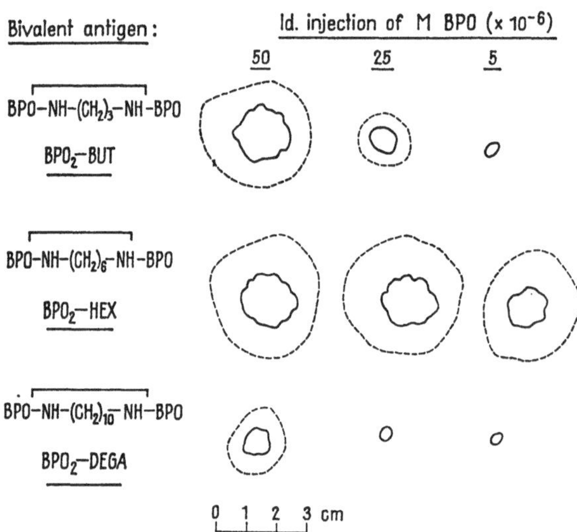

Fig. 4. Elicitation of immediate wheal ○ and erythema ○ skin reactions by low molecular weight penicilloyl dimers in a penicillin sensitive patient

ently monovalent antigens are capable of eliciting anaphylactic reactions, essentially the passive cutaneous anaphylaxis in the guinea pig. Such compounds have been p-azobenzenearsonate-tyrosine or -oligotyrosine (Borek *et al.*, 1965), some ε-DNP-lysines with acyl substituents of various chain length on the α-amino group (Amkraut *et al.*, 1963; Frick *et al.*, 1968) and α-DNP-oligolysines (Schlossman *et al.*, 1966). We have reported the same phenomenon with apparently monovalent penicilloyl-polylysine preparations (de Weck and Schneider, 1968). In all these cases, the preparations behaved *in vitro* as apparently monovalent, i.e. they specifically inhibited the precipitation of anti-hapten antibody by a plurivalent hapten-carrier conjugate. However, it is our contention that all these compounds are in fact "pseudomonovalent," their eliciting capacity being due to aggregation and electrostatic phenomena occuring *in vivo* and also to some extent *in vitro* (e.g. complement fixation). Arguments pleading for this view are developed elsewhere (de Weck and Schneider, 1969; de Weck and Schneider, 1968). In the case of the pseudomonovalent penicilloyl-polylysine preparation, it was striking to observe that complete substitution of the still free amino groups by succinyl groups, whereas leaving unchanged the affinity for anti-penicilloyl antibody and the capacity of inhibiting its precipitation, completely abolished the ability to elicit cutaneous anaphylactic reactions. This demonstrates that the positive

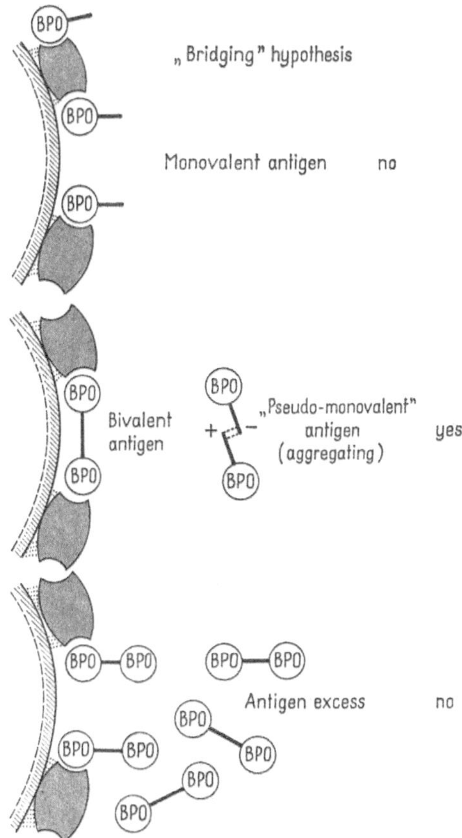

Fig. 5. Elicitation of anaphylactic reaction

charges of the amino groups on the polylysine carrier were responsible at least in part for the reaction.

The "bridging conception" of anaphylaxis has some practical implications:

1. It explains some of the clinical data encountered in the study of drug allergy, especially penicillin allergy. It has been noticed that the number of sensitized patients who may be demonstrated as possessing antibodies by immunological methods is much larger than the number of patients actually experiencing clinical allergic reactions upon administration of penicillin. The relative proportion of mono-, bi-, and plurivalent conjugates formed *in vivo* upon penicillin administration should play a decisive role on the outcome of penicillin

therapy in a sensitized individual. Monovalent conjugates compete for antibody combining sites with plurivalent conjugates and cause thereby an "inbuilt inhibition" phenomenon. This "inbuilt inhibition" is even fostered in the case of penicillin allergy by the fact that the unreacted penicillin molecule itself cross-reacts with the penicilloyl determinant and anti-penicilloyl antibodies.

2. The consistent inhibition of anaphylactic reactions by monovalent antigens may permit to achieve a specific inhibition of anaphylactic allergic reactions in the cases where the antigenic determinant is known. As will be seen below, it is even possible that by using non immunogenic monovalent haptens all types of allergic reactions would be inhibited.

3. We should pay increasing attention to the polymerization phenomena eventually occuring in solutions of allergenic drugs, e.g. the formation of eliciting antigens might eventually not require at all the formation of a conjugate with autologous proteins *in vivo*. In penicillin solutions, dimers and polymers may be

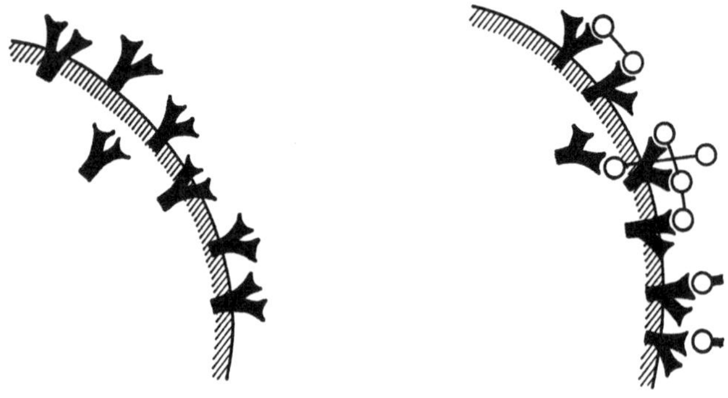

Fig. 6. Bridging

formed in several ways and this may represent an important aspect of penicillin anaphylaxis (de Weck *et al.*, 1968).

4. Theoretically, monovalent immunogenic molecules should be the ideal tool to achieve specific desensitization (or immunization) without risk of undesirable anaphylactic reactions by overdosage.

2. Elicitation of Arthus Reactions

Plurivalent antigens capable of precipitating antibody *in vitro* and of forming complement-fixing complexes are quite efficient in eliciting Arthus reactions in rabbits and guinea pigs, whether they are immunogenic or not (Table 3). In contrast with the observations made in anaphylaxis, bivalent antigens which may only form linear and soluble antigen-antibody complexes and do not fix complement *in vitro* (Ovary, 1963; de Weck and Schneider, 1969) were in our hands unable to elicit Arthus reactions in rabbits and guinea pigs possessing large amounts of anti-BPO antibodies and yielding massive Arthus reactions to plurivalent BPO antigens. Truly monovalent antigens were unable to elicit Arthus reactions.

On the other hand, the pseudomonovalent penicilloyl-polylysine (BPO_1 — PLL_{12}), which was inhibiting precipitation *in vitro* but fixed complement in

Table 3

Antigen			Immunogenicity	Elicitation of Arthus reactions			
			Induction of anti-BPO Ab	*in vitro*		*in vivo*	
				Ab precipitation	C'fixation	Rabbit	Guinea pig
Plurivalent immunogenic:	BPO BPO BPO BPO—(BGG)—BPO BPO BPO	BPO-BGG	$+++$	$+++$	$+++$	$+++$	$+++$
non immunogenic:	BPO BPO BPO $\dashv$ $\quad$ $\dashv$ $\quad$ $\dashv$ BPO BPO BPO	BPO_6-PLL_{12}	—	$+++$	$+++$	$+++$	$+++$
Bivalent non immunogenic:	BPO———BPO	BPO_2-HEX	—	—	—	—	—
Truly monovalent immunogenic:	□—BPO	BPO_1-BAC	$+++$	— inh	—	—	—
non immunogenic:	——— BPO	BPO-EACA	—	—	—	—	—
Pseudo monovalent immunogenic:	BPO	BPO_1-PLL_{12}	$+++$	—	$+++$[a]	$+++$[a]	$+++$[a]

[a] In part non specific: activity present at higher dose also in normal serum and normal animals; activity abolished by substitution of NH_2 groups.

presence of anti-BPO antibody, was very efficient in eliciting Arthus reactions. It soon became evident that some elements of the Arthus reaction elicited by such pseudomonovalent compounds are of non specific nature (de Weck and Schneider, 1968). First, in guinea pigs immunized with the monovalent penicilloyl-polylysine or with penicilloyl-bacitracin and possessing relatively low amounts of anti-BPO antibodies, Arthus reactions were elicited at equivalence of BPO determinants only by the monovalent preparation and not by the plurivalent. Furthermore, the Arthus eliciting ability was abolished by succinylation. The role of *in vivo* aggregation due to electrostatic interactions of the free ε-amino groups is made evident by the fact that similar reactions may be elicited at higher dosage even in normal guinea pigs ("Arthus-like" reaction) (de Weck and Schneider, 1968). The report by Schlossman *et al.* (1966) that Arthus reactions may be elicited in guinea pigs by supposedly monovalent α-DNP-oligolysines certainly rests in our opinion on a similar phenomenon. It is striking to notice that in Schlossman's experiments, Arthus reactions were not elicited by α-DNP-lysine or α-DNP-trilysine. Only α-DNP-oligolysines with at least 4 to 5 free amino groups appeared to be efficient Arthus elicitors.

3. Elicitation of Delayed Reactions

As may be seen in Table 4, the constellation of immunological responses elicited by various pluri-, bi- or monovalent antigens in the BPO system is different for delayed, anaphylactic or Arthus reactions. It is remarkable that non immunogenic antigens, whatever their number of antigenic determinants per molecule, are unable of eliciting delayed reactions. This appears to be the characteristic not only of that system but has been recognized also during the last years as well with α-DNP-oligolysines (Schlossman *et al.*, 1966), as with derivatives of the p-azobenzenearsonate group linked to various types of peptides or amino acids (Leskowitz, 1967). This has been apparent also in our experiments on more than 35 different DNP-amino acid preparations (Frey *et al.*, 1969). As a rule, only immunogenic preparations appear to be able to elicit delayed reactions in sensitized individuals. A special case appeared to be that of penicilloyl-bacitracin. This compound was able to induce a state of delayed hypersensitivity as demonstrated by marked delayed reactions to the pseudomonovalent penicilloyl-polylysines (de Weck and Schneider, 1968). However, penicilloyl-bacitracin itself was mostly unable of eliciting delayed reactions even in animals which had been immunized with that antigen. This phenomenon, which had for a while escaped our understanding, could now be explained if it would be admitted that the local delayed reaction represents in fact an anamnestic antibody response in situ.

The apparent absolute requirement for immunogenicity of antigens eliciting delayed reactions indicates that this reaction is probably an active process involving living sensitized lymphoid cells. As well as only immunogenic antigens are capable of eliciting delayed reactions *in vivo*, they alone also are able to induce the lymphoblastic transformation *in vitro*, the inhibition of macrophage migration and the induction of a secondary antibody response *in vivo* and *in vitro*. Furthermore, it is striking that the carrier specificity which appears to be a characteristic of delayed reactions *in vivo* is also encountered in lymphoblastic transformation, in the macrophage migration inhibition and in the induction of secondary antibody

Table 4

Antigen		Elicitation of Anaphylaxis	Arthus	Immunogenicity Induction of Ab formation	Induction of delayed hypers.	Secondary response in vitro	in vivo	Delayed reactions in vivo Local i.d.	Systemic i.v.	Flare up old tests
Plurivalent immunogenic:	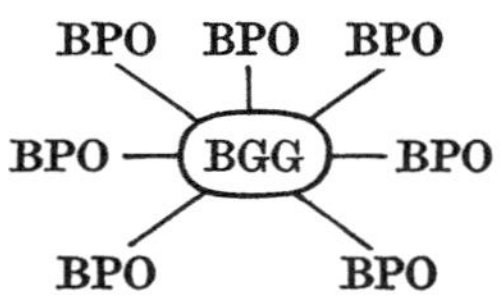 BPO_6-BGG	+++	+++	+++	+++	+++	+++	+++	+++	+++
non immunogenic:	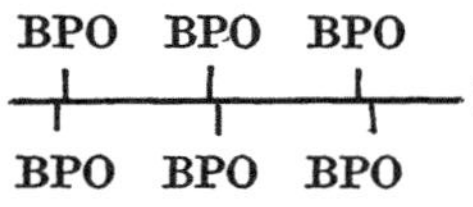 BPO_6-PLL_{12}	+++	+++	—	—	+++[a]	—[b]	—		
Bivalent non immunogenic:	BPO_2-HEX	+++	—	—	—		—[b]	—		
Truly monovalent immunogenic:	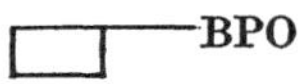 BPO_1-BAC	—	—	+++	+++		+++	—		
non immunogenic:	BPO-EACA	—	—	—	—	—	—	—	—[c]	—[c]
Pseudo monovalent immunogenic:	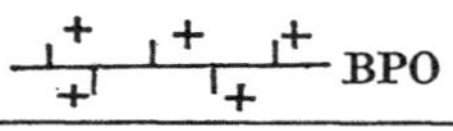 BPO_1-PLL_{12}	+++	+++	+++	+++		+++	+++	+++	+++

[a] By Ag-Ab complexes ?
[b] In animals primed by BPO-BGG.
[c] In the corresponding DNP system (α-DNP-lysine).

response *in vivo* and *in vitro*. Guinea pig antibodies appearing first during the immune response also appear to possess some carrier specificity. Some antibodies definitely demonstrate carrier specificity and it is therefore no longer tenable to distinguish immediate and delayed-type hypersensitivity on the basis of carrier specificity alone. Nevertheless, it is striking that the cellular elements responsible for the anamnestic or secondary antibody response share a common requirement for carrier specificity with the elements responsible for delayed reactions *in vivo*.

In recent years, a number of observations have supported the hypothesis that the delayed inflammatory reaction occuring at the site of local antigen deposition is due to an active antibody formation by lymphoid cells attracted to the reaction site (de Weck, 1969).

If the first stage of the delayed reaction could be considered as an anamnestic antibody response, a second stage might involve the formation of toxic antigen-antibody complexes. For the formation of such complexes, it would logically follow from what was discussed above that plurivalent antigens would be required. At that stage, the delayed reaction would ressemble somewhat the Arthus reaction and involve similar pathogenetic mechanisms. When considered from this point of view, it may be recalled how frequently difficult it is to distinguish sharply between the histology of Arthus and delayed reactions. The same cellular elements appear to be involved although with different timing and sequence. This is readily explainable if the antibodies required in delayed reactions are produced locally, appear at a different time and in different quantitative relationships. It would become readily understandable that truly monovalent penicilloyl-bacitracin is capable of inducing delayed type hypersensitivity but is unable of eliciting the delayed reaction. The elicitation of delayed reactions by pseudomonovalent antigens, as reported for dinitrophenyl or p-azobenzenearsonate derivatives will not be astonishing, as all these antigens were also capable of eliciting Arthus reactions.

However, this might be too simplistic a view. Experiments on inhibition of macrophage migration *in vitro* suggest that under the influence of antigen-protein substances are produced which will unspecifically act on the macrophages. It might be argued that these substances are precisely antigen-antibody complexes formed upon reaction of secreted antibody with antigen present in excess in the medium. Some reports (Svejcar *et al.*, 1968) indicate that supernates from antigen-sensitized lymphocytes mixtures obtained in presence of very little antigen will increase their inhibiting activity upon renewed addition of antigen. On the other hand, the macrophage inhibiting factor appears on gel chromatography to elute together with albumin and to have therefore a much smaller molecular weight as could be expected from antigen-antibody complexes (Bloom and Bennett, 1968).

Whatever will be the final answer, the use of synthetic antigens carrying one or a restricted number of antigenic determinants per molecule, taking advantage of the potentially unlimited number of immunogenic and non immunogenic peptide carriers at our disposal, will certainly increase in the near future our knowledge about the molecular mechanisms of delayed reactions.

References

Amkraut, H. A., L. T. Rosenberg, and S. Raffel: Elicitation of PCA univalent haptens. J. Immunol. **91**, 644 (1963).

Bloom, B. R., and B. Bennett: Migration inhibitory factor associated with delayed-type hypersensitivity. Fed. Proc. **27**, 13 (1968).

Borek, F., Y. Stupp, and M. Sela: Immunogenicity and role of size: response of guinea pigs to oligotyrosine and tyrosine derivatives. Science **150**, 1177 (1965).

Campbell, D. H., and G. E. McCasland: In vitro anaphylactic response to polyhaptenic and monohaptenic simple antigens. J. Immunol. **49**, 315 (1944).

Eisen, H. N., and G. W. Siskind: Variations in affinities of antibodies during the immune response. Biochemistry **3**, 996 (1964).

Farah, F. S., M. Kern, and H. N. Eisen: Specific inhibition of wheal and erythema responses with univalent haptens and univalent antibody fragments. J. exp. Med. **112**, 1211 (1960).

Frey, J. R., A. L. de Weck, H. Geleick, and W. Lergier: Immune responses to hapten-amino acid conjugates. I. The immunogenicity of dinitrophenyl (DNP)-amino acids. J. exp. Med. (under press).

Frick, O. L., W. Nye, and S. Raffel: Anaphylactic reactions to univalent haptens. Immunology **14**, 563 (1968).

Johner, R.: Antigenische Wirkung hoch- und niedermolekularer Komponenten von Insulinpräparaten in vitro und in vivo. Thesis, University of Bern, 1969.

Kaminski, M.: The analysis of the antigenic structure of protein molecules. Progr. Allergy **9**, 79 (1965).

Klopstock, A., u. G. E. Selter: Über chemospezifische Antigene. IV. Anaphylaxiereaktion mit chemospezifischen Antigenen. Z. Immun.-Forsch. **63**, 463 (1929).

Landsteiner, K.: The specificity of serological reactions. Boston: Harvard University Press 1945).

Leskowitz, S.: Mechanism of delayed reactions. Science **155**, 350 (1967).

Levine, B. B.: The nature of the antigen-antibody complexes which initiate anaphylactic reactions. I. A quantitative comparison of the abilities of non toxic univalent, toxic univalent, divalent and multivalent benzylpenicilloyl haptens to evoke passive cutaneous anaphylaxis in the guinea pig. J. Immunol. **94**, 111 (1965a).

— The nature of the antigen-antibody complexes which initiate anaphylactic reactions. II. The effect of molecular size on the abilities of homologous multivalent benzylpenicilloyl haptens to evoke PCA and passive Arthus reactions in the guinea pig. J. Immunol. **94**, 121 (1965b).

Ovary, Z.: In vitro and in vivo interactions of anti-hapten antibodies with monovalent and bivalent haptens. In: Conceptual advances in immunology and oncology, p. 206. New York: Hoeber-Harper 1963.

—, and F. Karush: Studies on the immunologic mechanism of anaphylaxis. I. Antibody-hapten interactions studied by passive cutaneous anaphylaxis in the guinea pig. J. Immunol. **84**, 409 (1960).

—, and A. Taranta: Passive cutaneous anaphylaxis with antibody fragments. Science **140**, 193 (1963).

Parker, C. W., M. Kern, and H. N. Eisen: Polyfunctional dinitrophenyl haptens as reagents for elicitation of immediate type allergic skin responses. J. exp. Med. **115**, 789 (1962a).

—, A. L. de Weck, M. Kern, and H. N. Eisen: The preparation and some properties of penicillenic acid derivatives relevant to penicillin hypersensitivity. J. exp. Med. **115**, 803 (1962b).

Schlossman, S. F., S. Ben-Efraim, A. Yaron, and H. A. Sober: Immunochemical studies on the antigenic determinants required to elicit delayed and immediate hypersensitivity reactions. J. exp. Med. **123**, 1083 (1966).

Sela, M.: Immunological studies with synthetic polypeptides. Advanc. Immunol. **5**, 29 (1966).

Standworth, D. R.: Reaginic antibodies. Advanc. Immunol. **3**, 181 (1963).

Svejcar, J., J. Pekarek, and J. Johanovsky: Studies on production of biologically active substances which inhibit cell migration in supernates and extracts of hypersensitive lymphoid cells incubated with specific antigen in vitro. Immunology **15**, 1 (1968).

Tillet, W. S., O. T. Avery, and W. F. Goebel: Active and passive anaphylaxis with synthetic sugar-proteins. J. exp. Med. **50**, 551 (1929).

Valentine, R. C., and N. M. Green: Electron microscopy of γG immunoglobulins. J. molec. Biol. **27**, 615 (1967).

de Weck, A. L.: Comparison of the antigen's molecular properties required for elicitation of
    various types of allergic tissue damage. In: Immunopathology, V, p. 295. (Miescher, P.,
    and G. MacMahon, Eds.). Basel: Schwabe 1968.
— The mechanism of delayed reactions (in preparation).
—, and C. H. Schneider: Immune and non immune response to monovalent low molecular
    weight penicilloyl-polylysines and penicilloyl-bacitracin in rabbits and guinea pigs.
    Immunology 14, 457 (1968).
— — Mono-, bi- and plurivalent antigens in the elicitation of anaphylactic reactions (in pre-
    paration).
— —, and J. Gutersohn: The role of penicilloylated protein impurities, penicillin polymers and
    dimers in penicillin allergy. Int. Arch. Allergy 33, 535 (1967).

Priv.-Doz. Dr. A. L. de Weck
Dermatologische Universitäts-Klinik,
Abteilung für Allergie
und klinische Immunologie,
3008 Bern, Schweiz, Inselspital

Discussion

Springer (Evanston): How did you prove that the haptens or the monovalent antigens actually polymerise or dimerise ? Did you carry out physical measurements ?

de Weck (Berne): This can be shown by centrifugation diffusion or chromatographic experiments.

Westphal (Freiburg): Polymerisates or aggregates are certainly much more easily obtained under these conditions than a monovalent substance. This difficulty must be specially emphasised.

Rajewsky (Cologne): I was especially attracted by the hypothesis you put forward that the bivalent hapten exerts its action by linking together two antibody combining sites. This is precisely what we and other people think about the induction of antibodies but I will go into this later. — I have a special question: Don't you think it could also be possible that the bivalent hapten is working by linking together the combining sites of the same antibody molecule which is bivalent itself ? What happens when one uses bivalent haptens with two different determinants in doubly sensitized animals ?

de Weck (Berne): This cannot be decided from our data. On the other hand, if you have a bivalent antigen, let us say with one antigenic determinant of one specificity and the other of another specificity, then you must have an animal which is doubly sensitised, in order to obtain a reaction. — To the antibody induction: these bivalent haptens are non-immunogenic.

Bayer-Symposium I, 47—62 (1969)

Mammalian Erythrocyte Receptors: Their Nature and their Significance in Immunopathology[1]

GEORG F. SPRINGER

With 3 Figures

Immunity reactions are interactions between the host and his environment. In this interaction "receptors" in the sense of Paul Ehrlich (1901) play a paramount role. The study of immunity reactions is not only important in itself but it furthers comprehension of other host-environment interactions including those of toxins, drugs or even live agents such as viruses. In all instances the agent or its products, be they noxious or beneficial, have first to attach to a receptor before they can begin to exert their influence.

Many of these interactions take place on cell surfaces and we have chosen the surface of the mammalian erythrocyte as a convenient and useful model for study of some of those surface receptors which show striking interactions with agents in the environment. We have isolated receptors with three different biological functions: first those which interact with antibodies, second those which interact with viruses and finally receptors which interact with toxins. Such investigations of isolated cell membrane components will ultimately allow integration of the findings on these isolated structures into the cell membrane as a whole and one may thus obtain a more accurate understanding of cell surfaces in general.

The first receptors to be discussed are those of the human blood-group MN system. They are fascinating in that the same terminal structure, sialic acid, is predominantly involved in both antibody binding and virus attachment. Furthermore, molecules carrying the receptor function occur in different stages of aggregation which profoundly influences their activities.

The Human MN Blood-Group Substances, Potent Myxovirus Receptors

The MN system was the second human blood-group system to be discovered (Landsteiner and Levine). The first conclusive evidence as to its chemistry was obtained in this laboratory (Springer and Ansell) and independently, a short while later by Finnish workers (Mäkelä and Cantell). It was shown that influenza viruses and Receptor Destroying Enzyme of *Vibrio cholerae* selectively destroy the main antigens of the MN system (Table 1). After publication of these results,

[1] This investigation has been supported by Atomic Energy Commission Contract No. At(11-1)1285, by National Institutes of Health Grant Nos. AI-05681 and AI-05682, by National Science Foundation Grant GB 8378, by The John A. Hartford Foundation Grant SD-340 and the Chicago Heart Association Grant RN 69-43.

Maintained by the Susan Rebecca Stone Found for Immunochemistry. The recent results described here were obtained in collaboration with Drs. J. Adye, W. Pollmann, S. V. Huprikar, A. Bezkorovainy and Mrs. H. Tegtmeyer.

other workers contributed significantly to the elucidation of the chemical nature of the MN blood-groups and influenza virus receptors of red blood cells (Klenk and Uhlenbruck; Baranowski *et al.*; Kathan *et al.*). We have succeeded in isolating highly active, homogeneous immunogenic MM, MN and NN substances from erythrocytes (Springer *et al.*, 1966a; Springer; Springer *et al.*, 1969a). In addition, these glycoproteins are together with the T and H urinary glycoprotein

Table 1. *Action of influenza viruses and "receptor destroying enzyme" on human red-cell antigens (2)*

The blood-group antigens A_1, B, H(0), Le^a, Le^b, S, s, P, Jk^a, K, k, Fy^a, Rh-, rh', rh'', hr', and hr'' are not inactivated

	Human erythrocyte agglutinogen			
	M	N	Lu^a	Lu^b
Influenza virus				
Type A				
Melbourne	+	+	+	+
Swine S_{15}	+	+	+	+
Type B				
Lee	+	+	+	+
Vibrio cholerae				
Receptor destroying enzyme	+	+	—	0

+ = inactivated; — = not inactivated; 0 = not tested.

Table 2. *Physical data on highly purified blood-group N-active human antigen*

	Erythrocyte antigen (NN) Ca 825
$S_{20, w}$ (S)	12.8 (c = 0)
$D_{20, w}$ (cm^2 sec^{-1})	1.67[a]
v (ml/g)	0.68
MW	595,000
f/f_o	2.34
$[\alpha]_D^{29}$ (H_2O, 1 dm)	—27.0° (c = 0.1)
η_{rel} (0.85% NaCl, 37.5°)	1.052[b], 1.099[c]
A 1%/274 mμ	10.90

[a] Average of values at 8.9 and 4.4 mg/ml; not concentration-dependent.
[b] c = 0.5%.
[c] c = 1.0%.

the most powerful inhibitors of hemagglutination by influenza viruses yet to be isolated (Springer *et al.*, 1969b).

These antigens and myxovirus receptors were isolated by gentle extraction of erythrocyte stroma of the appropriate type in the presence of electrolytes, differential centrifugation and fractionation on agar gel as well as Sephadex columns with preceding and subsequent precipitation by organic solvents followed by renewed differential centrifugation, gradient centrifugation and final electrodialysis.

We obtained the M and N antigens in physico-chemically homogeneous form, as determined by electrophoresis and ultracentrifugation. Table 2 contains physical data for the NN antigen (Bezkorovainy *et al.*). This particular preparation had a molecular weight of 600,000. The high f/f_0 values point to a marked asymmetry of the molecules. The strongly negative charge of the M and N glycoproteins was shown by their migration, as a single band, to the anode between pH 4.5 and 9.2.

Surprisingly the MN glycoproteins possess molecular weights which are multiples of 30,000 and the large molecules tend to disaggregate upon manipulation (Springer; Springer *et al.*, 1969a; Morawiecki). Blood-group as well as antiviral activities were highest for the largest molecules. The findings on sub-

Table 3. *In vitro activity of human MM and NN blood-group antigens: dependence on molecular size*

Antigen	Molecular weight	Smallest amount (µg/ml) completely inhibiting agglutination of human blood-group 0 erythrocytes by four agglutinating doses[a]		
		Human sera		Influenza virus
		Anti-M	Anti-N	PR8
MM				
Ca 979	12×10^6	1		0.05
Ca 980	6×10^6	3		0.2
Ca 1014	1.8×10^6	5		0.8
NN				
Ca 825	5.9×10^5		10	1.5
Ca 745	1.5×10^5		50	
M and N	3.1×10^4	500	3500	10

[a] Homologous, homozygous erythrocytes used for blood-group determination.

stances isolated in this laboratory under the gentle conditions described above are depicted in Table 3. It can be seen that blood-group and virus inhibitory capacity increase with molecular size. The difference in activity of the substances listed first and last respectively in the Table becomes even more striking if the activities are expressed on a molar basis: it is 10^4 to 10^6 fold.

Optical rotatory dispersion studies showed that the blood-group MN erythrocyte membrane antigens and virus receptors possess some conformational order (Fig. 1). Thus MM antigen Ca 1014 of molecular weight 1.8×10^6 and the NN antigen Ca 825 of molecular weight 5.95×10^5 contained 8 to 16% α-helical and extended β conformations. These conclusions were supported by determination of the Moffitt constants (b_0) and by measurements of circular dichroism. Conformational order decreased with decreasing molecular size (Jirgensons and Springer). Blood-group substances from secretions were largely disordered (Beychok and Kabat; Jirgensons and Springer). Our observation, that the blood-group substances and virus-receptors from cell membranes possess ordered structures to a significant degree are important in considerations

of cell membrane architecture. Ours appears to be the first observation of
the α and β conformations in blood-group glycoproteins, and the conformation
can be attributed to the peptide parts of the molecules. Also, these studies tempt
one to conclude that biological activities of the important cell-membrane glycoproteins depend not only on their terminal carbohydrates but in part on the conformation of their peptide constituents, since the disaggregation products showed
not only a lesser conformational order but also considerably lower blood-group and
antiviral activities than did the much larger aggregates from which they were
derived (Springer; Springer *et al.*, 1969a; Jirgensons and Springer).

In order to better assess the antiviral activity of the M and N antigens in comparison with the numerous other influenza virus inhibitors described (cf. Gott-

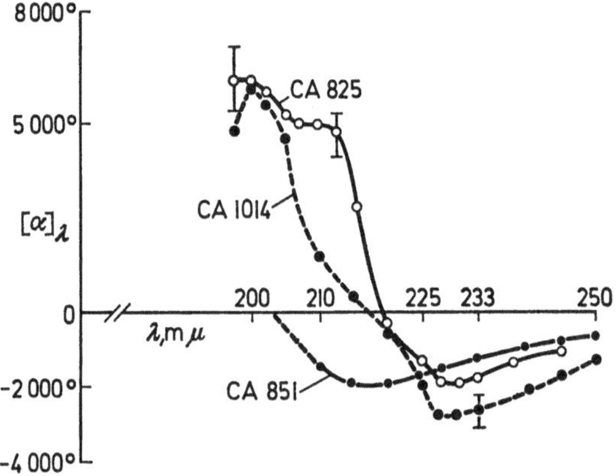

Fig. 1. Far-ultraviolet optical rotatory dispersion spectra of human blood-group antigens and
virus receptors. Ca 825, NN blood-group antigen and virus receptor from erythrocyte membranes. Ca 1014, MM blood-group antigen and virus receptor from erythrocyte membranes.
Ca 851, Vg blood-group antigen and virus receptor from meconium. The glycoproteins were
dissolved in 0.01 M sodium phosphate buffer, pH 7.2. The concentration of the substances was
from 0.020 to 0.038%; the optical path was 0.50, 0.20, or 0.10 cm. A symmetric angle at 5 deg.
was used for the oscillating prism

schalk) and in order to define the receptor truly complementary to these viruses,
activities of the M and N antigens towards various virus strains should be compared not only with one another but also with inhibitors from other sources.
Strict comparison is possible only if all inhibitors are tested in parallel since results
of serological titrations notoriously vary extensively from laboratory to laboratory (Kabat). As can be seen from Table 4 (Springer *et al.*, 1969a) human
blood-group MM glycoprotein Ca 979 was the most active substance with the
A/PR8 virus. The urinary glycoprotein (11/67) was the next most active preparation. There was a general dependence of activity on molecular size since glycoproteins with molecular weight $< 200{,}000$ even with sialic acid content of 7 to
12% had low activity. Also the number of inactive compounds increased with
decreasing molecular size.

Striking relations became demonstrable if molecular weight and sialic acid
residues of a given glycoprotein in Table 4 were expressed as per cent of reference
compound Ca 979. A ratio of approximately 1 for percent for molecular weight over

Table 4. *Influenza virus haemagglutination inhibition, molecular weight and sialic acid content of glycoproteins*

Glycoprotein	Molecular weight $\times 10^4$	Sialic acid (a)	(b)	Influenza virus inhibitory activity in % of human erythrocyte blood-group MM and myxovirus receptor substance Ca 979 Influenza virus strain			
				A/PR8		B/Md	
				weight	mole	weight	mole
Blood-group MM Ca 979	1200	11.5	4466	100	100	100	100
Urinary glycoprotein (11/67)	700	7.0	1586	60.0	35	400	234
γ-M globulin No. 2645	696[a]	1.8	405	1.5	0.870	25	14.51
Submax. mucin, bovine (J +, 2; 60—70)[b]	225	26.0	1667	7.5	1.404	12.5	2.343
α_2-macroglobulin No. 1067	82	1.8	48	N.A.[c]		5	0.342
Submax. mucin, ovine No. 3[b]	75	28.0	680	3.0	0.188	33.3	2.085
Blood-group NN Ca 825	59.5	16.2	312	4.17	0.207	12.5	0.622
Meconium-Vg Ca 851	52	9.3	157	3.75	0.163	100	4.340
γ-A globulin No. 662	25.4[a]	1.3	11	0.12	0.003	0.80	0.017
Sialomucopolysacch. Le[a] No. 350	23.7	18.0	138	7.5	0.148	200	3.950
Coeruloplasmin No. 2870	16	2.4	12	N.A.		0.80	0.011
Haptoglobin 1-1 (Co.)	8.5	5.2	14	0.12	0.001	25	0.177
Hemopexin No. 267	8.0	5.0	13	N.A.		10	0.067
α_{1x}-glycoprotein No. 1066	6.0	7.0	14	0.5	0.003	6.25	0.031
Tryptophan-poor glycoprotein No. 267	ca. 6.0	3.5	7	N.A.		0.4	0.002
α_1-antitrypsin No. 166	5.4	3.6	6	0.24	0.001	0.53	0.002
Fetuin, bovine I/III	4.5	6.0	9	0.24	0.001	12.5	0.047
α_1-acid glycoprotein No. 2507	4.4	12.1	17	N.A.		0.80	0.003
Zn-α_2-glycoprotein No. 1267	4.1	4.7	6	N.A.		0.80	0.003
β_2-glycoprotein I No. 466	4.0	4.5	6	N.A.		1.67	0.006
Blood-group MM subunit[d]	3.4	12	13	1	0.003	1	0.003

(a) Weight %. Determined and calculated as NANA except bovine submaxillary mucin as N, O-diacetyl derivative.

(b) Moles/Mole glycoprotein, nearest integer

[a] Mean molecular weights calculated from the weight distributions of different molecular species. γ-M globulin, molecular weights $\times 10^4$: 58, 100, 200, 1100, 2000 in percentages: 2, 41, 10, 34, 13. γ-A globulin, molecular weights $\times 10^4$: 16, 32, 48, 64 in percentages: 59, 28, 8, 5.

[b] Mean molecular weights, see text. Chemical data not corrected for ash and moisture.

[c] N.A. $<0.12\%$ inhibition for A/PR8 virus and $<0.4\%$ for B/Md virus. weight basis.

[d] Average values of two preparations tested.

per cent sialic acid existed for all but four glycoproteins with maximal deviations up to a factor of 3. There was also a relation of these two parameters to activity with the A/PR8 virus. The correlations became most readily evident if comparisons were made on a mole per cent basis for molecular weight and sialic acid and on a weight per cent basis for activity. Table 5 depicts the relations of these properties to Ca 979 and to one another. The ratios of molecular size and sialic acid over activity closely approaches 1, for nearly all of the glycoproteins listed, i.e., the decrease in activity is proportional to the decrease in molecular size (Springer *et al.*, 1969b). It follows that one may predict with a fair degree of accuracy the activity of glycoprotein of which the molecular weight and sialic acid content are known and conversely reasonable approximations may be made as to molecular weight and sialic acid content of a glycoprotein based on the extent of its inhibition of hemagglutination by the A/PR8 influenza virus.

If the activity of the inhibitors listed in Table 5 was also expressed on a molar basis as were the other properties with which it was compared, then decrease of molecular size and sialic acid content in the order of 1 decadic logarithm was accompanied by a decline in the potency of the active substances by 2 decadic logarithms, i.e., the decline in activity proceeded approximately with the square of the decrease of molecular weight and sialic acid content.

Nearly all glycoproteins tested were more active with the B/Md virus than with the A/PR8 virus. Also, two substances were more active on a weight basis against the B/Md virus than the reference compound, these were urinary glycoprotein and sialomucopolysaccharide Le[a]. Generally the decline of potency with decreasing molecular weight of the glycoproteins was less steep with the B/Md virus than that observed for the A/PR8 virus. For 13 of the 20 different glycoproteins compared with Ca 979 (Table 4) the ratio sialic acid over activity was < 0.3 and for 10 of these the ratio of molecular weight over activity was also < 0.3. This indicates that in contrast to its action with A/PR8 virus Ca 979 contains more sialic acid and has a larger molecular size than needed for an effect with the B/Md virus corresponding to that of the smaller molecules.

Influenza viruses and Receptor Destroying Enzyme (R. D. E.) of *Vibrio cholerae* and *Clostridium perfringens* as well as proteolytic enzymes destroy blood-group M and N activity and also the antiviral properties of the M and N antigens. It is remarkable that in addition galactose oxidase but not α- and β-galactosidase destroyed M and N specificities as measured with human anti-M and -N sera and, to a lesser extent, as measured with rabbit sera (Springer *et al.*, 1966a). Neither of the two latter enzymes affected the antiviral activity. The receptor properties of the M and N antigens determined with the plant extract from *Vicia graminea* were also inactivated by proteases but not by sialidases. The *Vicia* specificity of the NN antigen was inactivated by galactose oxidase (Krüpe and Uhlenbruck; Springer *et al.*, 1966a), galactose in β-glycopyranosidic linkage is most likely involved in *Vicia* specificity of the NN antigen since one of the two β-galactosidases tested inactivated the *Vicia* receptor (Springer *et al.*, 1966a).

Analysis of N-specific haptens isolated from the N antigen by mild acid or pronase hydrolysis supported the conclusion that galactose is present either in subterminal position or, less likely, as a branch adjoining sialic acid. These haptens possessed as carbohydrate components 1 to 2 N-acetylneuraminic acid residues per 1 to 2 galactose residues (Springer *et al.*, 1966a; Hotta and Springer). Therefore, sialyl, sialyl-galactopyranosyl and β-galactopyranosyl groups appear to be involved in the virus and/or blood-group specificities discussed here.

M and N antigens are glycoproteins. Chemical data obtained on the latter are given in Tables 6 and 7 (Springer *et al.*, 1966a). The composition values add up

Table 5. *Molecular weight and sialic acid content in relation to A/PR8 influenza virus inhibitory activity*

Glycoprotein	M_w[a]	Activity[b]	Sialic acid[c]	M_w[a] Activity[b]	Sialic acid[c] Activity[b]
Blood-group MM Ca 979	100	100	100	1.0	1.0
Urinary glycoprotein (11/67)	58.33	60.0	40.6	0.97	0.68
Submax. mucin, bovine (J+, 2; 60—70)	18.75 (4.17)[d]	7.5	37.3 (8.29)	2.50 (0.56)	4.97 (1.10)
Submax. mucin, ovine No. 3	6.25 (4.17)	3.0	15.2 (10.1)	2.08 (1.39)	5.07 (3.37)
Blood-group NN Ca 825	4.96	4.17	7.0	1.19	1.68
Meconium-Vg Ca 851	4.33	3.75	3.52	1.15	0.94
Sialomucopolysacch. Le[a] No. 350	1.98	7.50	3.09	0.26	0.41
Haptoglobin 1-1 (Co.)	0.71	0.12	0.31	5.92	2.58
α_{1x}-glycoprotein No. 1066	0.50	0.50	0.31	1.0	0.62
α_1-antitrypsin No. 166	0.45	0.24	0.13	1.89	0.54
Fetuin, bovine I/III	0.38	0.24	0.20	1.58	0.83
Blood-group MM subunit	0.28	1.0	0.29	0.28	0.29

[a] % of blood-group MM glycoprotein Ca 979.
[b] % of Ca 979 on weight basis.
[c] % of Ca 979 on molar basis.
[d] Figures in parentheses based on lowest possible molecular weight for these mucins; see text.

to approximately 100% since the NN antigen contains ca. 10% of water and 2.5% of ash. The molar ratio sialic acid: total hexosamine: galactose is close to 1:1:1 in the NN antigen. Galactose is the predominating carbohydrate (molar basis),

Table 6. *Carbohydrate components of highly purified NN antigen*

Structural units	NN-antigen Ca 825	
	(wt. %)	Moles per mole antigen
Acetylneuraminic acid	16.2	312
Galactosamine	4.3	144
Glucosamine	3.1	103
Galactose	11.1	367
Mannose	5.4	179
Glucose	0.3	10
Fucose	0.7	25

Table 7. *Amino acid analysis of NN antigen Ca 825*

Amino acid	(wt.%)	[a]	[b]
Aspartic acid	2.93	131	6.3
Threonine	4.26	213	10.3
Serine	3.58	203	9.8
Glutamic acid	4.21	170	8.2
Proline	2.93	151	7.3
Glycine	1.46	116	5.6
Alanine	2.21	148	7.2
Valine	3.07	156	7.5
Isoleucine	2.52	114	5.5
Leucine	4.07	185	8.9
Tyrosine	1.78	58	2.8
Phenylalanine	1.85	67	3.3
Lysine	2.31	94	4.5
Histidine	2.08	30	3.9
Arginine	2.54	87	4.2
Methionine	2.46	98	4.7
Sum	44.26	2071	
Tryptophan	0.00		
NH_4+	0.77	255	

[a] Moles of amino acid/mole of antigen (nearest whole number).

[b] Moles amino acid/100 moles amino acid.

see Table 6. However, in some earlier NN preparations sialic acid was the most abundant carbohydrate by a small margin. The ratio glucosamine: galactosamine is ca. 0.75, an extraordinarily low figure for a glycoprotein. In addition, fucose and glucose were found in low concentration. The antigen possessed components with chromatographic properties of N,O-diacetylneuraminic acid (Springer *et al.*, 1966a); these substances have hitherto not been found in man. They appear to be more abundant in the MM antigen and may be involved in M specificity.

Table 7 gives results of the quantitative analysis of amino acids in the NN antigen (Springer *et al.*, 1966a). Threonine, serine, leucine, and glutamic acid are the predominant amino acids in the NN substance. The sum of acidic amino acids amounts to approximately three quarters and that of the basic ones to two thirds of the hydroxyamino acids. The antigen is characterized by its low content of aromatic amino acids; tryptophan and cystine are absent. The amino acid composition of both antigens resembles that of the ABH (O) blood-group substances from ovarian cysts (Carsten and Kabat; Pusztai and Morgan).

Table 8. *Components of NN antigen. Destroyed by 0.5 NaOH (23°, 63 h)*[a]

Component	Quantitative determination by	% Destruction NN antigen, Ca 825
Hexosamine, total	Elson-Morgan	48
Galactosamine	A.A.A.[b]	80—90
Glucosamine	A.A.A.[b]	0
Galactose	P.J.[c] after chromatography	66
Threonine	A.A.A.[b]	48
Serine	A.A.A.[b]	39
Tyrosine	A.A.A.[b]	56

[a] For procedures and unaffected components see text: Springer *et al.* 1966a.

[b] Amino acid analyzer Beckman, 120 °C.

[c] Park-Johnson procedure.

It was attempted to elucidate the nature of the carbohydrate—peptide linkage in both antigens by alkali degradation following recently used procedures (Anderson *et al.*; Kabat *et al.*). The results are given in Table 8. Galactosamine and galactose as carbohydrates, and threonine and serine as amino acids are the constituents involved in this linkage in both antigens since they are destroyed by β-elimination (Springer *et al.*, 1966a). In addition amide linkages appear to be involved (Springer *et al.*, 1969c).

We have concluded from the sum of the chemical and biological results that the sugar chains may have a length of only 4 to 6 monosaccharides in the NN antigen. The immunological specificity is probably determined by small oligosaccharide groupings on these chains: multiple units of not more than 2 sugars for *Vicia* specificity and not more than 4 for human N specificity. The total number of chains with N specificity as determined with human anti-N serum is at most approximately 300 per molecule of antigen Ca 825 (Springer *et al.*, 1966a).

Heterogenetic Infectious Mononucleosis Receptors (I.M.R.s)

It is known since 1932 that powerful heterophile antibodies arise in patients suffering from infectious mononucleosis (Paul and Bunnell) a disease which may be caused by a virus. This antibody reacts with a variety of animal erythrocytes. It is likely that the anti-I.M. antibody is of cross-reacting nature. Infectious mononucleosis has had considerable attention since there have been recent reports (Henle *et al.*; Niederman *et al.*) which indicate that the agent causing infectious mononucleosis may be a herpes-type (E. B.) virus which occurs with remarkable frequency in cell lines derived from the malignant Burkitt's lymphoma. It is conceivable that the antibody of patients suffering from infectious mononucleosis is directed against a surface component of the agent causing I. M. or against a neoantigen induced by it.

---

1. *Cattle Erythrocyte Stroma* (act.^{a} 0.3)
   homogenize, pH 8.6
   centrifuge, 2000 g sediment

2. *Crude I. M. Receptor* (act. 0.05; 75% of 1.)
   reflux with 100% acetone and ethanol
   residue, extract with hot 75% ethanol
   centrifuge extract; 96,000 — 132,000 g interlayer
   ethanol fractionation, 77 to 92% precipitate

3. *Purified I. M. Receptor* (act. 0.002; 0.5% of 2.)
   gel filtration, Sepharose 2B
   main peak, centrifuged on sucrose density gradient (34 to 14%), 91,000 g, 15 h
   main peak, recentrifuged on sucrose density gradient
   main peak, dialysed

4. *Highly Purified I. M. Receptor* (act. 0.001; 0.005% of 2.)

---

^{a} act = mg/ml completely inhibiting the action of 4 hemagglutinating doses of I. M. serum.

Fig. 2. Extraction and purification of cattle I. M. receptor

Chemical characterization of the receptors which interact with the I. M. antibody has been confined to those located on beef and sheep erythrocytes (Springer and Rapaport; Callahan and Springer; Springer and Callahan, in preparation; Springer, in preparation). Fig. 2 shows our rather involved procedure of obtaining I. M. receptor from beef erythrocytes in highly specific and active form. The receptor material appears to be glycoprotein. On paper electrophoresis this material migrates as one homogeneous component to the anode between pH 3 and 9 but it is polydisperse in the ultracentrifuge.

This alkaline extraction procedure failed on sheep erythrocytes. The first observation pointing to the chemical nature of the I. M. receptor on sheep erythrocytes was its inactivation on treatment of sheep erythrocytes by influenza viruses and Receptor Destroying Enzyme (R. D. E.) from *Vibrio cholerae* (Springer and Rapaport). Recently we extracted I. M. R. from sheep erythrocyte stroma at 65 °C with 45% phenol in 0.45% aqueous NaCl. Active material was obtained and further purified by fractional centrifugation, gel filtration, ethanol fractionation and gradient ultracentrifugation. Again this highly active material appears to be of glycoprotein nature and migrates as one component on paper electrophoresis between pH 5.0 and 8.6. It has two closely similar components in the analytical ultracentrifuge and on disk electrophoresis (Callahan and Springer).

Table 9 shows that both the cattle and sheep receptors possess as high *in vitro* activities with anti infectious mononucleosis antibody as do the human blood-group glycoproteins isolated from either secretions or red cells measured with their respective antibodies. Both receptors cross-react with the type specific polysaccharides of pneumococcus XIV. The I. M. receptors possess only traces of serum sickness receptor activity. Forssman activity was even lower and usually not demonstrable in receptor preparations from beef erythrocytes, but in contrast to widely held opinion occasional preparations from cattle red cells did possess Forssman specificity. In addition some partly purified cattle I. M. receptor preparations cross-reacted with anti human blood-group B antibodies.

The sheep erythrocyte I. M. antigen is related biologically to the MN blood-group system of human erythrocytes as indicated by its blood-group M cross-

Table 9. *In vitro biological activities[a] of purified I.M.R.*

I.M.R. from	Hemagglutination inhibition				*Vicia graminea*	Precipitation[b]	
	Human anti					Anti — I.M.	Horse anti — pneumoc. XIV
	I.M.	Serum sick.	Forssman	M			
Sheep	0.01	0.6	1	0.01[c]	0.6	2.5	5
Beef	0.001	2.5	2.5—>5	>5	>5	0.3	1.2

[a] mg/ml, inhibiting or precipitating corresponding antibody.
[b] Capillary test.
[c] Active with 3 of 4 human anti-M sera.

activity, when determined with human antisera, and also by its *Vicia graminea* specificity. Both the I. M. and M activities are destroyed by plant proteases and R. D. E. treatment of the sheep I. M. R. The main difference of the I. M. R. from beef erythrocytes as compared to that from the sheep is the former's lack of notable cross-reactivity with human erythrocyte antigens and its relative resistance to proteases.

Analytical data are shown in Table 10. Sheep cell material had 7.5% N, ca. 7% sialic acid. The ratio N-glycolyl over N-acetyl was about 2:1 for these sialic acids. Hexosamine amounted to 11% with glucosamine predominating over galactosamine approximately 2:1. On paper chromatograms there was a predominance of galactose over both hexosamines combined as well as small amounts of fucose, glucose and mannose. A highly purified cattle receptor preparation contained 10.6% N, ca. 4.5% sialic acid with N-glycolyl neuraminic acid predominating over N-acetylneuraminic acid by about 3:1; 4.5% hexosamine was found colorimetrically and by paper chromatography about as much galactose as glucosamine with only a trace of galactosamine were detected. In addition small amounts of fucose, mannose and glucose were present. Paper chromatographic analyses for amino acid showed the I.M.R. preparations from both sources to contain significant

Table 10. *Analytical data for purified I.M.R.*

	Nitrogen %	Sialic acids %	Hexosamines %
Sheep:	7.5	7.0[a]	11.0
Cattle:	10.6	4.5[b]	4.5

Paper chromatography

Carbohydrates[c]

Sheep — gal, Nglu, Ngal, fuc, glu, man
Cattle — gal = Nglu, fuc, man, glu

Amino acids

Sheep and Cattle — leucine, valine, lysine, aspartic acid,
threonine, serine, alanine, glutamic acid, phenylalanine;
traces of glycine and proline

[a] N-glycolyl to N-acetyl neuraminic acid 2:1.
[b] N-glycolyl to N-acetyl neuraminic acid 3:1.
[c] Listed in order of decreasing intensity.

amounts of leucine, valine, lysine, aspartic acid, threonine, serine, alanine, glutamic acid and phenylalanine. Glycine and proline were found in small amounts.

Endotoxin Neutralizing Receptor Substance From Human Erythrocytes ("L.P.S.-Receptor")

Endotoxin of Gram-negative bacteria (L.P.S.) has to attach itself to host cell or tissue receptors before it can begin to exert its deleterious action. The attachment not only occurs *in vitro* (cf. Neter) but under severely pathological conditions also *in vivo* (Springer and Horton, 1964). Certain compounds of small molecular size, such as aldehydes, gangliosides and glycerophosphatides inhibit the irreversible L.P.S. attachment to red cells (Springer *et al.*, 1966b; Adye and Springer). The coating of red cells by L.P.S. is measured either by antisera directed against the serologically specific structures of the L.P.S. or by uptake of radioactively labelled L.P.S. (Lüderitz *et al.*; Adye and Springer). We have isolated material from human erythrocytes which carries the structures combining with the L.P.S. It possesses ca. 200 times the activity of washed, solubilized stroma (Springer *et al.*, 1966b; Springer *et al.*, 1969d). Activity was determined by the ability of the L.P.S. receptor preparations to inhibit erythrocyte sensitization by lipopolysaccharides with the micro-procedure described earlier (Springer and Horton; Springer *et al.*, 1966b). As can be seen from Table 11 the receptor material specifically inhibits 0 antigens of Gram-negative bacteria. Even the closely related common (Kunin) antigen of Gram-negative bacteria is barely inhibited in its coating action and the Vi antigens as well as antigens of Gram-positive bacteria are not inhibited by very large concentrations of L.P.S. Receptor. Thus we have isolated a highly specific structure.

Other substances such as the gangliosides and phospholipids inhibit L.P.S. fixation to a lesser extent than the L.P.S. Receptor and their action does not seem to be specific (Springer *et al.*, 1966b; Adye and Springer; Springer *et al.*, in preparation; Neter *et al.*, in preparation). The L.P.S. Receptor not only prevents the attachment of L.P.S. to red cells but is able to remove once attached lipopolysaccharide to a significant extent as do also certain glycolipids, as is shown in Table 12 (Adye and Springer). The L.P.S. Receptor is inactivated by the proteases papain and trypsin but not by numerous glycosidases.

Analysis of a typical L.P.S. Receptor preparation showed %: C, 48.2; H, 7.3; N, 10.8; S, 1.45; P, 0.14; hexosamine, 6; sialic acid, 6; methylpentose, 0.5. Total protein by the ninhydrin method was 54% and maximal reduction after hydrolysis

Table 11. *L.P.S.-Receptor: inhibitor of bacterial antigen fixation to erythrocytes*

Antigen	Antigen: Smallest amount coating maximally μg/ml	L.P.S.-receptor smallest amount inhibiting coating by >95% μg/ml
GRAM-NEGATIVE BACTERIA		
0 antigen	1—7.5	2—50
Kunin antigen	22	800
Vi antigen	1—2.5	700—>1000
GRAM-POSITIVE BACTERIA		
Rantz antigen	60—200	>1000
Staphylococcus pyogenes isolated group antigens, stearoyl derivatives	4	>1000

Table 12. *Removal of (^{32}P) L.P.S. from red cells by inhibitors of coating within 1 hr*

Inhibitor	Inhibitor (^{32}P) L.P.S. ratio[a]	% removed
Ganglioside	53	46
L.P.S.-Receptor	133	21
Phosphatidyl-ethanolamine	267	66

[a] Weight basis.

ca.15%. Paper chromatography of L.P.S. Receptor hydrolyzates revealed sugar spots migrating like sialic acid, galactosamine (2), glucosamine (2), galactose (2), mannose (1), and traces of glucose and fucose. Ninhydrin-positive spots like glycine, serine, threonine, aspartic acid, glutamic acid, alanine, valine, hydroxyproline, arginine, and (iso) leucine were also identified on paper chromatograms. The receptor material contained about 15% lipid.

This presentation began with blood-group substances and it will close with them since they serve to demonstrate that the receptors we have studied may be ubiquitous ones in nature. It is well known that all individuals possess antibodies against those antigens in the AB0 system which they do not possess themselves.

G. F. Springer

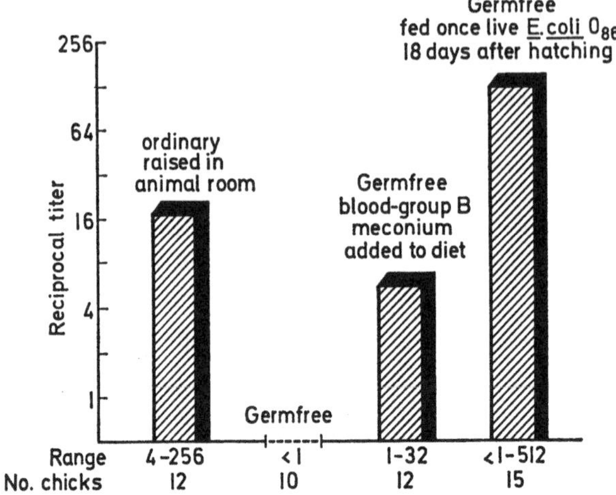

Fig. 3. Average titer — triplicate determination. Anti-human blood-group B agglutinins in White Leghorn chicks, 45 days old. Average weight of ordinary chicks 489 gm, of germfree 545 gm

Table 13. *Blood-group isoagglutinin stimulation in man by feeding killed or live blood-group active E. coli O_{86}*

Max. titer increase 1 mo. after start of E. coli feeding	Infants (2 weeks to 8 months old)			Adults	
	Diarrhea	Healthy	Not fed E. coli; Diarrhea or healthy	Intestinal lesions	Healthy
	16[a]	7	7	3	11
64—128 fold	3 (4)[b]				
16—32 fold	6 (1)	1 (3)		1 (2)	(3)
4—8 fold	2 (2)	1 (1)		1 (1)	4 (2)
<4 fold	5	5 (2)	7 (7)	1	7 (6)

[a] Number of cases.

[b] Values in parentheses = Coombs test; not all persons studied by this procedure.

Table 14. *Distribution of blood-group activity among gram-negative bacteria*

Genus	Strains tested	A_1	B	H(0)	A_1BH(0)	A_1B	A_1H(0)	BH(0)	Inactive
Escherichia	135	8	18	22	6	3	3	4	71
Salmonella	19	1	2	9	0	0	1	0	6
Arizona	3	0	1	1	0	0	0	1	0
Klebsiella	42	2	6	4	3	1	1	5	20
Citrobacter	24	2	2	2	0	2	2	3	11
Pasteurella	8	0	1	0	0	0	0	2	5
Proteus	20	0	6	2	0	0	0	1	11
Pseudomonas	15	1	1	2	0	0	1	0	10
Serratia	2	0	0	2	0	0	0	0	0
Alcaligenes	8	0	0	0	0	0	1	1	6
Shigella	5	0	0	0	0	0	0	0	5
Herrellea	1	0	1	0	0	0	0	0	0
Total	282	14	38	44	9	6	9	17	145

This fact necessitated the blood banks. Where do these antibodies come from if there was no immunization with red cells? For a long time they were thought to be inherited but Fig. 3 shows that in chickens these antibodies are due to immunogenic stimuli (Springer *et al.*) and we also found that in humans they can be stimulated by bacteria, Table 13 (Springer and Horton, 1969), which as Table 14 (Springer *et al.*) demonstrates are quite common.

It is evident then that study of receptors not only furthers knowledge of their structure and yields information about a specific interaction but also contributes to understanding of ubiquitous surface structure principles which nature has preserved throughout its phylogenetic development.

References

Adye, J. C., and G. F. Springer: Mode of inhibition of endotoxin coating of human red cells by compounds of known structure. Fed. Proc. **27**, Nr. 2, 267 (1968).

Anderson, B., P. Hoffman, and K. Meyer: The O-serine linkage in peptides of chondrotin 4- or 6-sulfate. J. biol. Chem. **240**, 156—167 (1965).

Baranowski, T., E. Lisowska, A. Morawiecki, E. Romanowska, and K. Strózecka: Studies on blood group antigens M and N; III. Chemical composition of purified antigens. Arch. Immunol. Terapii Dows. **7**, 15—27 (1959).

Beychok, S., and E. A. Kabat: Optical activity and conformation of carbohydrates. I. Optical rotatory dispersion studies on immunochemically reactive amino sugars and their glycosides, milk oligosaccharides of glucose, and blood group substances. Biochemistry **4**, 2565—2574 (1965).

Bezkorovainy, A., G. F. Springer, and K. Hotta: Some physical properties of the human NN- and Me-Vg blood-group antigens. Biochim. biophys. Acta (Amst.) **115**, 501—504 (1966).

Callahan, H., and G. F. Springer: Infectious mononucleosis receptor from sheep erythrocytes. Fed. Proc. **25**, Nr. 2, 435 (1966).

Carsten, M. E., and E. A. Kabat: Immunochemical studies on blood groups. XIX. The amino acids of blood group substances. J. Amer. chem. Soc. **78**, 3083—3087 (1956).

Ehrlich, P.: Reprinted in P. Ehrlich: Gesammelte Arbeiten, Vol. 2, p. 316 (1901). Berlin-Göttingen-Heidelberg: Springer 1957.

Gottschalk, A.: Glycoproteins, Vol. 5, pp. 434—438. Amsterdam, London, New York: Elsevier 1966.

Henle, G., W. Henle, and V. Diehl: Relation of Burkitt's tumor-association herpes-type virus to infectious mononucleosis. Proc. nat. Acad. Sci. (Wash.) **59**, 94—101 (1968).

Hotta, K., and G. F. Springer: Isolation and partial characterization of blood group N specific haptens from human blood group M and N substances. In: Proc. X. Congr. Int. Soc. Bl. Transf. Stockholm 1964, pp. 505—509. Basel-New York: Karger 1965.

Jirgensons, B., and G. F. Springer: Conformation of blood-group and virus receptor glycoproteins from red cells and secretions. Science **162**, 365—367 (1968).

Kabat, E. A.: Blood-group substances. New York: Academic Press, Inc. 1956.

—, E. W. Bassett, K. Pryzwansky, K. O. Lloyd, M. E. Kaplan, and E. J. Layug: Immunochemical studies on blood groups. XXXIII. The effects of alkaline borohydride and of alkali on blood group A, B, and H substances. Biochemistry **4**, 1632—1638 (1965).

Kathan, R. H., R. J. Winzler, and C. A. Johnson: Preparation of an inhibitor of viral hemagglutination from human erythrocytes. J. exp. Med. **113**, 37—45 (1961).

Klenk, E., u. G. Uhlenbruck: On the isolation of mucoids containing neuraminic acid from human erythrocyte stroma, a contribution to the chemistry of agglutinogens. Z. physiol. Chem. **319**, 151—160 (1960).

Krüpe, M., u. G. Uhlenbruck: Zur Natur der Phytagglutininrezeptoren an einigen Erythrozytenmucoiden von Mensch, Rind und Pferd. Z. Immun-Forsch. **126**, 408—414 (1964).

Landsteiner, K., and P. Levine: Inheritance of agglutinogens of human blood demonstrable by immune agglutinins. J. exp. Med. **48**, 731—749 (1928).

Lüderitz, O., O. Westphal, K. Sievers, E. Kröger, E. Neter u. O. H. Braun: Über die Fixation von P³²-markiertem Lipopolysaccharid (Endotoxin) aus *Escherichia coli* an menschlichen Erythrozyten. Biochem. Z. **330**, 34—46 (1958).

Mäkelä, O., and K. Cantell: Destruction of MN blood group receptors of human red cells by some influenza viruses. Ann. Med. exp. Fenn. **36**, 366—374 (1958).

Morawiecki, A.: Dissociation of M- and N-group mucoproteins into subunits in detergent solutions. Biochim. biophys. Acta (Amst.) **83**, 339—347 (1964).

Neter, E.: Bacterial hemagglutination and hemolysis. Bact. Rev. **20**, 166—188 (1956).

Niederman, J. C., R. W. McCollum, G. Henle, and W. Henle: Infectious mononucleosis. Clinical manifestations in relation to EB virus antibodies. J. Amer. med. Ass. **203**, 205—209 (1968).

Paul, J. R., and W. W. Bunnell: The presence of heterophile antibodies in infectious mononucleosis. Amer. J. med. Sci. **183**, 90—104 (1932).

Pusztai, A., and W. T. J. Morgan: Studies in immunochemistry 22. The amino acid composition of the human blood-group A, B, H, and Leᵃ specific substances. Biochem. J. **88**, 546—555 (1963).

Springer, G. F.: Human MN glycoproteins: dependence of blood-group and anti-influenza virus activities on their molecular size. Biochem. biophys. Res. Commun. **28**, 510—513 (1967).

—, and N. J. Ansell: Inactivation of human erythrocyte agglutinogens M and N by influenza viruses and receptor-destroying enzyme. Proc. nat. Acad. Sci. (Wash.) **44**, 182—189 (1958).

—, M. A. Fletcher, and J. Gregersen: Amide content of erythrocyte blood-group and virus inhibitory glycoproteins. Fed. Proc. **28**, Nr. 2, 899 (1969 c).

—, and R. E. Horton: Erythrocyte sensitization by blood group specific bacterial antigens. J. gen. Physiol **47**, Nr. 6, 1229—1250 (1964).

— — Blood-group isoantibody stimulation in man by feeding blood-group active bacteria. J. Clin. Invest. July, 1969.

— —, and M. Forbes: Origin of anti-human blood group B agglutinins in white leghorn chicks. J. exp. Med. **110**, Nr. 2, 221—244 (1959).

—, S. V. Huprikar, and E. Neter: Specific endotoxin neutralization by human erythrocyte receptor substance. Submitted for publication, 1969 d.

—, Y. Nagai, and H. Tegtmeyer: Isolation and properties of human blood-group NN and Meconium-Vg antigens. Biochemistry **5**, 3254—3272 (1966 a).

—, W. Pollmann (1) and C. S. Wang: In preparation (1969 a).

—, and M. J. Rapaport: Specific release of heterogenetic "mononucleosis receptor" by influenza viruses, receptor destroying enzyme and plant proteases. Proc. Soc. exp. Biol. (N. Y.) **96**, 103—107 (1957).

—, H. G. Schwick, and M. A. Fletcher: The relationship of the influenza virus inhibitory activity of glycoproteins to their molecular size and sialic acid content. Proc. nat. Acad. Sci. (Wash.) June, 1969 b.

—, E. T. Wang, J. H. Nichols, and J. M. Shear: Relations between bacterial lipopolysaccharide structures and those of human cells. Ann. N.Y. Acad. Sci. **133**, 2, 566—579 (1966 b).

—, P. Williamson, and W. C. Brandes: Blood group activity of gramnegative bacteria. J. exp. Med. **113**, Nr. 6, 1077—1093 (1961).

Prof. Dr. G. F. Springer
Department of Immunochemistry Research,
Evanston Hospital, Northwestern University,
2650 Ridge Avenue, Evanston,
Illinois 60201, U.S.A.

Bayer-Symposium I, 63—68 (1969)

Studies on the Structure and Formation of Antibodies

Felix Haurowitz

When we began to work on antibodies in 1929, we found soon that the non-antigen portion of the antigen-antibody precipitate had a composition similar to that of the serum globulins and that it was free of any non-protein prosthetic group. We drew the following conclusions: (1) the globulin found in the antigen-antibody precipitates is indeed antibody and not a contaminant of antibody molecules of unknown composition as suspected by many scientists at that time; (2) the formation of the antigen-antibody complex is caused by a close complementary fit between the peptide chains of the antibody molecule and the determinant groups of the antigen; and finally, (3) the complementary fit of the antibody molecule might be accomplished by interference of the administered antigen with the biosynthesis of the antibody globulins and with changes in the amino acid composition of the antibody molecules. According to this view the antigen acted as a template which instructed the cell what antibody it has to form. While conclusions (1) and (2) have been confirmed and are now widely accepted, the template hypothesis is at present less attractive than other views on the role of the antigen, although some instructive action of the antigen cannot yet be excluded. The principal reason for this change in our views is the enormous heterogeneity of the immunoglobulin population. Each of us may indeed have many thousands if not millions of different immunoglobulin molecules. Their number may be so high, that almost any injected antigen may encounter a molecule complementarily adapted to the antigenic determinants. The great heterogeneity of the immuno-globulin population has prevented complete elucidation of their amino acid sequence and has also made difficult the elucidation of the mechanism of antibody formation.

In my laboratory we have first tried to detect differences in the amino acid composition of antibodies of different specificity (Fleischer *et al.*, 1961). We used as antigens two azoproteins injected into different rabbits. One of these azoproteins contained the p-azophenylarsonate (As) determinant, the other the analogous p-azophenyl-N-trimethylammonium (R_4N) determinant. We precipitated from the serum of the rabbits the anti-As and anti-R_4N antibodies by the homologous antigens, isolated the antibodies and determined their amino acid composition. We found only very small differences which we considered as insignificant. These experiments were repeated by Koshland and Englberger (1963) who injected As-BGG and R_4N-BSA into the same rabbit and thus eliminated the possibility of genetic differences between rabbits. They found that the amino acid content in 16 of the 20 amino acids was identical, but that the anti-As antibodies contained more arginine and isoleucine, and less aspartic acid (or asparagine) and leucine than the anti-R_4N antibodies. Since BGG (= bovine γ globulin) has a much higher molecular weight than BSA (= bovine serum albumin), it seemed to us that the organ distribution of the two antigens in the rabbit organism might be different. In order to eliminate this possibility, we coupled equivalent amounts of the two haptens to BSA and injected the animals with doubly substituted As-R_4N-BSA. The serum of the injected rabbits contained at least three types of antibody, namely the two hapten-specific antibodies anti-As and anti-R_4N, and the mixture of anti-BSA antibodies directed against the various unknown determinants of the BSA molecule. There was no cross-reactivity between these three types of antibody so that they were easily separated from each other (Knight *et al.*, 1966).

When we isolated anti-As and anti-R_4N from individual rabbits and compared their amino acid composition, we found values very close to those found by Koshland and Englberger (1963). Whereas these authors had claimed that their amino acid equivalents correspond to integral numbers for each of the amino acids, we find that many of the amino acids occur in fractions of integral numbers. This would indicate that our preparations are heterogeneous mixtures of very similar, but not identical, antibodies directed against either the As or the R_4N determinant, respectively. Analyses of Koshland *et al.* (1966) on the isolated heavy and light chains of their purified antibodies have led them to the same conclusion since the amino acid equivalents per light or heavy chain obtained in these analyses were not integers. Evidently, the antibody preparations of Koshland *et al.* were just as heterogeneous as ours. Their finding of integral numbers in their earlier analyses may have been accidental.

Since the sensitivity of the fingerprint method is much higher than that of amino acid analyses, we digested the purified antibodies with trypsin and prepared peptide maps by electrophoresis in one dimension and chromatography in butanol-acetic acid in the second dimension. To our surprise, we failed to find any significant difference between the fingerprints. Occasionally, we found a small difference in one or two spots. However, this finding was not related to the hapten-specificity because it was not reproducible in other rabbits injected with the same As-R_4N-BSA preparation. Similar negative results have been obtained in other antibodies by Givol and Sela (1964), by Seijen and Gruber (1963) and by other authors. Our failure of finding any differences between the peptide maps of anti-As and anti-R_4N from rabbit serum cannot be attributed to insensitivity of the method. We find very clearcut differences between anti-As (or anti-R_4N) of two different species, rabbit and chicken. They reflect large differences in the amino acid composition of rabbit and chicken antibodies. However, we find no differences between the peptide maps of anti-As and anti-R_4N from the serum of chickens (Gold *et al.*, 1966).

Our failure to detect differences between the peptide maps of anti-As and anti-R_4N leads us to the conclusion that the specific combining sites of antibodies are highly heterogeneous. Heterogeneity of the purified antibody molecules can be demonstrated easily by gel electrophoresis of their reduced and alkylated peptide chains. We find in anti-As and anti-R_4N at least 2 bands of the heavy chains which at pH 8.2 migrate cathodically, and at least 6 to 8 bands of the light chains which migrate anodically. The electropherograms show small differences in the position and the intensities of the light chain bands; they also show that the heavy chains of anti-As migrate slightly faster toward the cathode than those of anti-R_4N. This is in agreement with the higher arginine content of anti-As antibodies.

Our statement that the specific combining sites of anti-As (and of anti-R_4N) are heterogeneous and yet complementarily adapted to the As- and R_4N-determinant, respectively, seems at first sight to contradict the view that the amino acid sequence determines the conformation of the peptide chain. However, this statement must not be reversed. One and the same conformation fitting complementarily to the As- or R_4N-determinant may be accomplished by many quite different amino acid sequences. It must be remembered that the complementariness needs to be only approximate. We know from affinity measurements that a serologically homogeneous antibody preparation consists of a population of antibodies with very different affinities for the antigenic determinant. We also know that the specificity of antibodies is usually not absolute and that most antibodies cross-react i.e., combine with antigens which carry determinant groups similar to but slightly different from the determinant group of the antigen used for sensitization.

The high heterogeneity of purified antibodies has rendered sequence analyses extremely difficult. They would be almost impossible if Edelman and Gally (1963) had not discovered that the Bence-Jones proteins are the light chains of very homogeneous immunoglobulins produced by myeloma cells. Dr. Hilschmann with Craig (1965) were the first to analyse the amino acid sequence of a Bence-Jones protein and thus made possible the comparison of their values with those obtained for the light chains of normal immunoglobulins and antibodies. Normal immunoglobulins and antibodies, according to these findings are mixtures of many hundreds or thousands of similar immunoglobulins, each of them probably produced in a different cell. If we consider the 8 to 10 bands of light chains as primary products, there should be at least 8 to 10 different types of immunocompetent, i.e., antibody forming cells. We have investigated immunoglobulin production and also antibody production in splenectomized rabbits and also in rabbits which were irradiated by heavy doses of X-rays but whose spleen was protected by a lead shield (Knight, 1967). We did not find any essential difference in the banding of the light chains, and conclude that the splenectomized rabbits have still the ability to produce all of the 8 to 10 different types of light chains. Hence, the 8 to 10 bands do not correspond to 8 to 10 different organs, but to 8 to 10 types of cells as claimed by Cohen and Porter (1964).

Analyses of Hill *et al.* (1966) and Cebra *et al.* (1968) have demonstrated that not only the light chains contain a heterogeneous variable portion but that a variable and heterogeneous amino acid sequence is also found in a part of the Fd portion of the heavy chains. Whereas almost all of the amino acid sequences of the Fc portion of the heavy chain in man and rabbit have been clarified, very little is known concerning the composition of the specific combining sites. Cebra *et al.* (1968) who investigated the Fd portion of the heavy chains of rabbit immunoglobulins, did not find any differences between the isolated tryptic peptides of normal immunoglobulin and anti-DNP antibodies, in agreement with our negative findings in fingerprints. Obviously, there must be a difference. However, the fingerprint method fails if a peptide occurs in less than about 20% of the molecules of a protein mixture. Such a peptide would not be detectable by the fingerprint method because the spot given with ninhydrin would be so weak that it would be impossible to differentiate it from the background of the peptide map.

The enormous heterogeneity of the immunoglobulins is satisfactorily explained by the variability of the N-terminal half of the light chains and similar variability of parts of the Fd portion of the heavy chains. Since both, heavy and light chains are variable, each of them possibly occurring in thousands of amino acid sequences, millions of different immunoglobulins could be formed. This makes the selective theories of antibody formation much more attractive, and makes it unnecessary to postulate a direct template action of the antigen (Breinl and Haurowitz, 1930; Haurowitz, 1952 and 1968). On the other hand, it is difficult to reconcile the heterogeneity of serologically pure, haptenspecific antibodies with Burnet's claim that all these antibodies are produced by clonal selection, i.e., by the selection of cells which after stimulation by the antigen multiply and produce clones of genetically identical daughter cells (Burnet, 1959). Burnets clonal selection theory is based on the assumption that each cell is predestined to produce only *one* definite type of immunoglobulin.

It seems to me that the heterogeneity of a preparation of haptenspecific antibodies produced in an individual rabbit is better explained by the assumption that the immunocytes or their immediate precursors are endowed with multipotentiality, but that they become actually unipotent after contact with the antigen. This idea was first advanced by Szilard (1960) who assumed that many if not most of the genes in immunocytes are repressed and silent, and that the antigen derepresses those of the genes which produce antibodies complementarily adapted to the antigenic determinants. According to this view, the antigen would not select among different cells but rather among different intracellular units of mRNA or DNA. Similar views were advanced by Gurvich and Nezlin (1965) and by Finch (1964).

Multipotentiality of the immunocytes is supported by the observation that in mice injected with sheep red blood cells all of the lymphoid cells of the spleen were able to lyse added sheep erythrocytes (Möller, 1968). Multipotentiality of a clone of lymphoid cells from a normal mouse was also demonstrated after transfer of these cells to irradiated mice injected with three different antigens; the transferred cells produced antibodies against all three antigens (Trentin *et al.*, 1967). The problem of multipotentiality versus unipotentiality is not yet solved. It is complicated by the fact that antibody formation seems to be a cooperative process in which two or more cell types take part, namely the macrophages in which we find most of the injected antigen, and the lymphocytes and plasma cells which produce antibody. It seems that the macrophages 'process' the antigen in some way and that a complex of RNA with the processed antigen is transferred from the macrophages to lymphoid cells and stimulates the latter to produce antibodies (Fischman, 1961; Fischman and Adler, 1963).

If the antigen acts indeed as a derepressor and thus selects between numerous genes or their mRNA products, the question may be raised whether the immunocytes contain a sufficient number of genes which would code for a large number of similar immunoglobulins. Recent work of Britten and Kohne (1968) and other authors has indeed demonstrated that mammalian cells contain a large number, probably more than 10^6, of similar nucleotide sequences in their DNA. The great variety of these nucleotide sequences, the genes, indicates a high rate of mutations of these genes during the phylogenetic evolution (Dreyer *et al.*, 1967). Although this is in excellent agreement with the view of intracellular selection, this view cannot yet be considered as definitely proved.

What are the alternatives? One of them suggested by Smithies (1968), Whitehouse (1967), and Edelman and Gally (1967), is the assumption of somatic mutations, for instance by crossing-over between DNA strands, or between different loops of a single DNA strand. Hypermutability of the antibody producing cells has been postulated first by Lederberg (1959). The idea was taken over by Burnet (1959) who postulated selective action of the antigen in a population of lymphoid cells undergoing rapid random mutations. It is at present impossible to prove convincingly that somatic mutations take place since the basic experiment of genetics, the mating of male and female cells, cannot be applied to somatic cells.

The idea of random mutations does not appeal to me because antibody formation is a predictable reaction which does not seem to depend on random events. I would rather believe in an orderly, predictable somatic process such as differentiation. We know that the precursors of the immunocytes undergo differentiation from lymphocytes to blast cells and finally to plasmacytes. This drastic change in morphology is certainly accompanied by changes in the function. Contact of a dormant lymphoid cell with the antigen as derepressor may trigger the multiplication and differentiation of the cell, and might thus convert the cell which is endowed with multipotentiality into a unipotent immunocyte which, on reinjection of the same antigen, would rapidly divide and multiply, and produce a large amount of the homologous antibody. The end product of this differentiation would be the plasma cell in whose cytoplasm we indeed see large quantities of antibody. One might designate such a process as selective or instructive differentiation.

I hope to have given you a short review on our present views on structure and formation of antibodies. Neither of these problems is solved. Both are of the utmost importance for our understanding of protein biosynthesis in general and particularly for our views on the mechanism of antibody formation.

The experimental work of my laboratory was supported by grants of the National Institutes of Health (GM 01852) and the National Science Foundation (GB 7850), and by contracts of Indiana University with the Office of Naval Research (NR 106-035) and the Atomic Energy Commission (AT 11-1) 209.

References

Breinl, F., u. F. Haurowitz: Z. physiol. Chem. **192**, 45 (1930).

Britten, R. J., and D. E. Kohne: Science **161**, 259 (1968).

Burnet, F. M.: The clonal selection theory of acquired immunity. Vanderbilt Univ. Press 1959.

Cebra, J. J., D. Givol, and R. R. Porter: Biochem. J. **107**, 69 (1968).

—, L. A. Steiner, and R. R. Porter: Biochem. J. **107**, 79 (1968).

Cohen, S., and R. R. Porter: Biochem. J. **90**, 268 (1964).

Dreyer, W., W. R. Gray, and L. Hood: Cold Spr. Harb. Symp. quant. Biol. **32**, 353 (1967).

Edelman, G. M., and J. A. Gally: J. exp. Med. **118**, 41 (1963).

— — Proc. nat. Acad. Sci. (Wash.) **57**, 353 (1967).

Finch, I. R.: Nature (Lond.) **201**, 1288 (1964).

Fischman, M.: J. exp. Med. **114**, 837 (1961).

—, and F. L. Adler: J. exp. Med. **117**, 595 (1963).

Fleischer, S.: Arch. Biochem. **92**, 329 (1961).

Givol, D., and M. Sela: Biochemistry **3**, 451 (1964).

Gold, E. F., S. Cordes, M. A. Lopez, K. L. Knight, and F. Haurowitz: Immunochemistry **3**, 433 (1966).

Gurvich, A. E., and R. S. Nezlin: Usp. biol. Khim. **7**, 150 (1965).

Haurowitz, F.: Biol. Rev. **27**, 247 (1952).

— Immunochemistry and the biosynthesis of antibodies. New York: J. Wiley and Sons 1968.

Hill, L. R., R. Delaney, H. E. Lebovitz, and R. E. Fellows: Proc. Roy. Soc. B, **166**, 159 (1966).

Hilschmann, N.: Z. physiol. Chem. **348**, 1718 (1967).

—, and L. C. Craig: Proc. nat. Acad. Sci. (Wash.) **53**, 1403 (1965).

Knight, K. L.: Proc. Soc. exp. Biol. (N. Y.) **124**, 1122 (1967).

—, M. A. Lopez, and F. Haurowitz: J. biol. Chem. **241**, 2286 (1966).

Koshland, M. E., and F. M. Englberger: Proc. nat. Acad. Sci. (Wash.) **50**, 61 (1963).

— —, and R. Shapanka: Biochemistry 5, 641 (1966).

Lederberg, J.: Science **129**, 1649 (1959).

Möller, G.: J. exp. Med. **127**, 291 (1968).

Seijen, H. G., and M. Gruber: J. molec. Biol. **6**, 209 (1963).

Smithies, O.: Cold Spr. Harb. Symp. quant. Biol. **32**, 161 (1968).

Szilard, L.: Proc. nat. Acad. Sci. (Wash.) **46**, 293 (1960).

Trentin, J., N. Wolf, V. Cheng, W. Fahlberg, D. Weiss, and R. Bonhag: J. Immunol. **98**, 1326 (1967).

Whitehouse, H. L. K.: Nature (Lond.) **215**, 371 (1967).

Prof. Dr. F. Haurowitz
Indiana University, Department of Chemistry,
Chemistry Building, Bloomington,
Indiana 47401, U.S.A.

Bayer-Symposium I, 69—89 (1969)

Structure and Formation of Antibodies

N. Hilschmann, H. U. Barnikol, M. Hess, B. Langer, H. Ponstingl,
M. Steinmetz-Kayne, L. Suter, and S. Watanabe

With 10 Figures

Antibodies are proteins which are produced in vertebrates after stimulation with an antigen. They are specifically directed against the antigen which has caused their production.

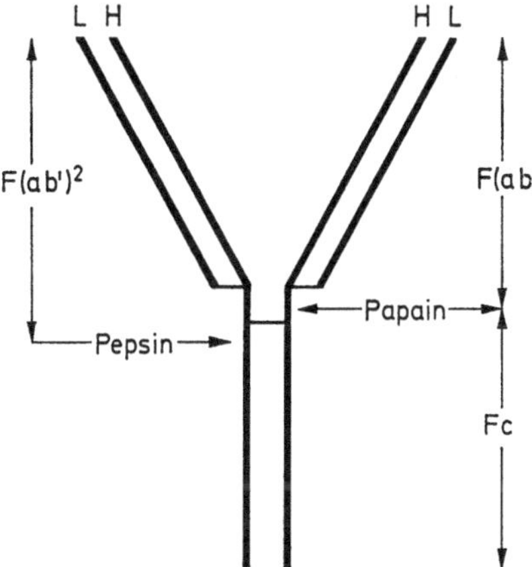

Fig. 1. Schematic representation of the 4-chain structure of IgG. L-(light) and H-(heavy) chains are linked by disulphide bonds. Indicated by arrows are the sites susceptible to enzymatic digestion. The combining sites are at both ends of the freely movable F(ab)-fragments

Antibodies consist of subunits. The smallest subunit of an immunoglobulin molecule has two identical L- and H-chains, which are connected by disulphide bridges and non-covalent bonds as shown in Fig. 1 (Fleischman *et al.*, 1963; Edelman and Gally, 1964). Several types of chains can be distinguished: $\varkappa$- and λ-type L-chains, and γ, α and μ-H-chains. The H-chain types determine the classification into the main immunoglobulin classes IgG, IgA and IgM, respectively. The outer shape of the IgG molecule is that of an Ypsilon, the two combining sites being at the ends of the two freely movable arms (Valentine and Greene, 1967). These combining sites comprise only a small percentage of the surface of the antibody molecule (Kabat, 1961).

The specificity of the antibody molecule is not determined by a different folding of one unique primary structure of the protein (Pauling, 1940), but by the different primary structures in the constituent chains: different antibodies having different amino acid sequences (Koshland and Engelberger, 1963; Haber, 1964; Whitney and Tanford, 1965).

Normally the information for the sequence of a protein is laid down in the genes. The question arises, whether the information for presumably 10^6 different antibodies is genetically transferred in the usual manner or if it is acquired during individual development. Does the germ-cell already have all the information for all possibly needed antibodies (multiple germ line), or is the information newly formed during the differentiation of the immuno-competent cells (somatic hyper-mutation)?

Whatever genetic mechanism is responsible for antibody formation, it should be reflected in the primary structure of the antibody molecule. A comparison between the primary structure of two antibodies of different specificity should show what kind of structural differences cause different specificities. Interpretation of these structural differences should give insight into the genetic mechanism which causes these structural differences.

However, one of the prerequisites of sequence analysis is that the substance under investigation must be chemically homogeneous and this unfortunately is not true in the case of antibodies even those made against one specific hapten.

Antibodies are produced in lymphoid or plasma cells. It has been shown by several investigators, although not quite univocally, that one single cell produces one single type of antibody (Pernis *et al.*, 1965; Pernis, 1967; Cebra *et al.*, 1966; Green *et al.*, 1967a; Green *et al.*, 1967b). When stimulated by antigen these cells or their precursors proliferate and form a cell clone. Since the antigen triggers the proliferation of various of these cells, a population of clones results, which produces a variety of chemically different antibodies with varying affinity for the antigen.

Homogeneous clones, however, do exist in multiple myeloma, or in macro-globulinaemia Waldenström, tumors which are derived from one single cell. The proteins produced by these tumors are the myeloma globulins, the Waldenström's macroglobulins and the Bence-Jones proteins, the latter being L-chains produced in excess and excreted in the urine (Edelman and Gally, 1962).

These monoclonal proteins are chemically homogeneous and therefore suitable for sequence analysis. Comparative sequence studies with these proteins made it possible to understand the complexity of antibody molecules. It has been determined which part of the immunoglobulins was responsible for antibody specificity and what kind of structural differences caused this specificity. In combination with genetic investigations we gained insight in the genetic mechanism of antibody formation. These studies also demonstrated that monoclonal immunoglobulins are not para- or abnormal proteins, but rather normal constituents of the immuno-globulin spectrum. They confirmed earlier serological data pointing in the same direction (Waldenström, 1961; Kunkel, 1965).

For the most part these conclusions were deduced from structural studies with L-chains which have a molecular weight of 23,000 and consist of 211 to 221 amino acid residues. They are composed of two covalently bound parts of equal length: an N-terminal variable and C-terminal constant half, i.e. structural differences which exist between different L-chains, are limited to the N-terminal half of the molecule, and consist of multiple amino acid exchanges and some deletions. These structural differences resemble homologies in proteins of different animals which are phylogenetically related. The constant half is identical in chains of the same antigenic type (Fig. 2) (Hilschmann and Craig, 1965; Hilschmann, 1967a). A genetic factor (inv) which is an allele, inherited codominantly in a simple Mendelian manner, was found to be localized in position 191 of the constant part of human $\varkappa$-type L-chains, inv a+ having Leucine and inv b+ having Valine in this position (Hilschmann and Craig, 1965; Milstein, 1966a; Baglioni et al., 1966; Hilschmann, 1966).

The general validity of these observations was soon confirmed with several monoclonal human (Titani et al.; Milstein, 1966b) and murine (Gray et al., 1967) $\varkappa$-type L-chains, with human λ-type L-chains (Putnam et al., 1967; Ponstingl et al., 1968; Langer et al., 1968; Milstein et al., 1967a) and with so called normal L-chain preparations (Milstein, 1965).

The H-chains, having just double the size of the L-chains, seem to be constructed according to the same principle. The length of the variable part is not yet exactly known; in all probability it is as long as that of the L-chains which

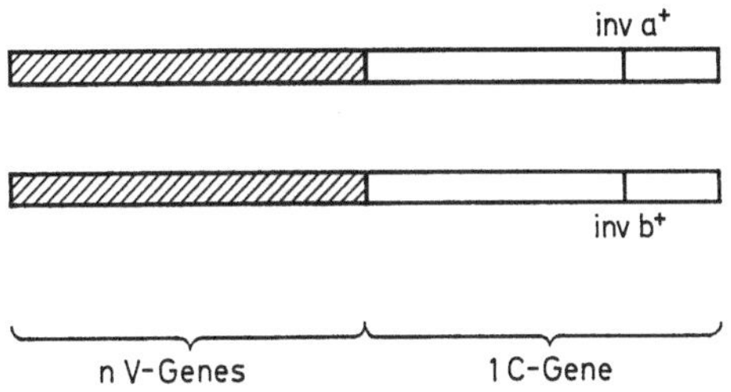

Fig. 2. Variable and constant halves of immunoglobulin L-chains. Variability is caused by homologous sequences, constancy by identical sequences in L-chains of the same antigenic type. This, together with the location of the allotypes on the constant part, indicates that variable and constant part must be under different genetic control: several genes for the variable and one gene for the constant part. For hypotheses on this phenomenon see text

would be one quarter of the molecule (Frangione and Milstein, 1967; Press and Piggot, 1967; Gottlieb et al., 1968).

These structural peculiarities had never been observed with other proteins. In accordance with the one gene one polypeptide chain dogma and because of the homology between the variable parts of different L-chains, several evolutionarily related genes (the V-genes) had to be assumed to control these different variable parts. For the constant part, however, the findings were only compatible with the assumption of one gene (the C-gene). This was concluded from the constancy of the sequence of the C-terminal half of L-chains of one chain type, and also from the localization of the allotypes on this part of the $\varkappa$-chains. When there is allelism, then this is an indication that this particular gene occurs only once in one haploid chromosome set. If there were as many C-genes as V-genes in one chromosome, these allotypes would not seggregate in a simple manner as they do (Steinberg, 1962). Also they would have to be introduced in several C-genes in exactly the same position during evolution, because these allotypes are not present in the mouse $\varkappa$-type L-chains (Gray et al., 1967).

From these considerations it was concluded that the variable and constant parts of the immunoglobulin chains must be under different genetic control: several genes for the variable and one for the constant part (Fig. 2).

Since both variable and constant parts are covalently bound in one L-chain protein, and since the size of mRNA and polysomes involved in antibody synthesis corresponds to that expected for the synthesis of a complete L- or H-chain, (Becker and Rich, 1966; Shapiro *et al.*, 1966; Williamson and Askonas, 1967) somatic gene fusion during individual development for the C- and V-genes had to be assumed.

A controversy arose concerning the number of V-genes which had to be inherited. The multiple germ line hypothesis postulated as many V-genes as variab-

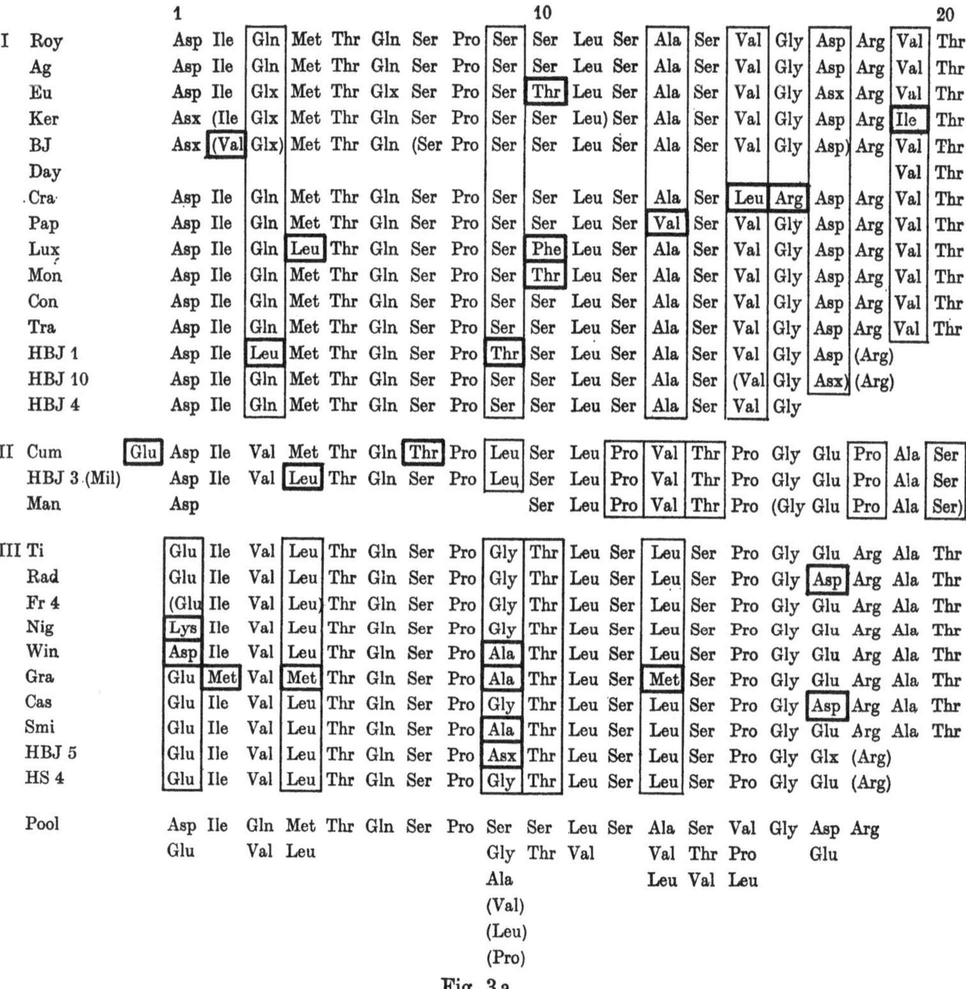

Grp	Name	ins	1	2	3	4	5	6	7	8	9	10	11	12	13	14	15	16	17	18	19	20
I	Roy		Asp	Ile	Gln	Met	Thr	Gln	Ser	Pro	Ser	Ser	Leu	Ser	Ala	Ser	Val	Gly	Asp	Arg	Val	Thr
	Ag		Asp	Ile	Gln	Met	Thr	Gln	Ser	Pro	Ser	Ser	Leu	Ser	Ala	Ser	Val	Gly	Asp	Arg	Val	Thr
	Eu		Asp	Ile	Glx	Met	Thr	Glx	Ser	Pro	Ser	Thr	Leu	Ser	Ala	Ser	Val	Gly	Asx	Arg	Val	Thr
	Ker		Asx	(Ile	Glx	Met	Thr	Gln	Ser	Pro	Ser	Ser	Leu)	Ser	Ala	Ser	Val	Gly	Asp	Arg	Ile	Thr
	BJ		Asx	(Val	Glx)	Met	Thr	Gln	(Ser	Pro	Ser	Ser	Leu	Ser	Ala	Ser	Val	Gly	Asp)	Arg	Val	Thr
	Day																				Val	Thr
	Cra		Asp	Ile	Gln	Met	Thr	Gln	Ser	Pro	Ser	Ser	Leu	Ser	Ala	Ser	Leu	Arg	Asp	Arg	Val	Thr
	Pap		Asp	Ile	Gln	Met	Thr	Gln	Ser	Pro	Ser	Ser	Leu	Ser	Val	Ser	Val	Gly	Asp	Arg	Val	Thr
	Lux		Asp	Ile	Gln	Leu	Thr	Gln	Ser	Pro	Ser	Phe	Leu	Ser	Ala	Ser	Val	Gly	Asp	Arg	Val	Thr
	Mon		Asp	Ile	Gln	Met	Thr	Gln	Ser	Pro	Ser	Thr	Leu	Ser	Ala	Ser	Val	Gly	Asp	Arg	Val	Thr
	Con		Asp	Ile	Gln	Met	Thr	Gln	Ser	Pro	Ser	Ser	Leu	Ser	Ala	Ser	Val	Gly	Asp	Arg	Val	Thr
	Tra		Asp	Ile	Gln	Met	Thr	Gln	Ser	Pro	Ser	Ser	Leu	Ser	Ala	Ser	Val	Gly	Asp	Arg	Val	Thr
	HBJ 1		Asp	Ile	Leu	Met	Thr	Gln	Ser	Pro	Thr	Ser	Leu	Ser	Ala	Ser	Val	Gly	Asp	(Arg)		
	HBJ 10		Asp	Ile	Gln	Met	Thr	Gln	Ser	Pro	Ser	Ser	Leu	Ser	Ala	Ser	(Val)	Gly	Asx)	(Arg)		
	HBJ 4		Asp	Ile	Gln	Met	Thr	Gln	Ser	Pro	Ser	Ser	Leu	Ser	Ala	Ser	Val	Gly				
II	Cum	Glu	Asp	Ile	Val	Met	Thr	Gln	Thr	Pro	Leu	Ser	Leu	Pro	Val	Thr	Pro	Gly	Glu	Pro	Ala	Ser
	HBJ 3 (Mil)		Asp	Ile	Val	Leu	Thr	Gln	Ser	Pro	Leu	Ser	Leu	Pro	Val	Thr	Pro	Gly	Glu	Pro	Ala	Ser
	Man		Asp									Ser	Leu	Pro	Val	Thr	Pro	(Gly	Glu	Pro	Ala	Ser)
III	Ti		Glu	Ile	Val	Leu	Thr	Gln	Ser	Pro	Gly	Thr	Leu	Ser	Leu	Ser	Pro	Gly	Glu	Arg	Ala	Thr
	Rad		Glu	Ile	Val	Leu	Thr	Gln	Ser	Pro	Gly	Thr	Leu	Ser	Leu	Ser	Pro	Gly	Asp	Arg	Ala	Thr
	Fr 4		(Glu	Ile	Val	Leu)	Thr	Gln	Ser	Pro	Gly	Thr	Leu	Ser	Leu	Ser	Pro	Gly	Glu	Arg	Ala	Thr
	Nig		Lys	Ile	Val	Leu	Thr	Gln	Ser	Pro	Gly	Thr	Leu	Ser	Leu	Ser	Pro	Gly	Glu	Arg	Ala	Thr
	Win		Asp	Ile	Val	Leu	Thr	Gln	Ser	Pro	Ala	Thr	Leu	Ser	Leu	Ser	Pro	Gly	Glu	Arg	Ala	Thr
	Gra		Glu	Met	Val	Met	Thr	Gln	Ser	Pro	Ala	Thr	Leu	Ser	Met	Ser	Pro	Gly	Glu	Arg	Ala	Thr
	Cas		Glu	Ile	Val	Leu	Thr	Gln	Ser	Pro	Gly	Thr	Leu	Ser	Leu	Ser	Pro	Gly	Asp	Arg	Ala	Thr
	Smi		Glu	Ile	Val	Leu	Thr	Gln	Ser	Pro	Ala	Thr	Leu	Ser	Leu	Ser	Pro	Gly	Glu	Arg	Ala	Thr
	HBJ 5		Glu	Ile	Val	Leu	Thr	Gln	Ser	Pro	Asx	Thr	Leu	Ser	Leu	Ser	Pro	Gly	Glx	(Arg)		
	HS 4		Glu	Ile	Val	Leu	Thr	Gln	Ser	Pro	Gly	Thr	Leu	Ser	Leu	Ser	Pro	Gly	Glu	(Arg)		

Pool:

Name	1	2	3	4	5	6	7	8	9	10	11	12	13	14	15	16	17	18
Pool	Asp	Ile	Gln	Met	Thr	Gln	Ser	Pro	Ser	Ser	Leu	Ser	Ala	Ser	Val	Gly	Asp	Arg
	Glu		Val	Leu					Gly	Thr	Val		Val	Thr	Pro		Glu	
									Ala				Leu	Val	Leu			
									(Val)									
									(Leu)									
									(Pro)									

Fig. 3 a

Fig. 3a—b. Comparison of the variable parts of ϰ-type L-chains of Roy (Hilschmann, 1967a), Cum (Hilschmann, 1967c), Ti [Suter *et al.* (in preparation)], Ag (Titani *et al.*, 1966), Eu (Cunningham *et al.*, 1968) Ker, BJ, Day, Man, Rad, Fr. 4 (Milstein, 1967b; Milstein, 1966c), HBJ 1, HBJ 10, HBJ 4, HBJ 5, HS 4 (Hood *et al.*, 1967), HBJ 3 (Mil) (Dreyer *et al.*, 1967), Cra, Pap, Lux, Mon, Con, Tra, Nig, Win, Gra, Cas, Smi, and Pool (Niall and Edman, 1967). On the basis of their chemical homology the proteins are divided into groups I to III. Group specific exchanges against the basic sequence (identical residues in at least two groups) are marked by light boxes, individual specific exchanges by dark boxes, deletions by —. Not determined sequences are within brackets

le parts (Dreyer and Bennett, 1965), therefore restricting the somatic process to a fusion of the C-with one of the V-genes. In opposition to this the somatic hypermutation hypotheses assumed only a limited number of V-genes in the germ line (Smithies, 1967; Hilschmann, 1967b; Edelman and Gally, 1967; Whitehouse, 1967). In order to cope with the observed diversity of the variable parts, the somatic process was extended also to somatic recombination between the V-genes. Some of the findings in L-chain structure could in fact be interpreted as being such a hybridization process (Hilschmann and Craig, 1965; Hilschmann, 1967b),

```
             23                              29  29a                   29f  30
Ile  Thr Cys Gln Ala Ser Gln Asp (Ile  —  —  —  —  —  —   Ser) Ile  Phe Leu Asn
Ile  Thr Cys Glx Ala Ser Glx (Asx Ile  —  —  —  —  —  —   Ser  Asx Phe) Leu Asn
Ile  Thr Cys Arg Ala Ser Glx Ser  Ile  —  —  —  —  —  —   Asx  Thr Trp Leu Ala
Ile  Thr Cys Gln Ala Ser Gln Asp  Ile  —  —  —  —  —  —   Lys  (Asn Phe)
Ile  Thr Cys Gln Ala Ser Gln Asp  Ile  —  —  —  —  —  —   Asn  Lys Tyr
Ile  Thr Cys Gln (Ala Ser Glx Asx Ile  —  —  —  —  —  —   Ser  Asx Phe Leu)
Ile  Thr
Ile  Ala
Ile  Thr
Ile  Thr
Ile  Thr
```

```
Ile  Ser Cys Arg Ser Ser Gln Ser Leu Leu Asp Ser Gly Asp Gly Asn Thr Tyr Leu Asn
Ile  Ser Cys Arg Ser Ser Gln Asn Leu Leu Glx Ser     Asx Gly (Asx)    Tyr Leu Asp
Ile  Ser Cys Arg
```

```
Leu Ser Cys Arg Ala Ser Gln Ser Val —  —  —  —  —     Ser Asn Ser Phe Leu Ala
Leu Ser Cys Arg Ala Ser Gln     Val —  —  —  —   Ser  Ser Asn Ser Tyr Leu
Leu Ser Cys Arg
Leu Ser
Leu Ser
Leu Ser
Leu Ser
Leu Ser
```

Fig. 3a (continuation)

but data were too little and too fragmentary to prove or disprove these recombination models. What was needed was a greater number of completely sequenced L-chains.

Comparison of L-Chain Structures

Recently the number of completely or almost completely sequenced κ- and λ-chains has considerably increased, giving a much more detailed insight into the variable or specificity region of these proteins (Hilschmann et al., 1968). Figs. 3 and 4 show all the variable parts of the human κ- and λ-type proteins, whose structure has thus far been determined. Variable parts consist of 106 to 115 residues, comprising the N-terminal half of the L-chains. The switch from the variable to the constant part of the molecule occurs in κ- and in λ-chains in identical positions.

As has already been mentioned, the variable parts of ϰ- as well as λ-chains are homologous proteins, i.e., all proteins have the same basic sequence. Differences between these proteins are caused by single or accumulated amino acid exchanges. The chains in Figs. 3 and 4 are arranged in such a way that this homology can clearly be recognized: identical or similar residues are in identical positions in every chain. Deviations from the basic sequence, caused by amino acid exchanges, are indicated by boxes. These exchanges are scattered equally all over the chains. Not only amino acid exchanges are observed, but also so called sequence gaps are found which are caused by the unequal length of the individual chains at certain positions. In both types of L-chains these sequence gaps have been observed to

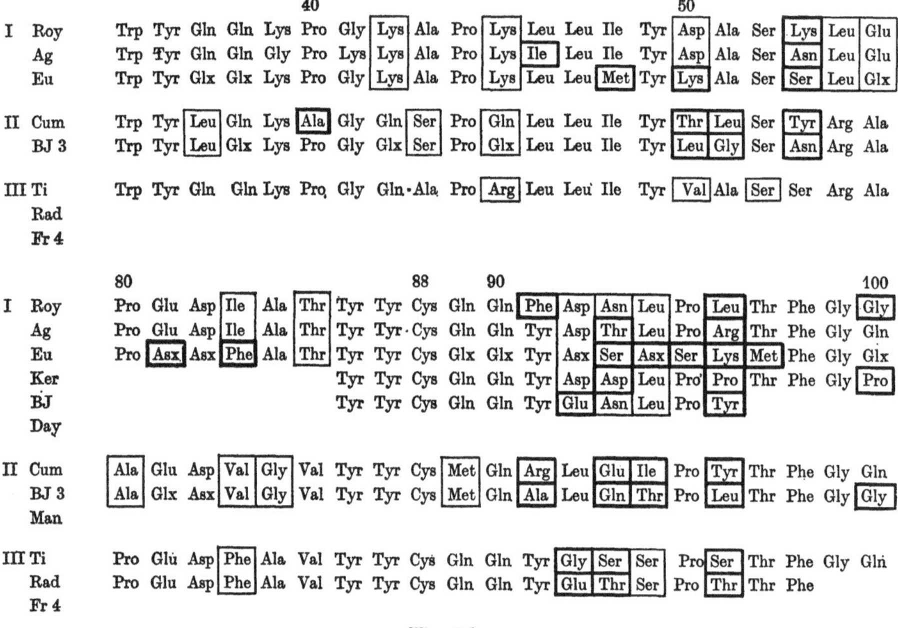

Fig. 3 b

occupy a position a few residues C-terminal of the first cysteine residue; in some λ-chains there is an additional gap after the second cysteine residue of the variable part.

The more data on primary structures of different L-chains became available, the more it became evident, that there was not only one basic sequence for the variable parts of one chain type, but several. Although all individual chains were homologous, some of these were chemically more similar than others. On the basis of this differing homology three clearcut groups could be recognized in the ϰ-chains, and four in the λ-chains. The light boxes in Figs. 3 and 4 indicate the positions where the group specific sequences deviate from the overall basic sequence. These group specific sequences or exchanges amount to about 40 to 50% of the residues of the variable part and are equally distributed all over the chain. They are mostly paralleled with a characteristic number of deleted amino acids in the sequence gaps in positions 28, 29 or 95/96 respectively. Proteins of one group have, in most cases, the same number of deleted amino acid residues. These sequence gaps were explained by deletions in the corresponding gene which have occured during evolution.

Superimposed in these specific sequences are single amino acid exchanges characteristic for one individual chain. Where these individual specific sequences differ from the group specific sequences, these exchanges have been marked by dark boxes in Figs. 3 and 4. Since these individual specific sequences do not exceed 25% of the group specific sequences, they do not disturb the classification into groups. The clear distinction between these groups is extremely important for the question of whether the variability of the immunoglobulins is caused by evolution or somatic hypermutation. The conclusions which can be drawn from

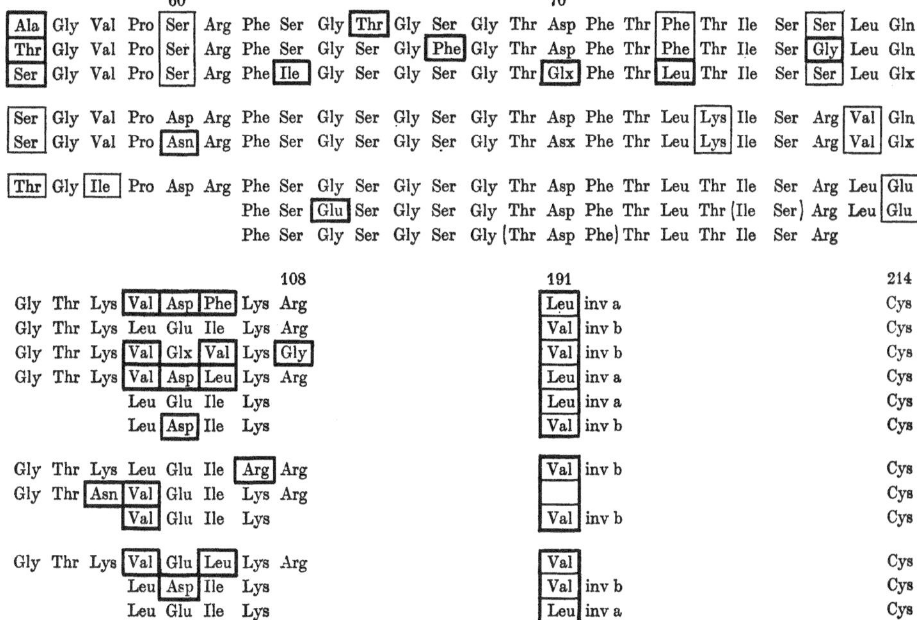

Fig. 3 b (continuation)

these structural studies in this respect had recently been discussed (Hilschmann et al., 1968 a), and will be described in detail later.

At first it should be recalled that diversity of immunoglobulin structure as depicted in Figs. 3 and 4 is responsible for the specificity of antibodies. This can be concluded from the earlier observation that the F(ab)-fragments (Porter, 1959) which, as we now know, comprise the variable parts of the L- as well as of the H-chain, also contain the combining sites of the antibody molecule. More direct evidence was obtained by more recent experiments in which it was possible to mark a tyrosine residue in or near the combining site of a specific antibody by the method of affinity labelling. Comparison of several isolated small enzymatic fragments containing this label with the known structure of monoclonal L-chains demonstrated, that this tyrosine residue occupied position 86 of the variable part of the L-chains (Singer and Thorpe, 1968).

Fig. 5 shows the constant parts of the $\varkappa$- and λ-type L-chains. As already mentioned sequences in the constant half are identical for every chain type. A single amino acid exchange in position 191 of the $\varkappa$-type proteins has been correlated with the corresponding allotypes inv a+ and inv b+. Several single amino acid exchanges could be observed in the constant part of different λ-chains (Ein and Fahey, 1967; Appella and Ein, 1967; Ponstingl *et al.*, 1967; Milstein, 1967 d).

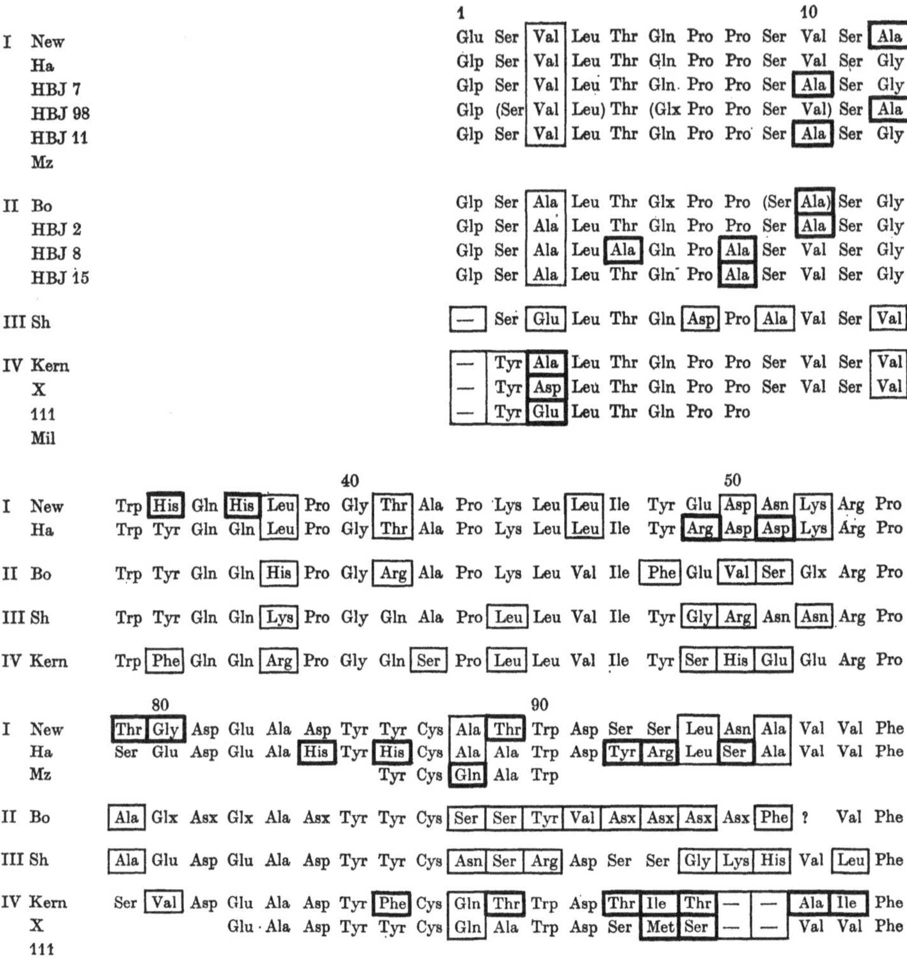

Fig. 4. Comparison of the variable parts of λ-type Bence-Jones Proteins Kern (Ponstingl *et al.*, 1968), New (Langer *et al.*, 1968), Sh, Ha, Bo (Putnam *et al.*, 1967), X, Mil, Mz [Milstein, 1967 (3); Cohen and Milstein (1967)], HBJ 2, HBJ 7, HBJ 11, HBJ 15 (Hood *et al.*, 1967), and BJ 98 (Baglioni 1967). On the basis of their chemical homology the proteins are divided in groups (I to IV). For symbols used see legend to Fig. 3. Exchanged amino acids in the constant part are shown for the Kern (Ponstingl *et al.*, 1967), the Oz (Ein and Fahey, 1967; Appella and Ein, 1967), and the Mz (Milstein, 1967 d) proteins

For one of these exchanges non allelic behaviour has been demonstrated using genetic analysis (Ein, 1968). It might be possible that these exchanges are an expression of the beginning subtyping of λ-type genes. This means that there might be more than one gene for the C-terminal part of λ-chains.

Fig. 5 also shows that the constant parts of $\varkappa$- and λ-chains are homologous proteins. Sequences which are identical in both chain types are marked in the figure by boxes. They account for 37% of the overall sequences. Similar values are obtained, when the variable parts of $\varkappa$- and λ-chains are compared, indicating a similar phylogenetic distance for both the variable and the constant parts from a common precursor.

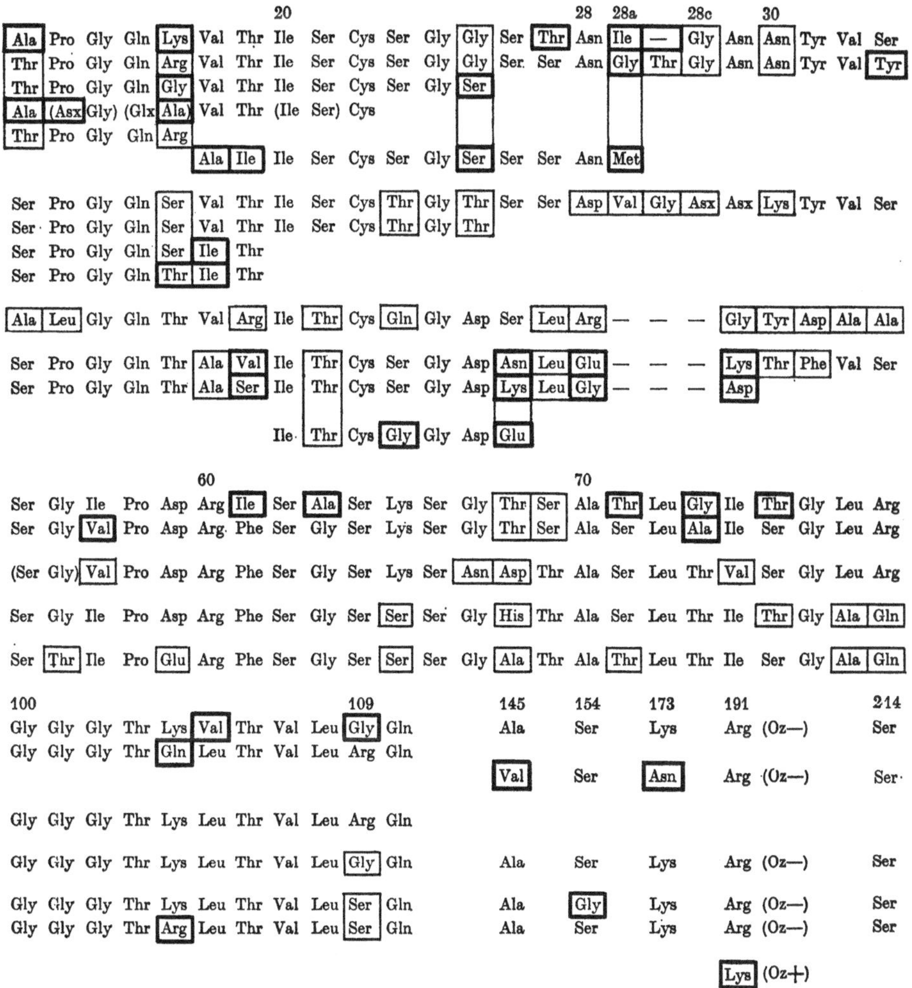

Fig. 4

Evolution of the Immunoglobulins

Homology does not only exist between different chain types, but also within the variable and constant parts of one chain. This internal homology can easily be recognized, when the sequences of the variable and constant part are compared as in Fig. 6. A similar comparison was drawn between the known sequences of the L-chains and the sequences of the Fc-fragment of rabbit IgG, including the constant half of the H-chain. From these data, the following scheme for the evolution of the immunoglobulin chains was drawn (Hill *et al.*, 1966) (Fig. 7).

According to this scheme the precursor gene of the immunoglobulins was most likely only half as large as an L-chain gene. It might have corresponded in size to a gene for the constant or variable part. From this precursor gene the L-chain gene has arisen by gene duplication and gene fusion. Gene duplication and translocation of this primitive L-chain gene followed by independent evolution has given rise to the ϰ- and λ-chains. In a similar fashion, the H-chain genes may be the product of

ϰ-Typ
λ-Typ

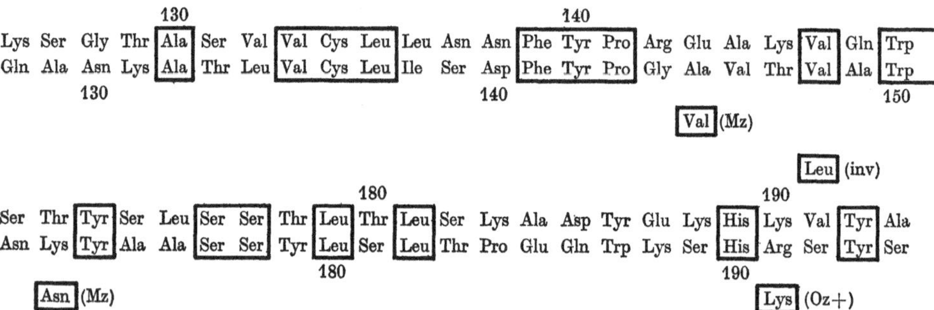

Fig. 5. Comparison of the constant parts of ϰ- and λ-chains (Hilschmann, 1967a; Hilschmann, 1966; Titani *et al.*, 1966; Milstein, 1966b; Putnam *et al.*, 1967; Ponstingl *et al.*, 1968; Langer *et al.*, 1968; Milstein, 1967a). Homologous positions between the two chain types are marked by boxes. Also indicated are amino acid exchanges in the constant parts of both chains. For λ-chains exchanges have been found in the Oz (Ein and Fahey, 1967; Apella and Ein, 1967), the Kern (Ponstingl *et al.*, 1967) and the Mz (Milstein, 1967d) protein. In ϰ-chains only the Val-Leu exchange in position 191 was shown to be an allotypic variant (Hilschmann and Craig, 1965; Milstein, 1966a; Baglioni, 1966)

gene duplication and gene fusion of the primitive L-chain gene. From this, also by gene duplication, the genes of the different H-chain types might have developed.

It is known that the H-chains of the IgG class exist in 4 subtypes which are serologically distinguishable, but chemically very similar: γG1, γG2, γG3 and γG4. From progeny studies it was concluded that at least 3 of the 4 corresponding γ-chain genes are genetically linked; this means that they are all located in the same general area on one chromosome (Kunkel, 1965; Natvig *et al.*, 1967; Martensson, 1966). Obviously gene duplication was not followed by gene translocation.

Gene duplication and gene fusion or translocation seem to be a general principle of the evolution of the immunoglobulin chains. It leads to various chain types of L- and H-chains, which combine to form the different immunoglobulin classes. This principle is not restricted to immunoglobulins. It has also been observed with other phylogenetically related proteins.

Discussion of Hypotheses of Antibody Diversity

As already mentioned and clearly demonstrated in Figs. 3 and 4, the variable parts of different L-chains of one chain type are homologous. The question is whether this homology has been acquired during the evolution of genes separated in the germ line or by the somatic hypermutation of genes outside the germ line during individual development.

Very interesting in this respect is a comparison of the different variable parts of L-chains with other homologous proteins whose evolutionary origin, deriving from one single precursor gene, has been well established. This relationship between chemical structure and phylogeny has been extensively studied in the

```
              110                                        120
Arg Thr Val  [Ala Ala Pro Ser Val]  Phe Ile  [Phe Pro Pro Ser]  Asp [Glu] Gln [Leu]
Gln Pro Lys  [Ala Ala Pro Ser Val]  Thr Leu  [Phe Pro Pro Ser]  Ser [Glu] Glu [Leu]
              110                                        120

      150                                 160                                    170
[Lys [Val [Asp] Asn Ala Leu Gln Ser Gly Asn Ser Gln [Glu] Ser Val [Thr] Gln Gln Asp Ser Lys Asp
[Lys [Ala [Asp] Ser Ser Pro Val Lys Ala Gly Val  —  [Glu] Thr Thr [Thr] Pro Ser Lys Gln Ser Asn
                                        160                                    170
      [Gly] (Kern)

                          200                         210          214
[Cys] Glu [Val Thr His] Gln [Gly] Leu Ser [Ser] Pro [Val] Thr [Lys] Ser Phe Asn Arg Gly [Glu Cys]  —
[Cys] Gln [Val Thr His] Glu [Gly]  —   —  [Ser] Thr [Val] Glu [Lys] Thr Val Ala Pro Thr [Glu Cys] Ser
                          200                         210          214
```

Fig. 5

haemoglobins (Braunitzer *et al.*, 1964; Braunitzer, 1967) and can be schematically summarized in an evolutionary tree shown in Fig. 8a. According to this scheme the variety of haemoglobin chains present in the human can be explained by a number of consecutive gene duplications occurring during evolution, followed by

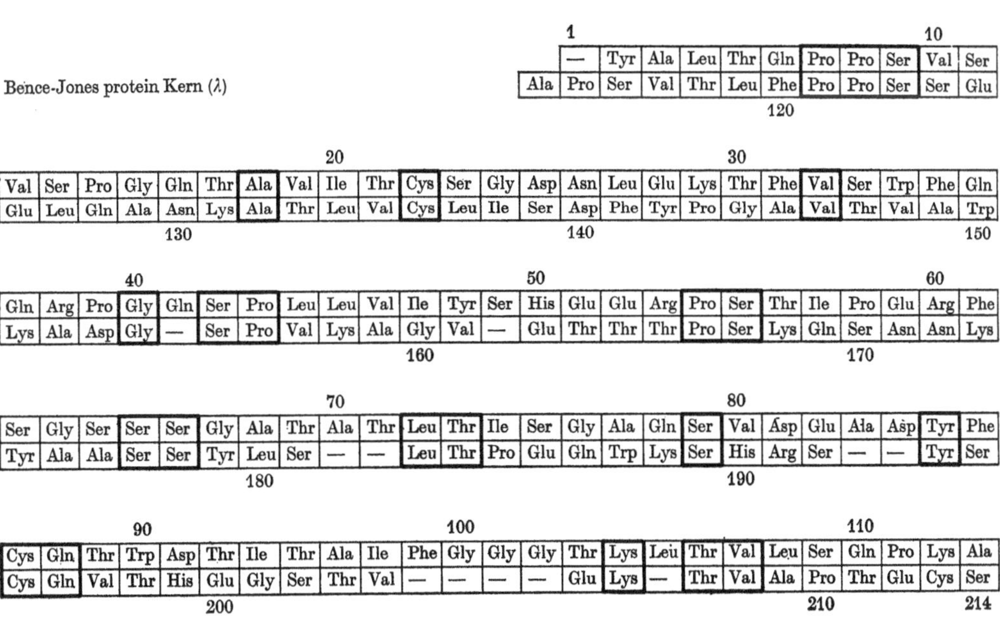

Bence-Jones protein Kern (λ)

```
                1                                                    10
      [ —  | Tyr | Ala | Leu | Thr | Gln |[Pro | Pro | Ser]| Val | Ser]
  Ala | Pro | Ser | Val | Thr | Leu | Phe |[Pro | Pro | Ser]| Ser | Glu
                                      120

                              20                                    30
Val | Ser | Pro | Gly | Gln | Thr |[Ala]| Val | Ile | Thr |[Cys]| Ser | Gly | Asp | Asn | Leu | Glu | Lys | Thr | Phe |[Val]| Ser | Trp | Phe | Gln
Glu | Leu | Gln | Ala | Asn | Lys |[Ala]| Thr | Leu | Val |[Cys]| Leu | Ile | Ser | Asp | Phe | Tyr | Pro | Gly | Ala |[Val]| Thr | Val | Ala | Trp
                              130                                   140                                                 150

                              40                                    50                                    60
Gln | Arg | Pro |[Gly]| Gln |[Ser | Pro]| Leu | Leu | Val | Ile | Tyr | Ser | His | Glu | Glu | Arg |[Pro | Ser]| Thr | Ile | Pro | Glu | Arg | Phe
Lys | Ala | Asp |[Gly]|  —  |[Ser | Pro]| Val | Lys | Ala | Gly | Val |  —  | Glu | Thr | Thr | Thr |[Pro | Ser]| Lys | Gln | Ser | Asn | Asn | Lys
                                                            160                                         170

                              70                                    80
Ser | Gly | Ser |[Ser | Ser]| Gly | Ala | Thr | Ala | Thr |[Leu | Thr]| Ile | Ser | Gly | Ala | Gln |[Ser]| Val | Asp | Glu | Ala | Asp |[Tyr]| Phe
Tyr | Ala | Ala |[Ser | Ser]| Tyr | Leu | Ser |  —  |  —  |[Leu | Thr]| Pro | Glu | Gln | Trp | Lys |[Ser]| His | Arg | Ser |  —  |  —  |[Tyr]| Ser
                              180                                   190

                              90                                    100                                   110
[Cys | Gln]| Thr | Trp | Asp | Thr | Ile | Thr | Ala | Ile | Phe | Gly | Gly | Gly | Thr |[Lys]| Leu |[Thr | Val]| Leu | Ser | Gln | Pro | Lys | Ala
[Cys | Gln]| Val | Thr | His | Glu | Gly | Ser | Thr | Val |  —  |  —  |  —  |  —  | Glu |[Lys]|  —  |[Thr | Val]| Ala | Pro | Thr | Glu | Cys | Ser
                              200                                                      210                214
```

9

Fig. 6. Internal homology between the variable and constant part of a λ-chain. Identical residues are marked by boxes

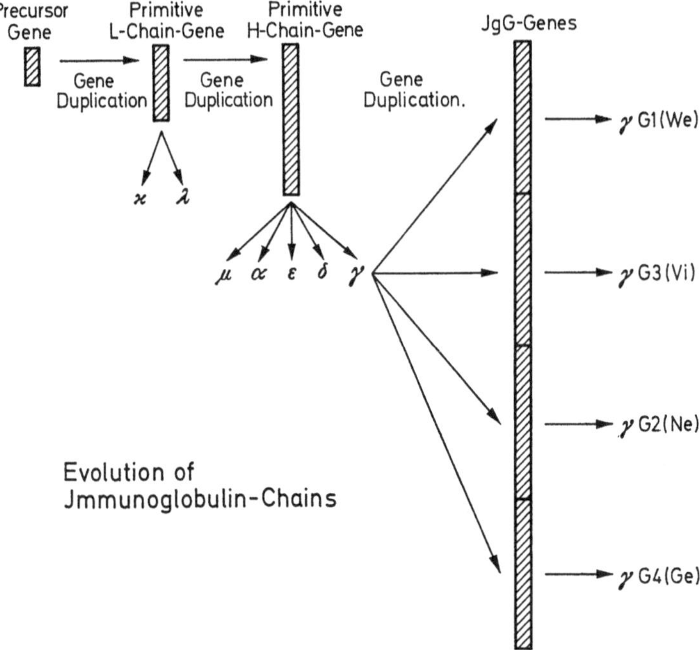

Fig. 7. Scheme for the evolution of the immunoglobulin chains by multiple gene duplication and gene fusion (see text)

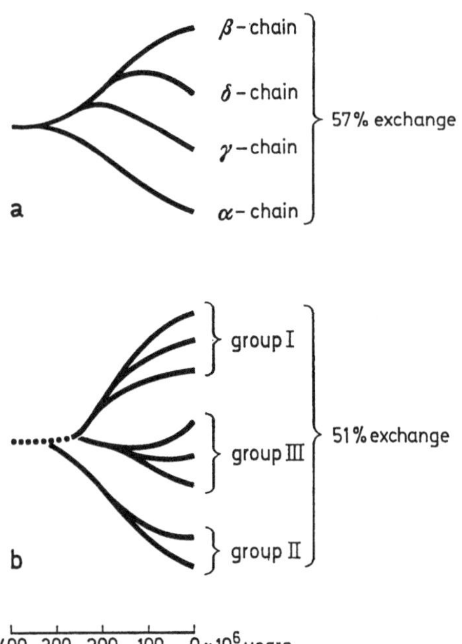

Fig. 8. Schematic phylogenetic trees for human haemoglobin and the variable parts of immunoglobulin L-chains. The exchange rate of amino acids between the α- and β-chains of haemoglobin and between group specific sequences (groups I and II) of one antigenic type ($\varkappa$) is compared

an accumulation of single point mutations on these duplicated genes. The distance from a common precursor is reflected by the differing chemical homology between the different genes: chains having branched off a common precursor relatively late during evolution being more similar in structure than others. The point of convergence is reached at the lower vertebrates. The lamprey, a Cyclostoma, has only one haemoglobin chain with a molecular weight of 17,000 and one unique amino acid sequence (Rudloff *et al.*, 1966).

Chemically the homology of the variable parts of the immunoglobulins exactly resembles that of the haemoglobins. This resemblance is not only qualitative; the number of exchanged amino acids between two variable parts of different grouping is comparable to that between the α- and β-chain of human haemoglobin. According to their varying degree of homology, the variable parts of the $\varkappa$- and λ-chains can be comprehended as the end points of an evolutionary tree similar to that of the haemoglobins, the groups representing the main branches, the individual chains the terminal ramifications of this evolutionary tree, as shown in Fig. 8 b (Hilschmann *et al.*, 1968 a). A similar arrangement can be concluded for λ-type L-chains.

Amino acid exchanges which exist between proteins of one group can be explained in the most cases by single point mutations, i.e., the exchange of just one base in the triplet coding for this particular amino acid. This also corresponds with the amino acid exchanges of phylogenetically closely related haemoglobins. Consistently the number of amino acid exchanges requiring at least two base exchanges increases, when proteins of different groups are compared.

Assuming a phylogenetic origin for antibody variability, it should be expected that at the point of convergence the N-terminal parts of the immunoglobulins are no longer variable, but possess one amino acid sequence. Unfortunately an immunoglobulin with a completely unique sequence has not yet been isolated. If, however, the immune response depends on the ability of the organism to select between differences in structure, animals beyond the convergence point should have no antibody activity. The lampreys which have been examined in this respect, still have antibodies which show differences in structure, as they should (Marchalonis and Edelman, 1968). In the hagfish, their somewhat older relations, no antibody activity could be detected, but also no band comparable to γ-globulin was present in serum electrophoresis (Good and Papermaster, 1964). All lower vertebrates which can produce antibodies, like the leopard shark and the paddlefish, already show diversity in structure in the L-chains comparable to that found in the different groups of human and murine L-chains (Suran and Papermaster, 1967; Pollara *et al.*, 1968). It should, however, be mentioned that the H-chains of these different animals each have one unique structure for the N-terminal five amino acid residues which have been determined. From these data, the point of convergence has to be assumed beyond the branching off of the lampreys, but probably not very much considering the similar exchange ratio for the variable parts of the immunoglobulins and the haemoglobins, provided the mutation rate is the same for both proteins.

So far all data are in agreement with and can easily be explained by an evolutionary origin of antibody variability. This implies that there must be many genes separated in the germ line carrying all the information needed for the antibody response with every possible antigen. This information must already be present in the germ cell (Fig. 9).

This multiplicity of genes can, however, not be assumed for the constant part. Contrary to the variable part, this section of the protein chain is controlled by only one gene. This conclusion can be drawn from their identical sequence, and the localization of the allotypes on their constant part. Only one allotype can be present in one chromosome. In heterozygotes these allotypes segregate in a simple Mendelian manner. This is only compatible with the existence of one gene for the constant part, necessarily being separated from the multiple genes for the variable parts.

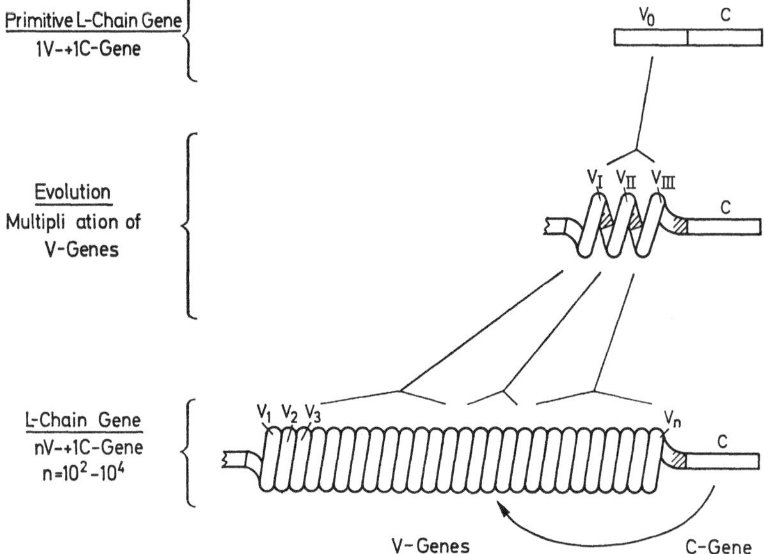

Fig. 9. The genetic control of L-chain structure. The germ cell has most likely all the information for the possibly needed antibodies. The gene for the L-chains of one antigenic type has presumably a great number of serially repeated V-genes for the different variable parts and one C-gene for the constant part. The different structures of the V-genes and the corresponding variable parts of the L-chains can best be explained by an evolutionary process in the germ line. The different V-genes would then represent the terminal ramifications, the V_I, V_{II} and V_{III} genes the main branches of the evolutionary tree, giving rise to the groups of varying homology in the variable parts. The final L-chain gene is produced by fusion of the C-gene with one of the V-genes. This gene fusion must occur by a somatic process outside the germ line, thereby reducing the multipotency of the germ cell to the unipotency of the plasma cell. The area of gene fusion is indicated by hatched lines

Since the gene for the constant part as well as one for the variable part express themselves in one immunoglobulin chain, it has to be assumed that this somatic gene fusion between the C-gene and one of the V-genes takes place during the time when the germ cell is developing into the immune competent cell. This gene fusion must be very specific, since a C-gene of a λ-chain never fuses with one of the $\varkappa$-chain V-genes or vice versa. One of the prerequisites of this gene fusion might be base complementarity between certain sections of the V- and C-genes, indicated by the hatched areas in Fig. 9. Whether in addition to this genetic linkage plays a role is not yet known. It is also not known why in the case of immunoglobulins nature works in such a complicated manner. It can, however, be imagined that it may have something to do with the fact that multipotency of the germ cell has to be reduced to the perspective unipotency of the plasma cell.

While for the multiple germ line models (Dreyer and Bennett, 1965) this gene fusion is the only somatic step which occurs during antibody formation, somatic hypermutation models assume that antibody diversity itself is caused by somatic hypermutation processes. These models shifted the "generator of diversity" from evolution to individual development and therefore reduced the number of genes to be carried in the germ line. The recombination models for instance do not repeat evolution in every single step, but explain antibody variability by somatic recombination between a limited number of preexisting and inherited genes. The variable parts were assumed to be recombination products of these few basic genes, the constancy of the C-terminal part being ensured by exclusion from the recombination process. The outer limits of variability were guaranteed by the evolutionary differences between the basic genes.

These hypermutation models (Smithies, 1967; Hilschmann, 1967b; Edelman and Gally, 1967; Whitehouse, 1967) discussed some time ago were based on early observations that some parts of L-chain structure could be perceived as hybrids between other structures, similar to the haemoglobins Lepore which were explained as crossover products between the δ- and β-chain-genes of haemoglobin, (Baglioni, 1962). This observation was made when only partial formulas of a few L-chains were known. The recently available larger number of completely sequenced L-chains does not support these recombination models (Hilschmann et al., 1968a).

Minimum models (Smithies, 1967) assuming recombination or "scrambling" between only 2 of these basic genes can not explain the 3 or 4 basic sequences into which $\varkappa$- or λ-chains can be classified. But even if one extends these minimum models to 3 or 4 basic genes (Hilschmann, 1967b) the observed structural differences in the variable parts of immunoglobulin chains do not support a recombination hypothesis between these few basic genes.

Let us suppose that the 3 or 4 basic sequences of the groups into which the variable parts can be classified are an expression of 3 or 4 basic genes and that antibody variability is caused by recombination between these genes. What we should expect then is that a protein might belong to one group in one part of the molecule and to another group in another part of the molecule. Blocks of sequences belonging to different groups should be observed in one protein. This, however, is not the case. The groups are remarkably constant throughout the entire variable part. This can not only be observed for the group specific sequences, but also for the deletions.

It also has to be kept in mind that with any recombination model the analyzed sequences in the variable part are not reprints of the basic genes, but are already the recombinants of these hypothetical basic genes. The situation might be more complex when "scrambling" occurs with a high recombination frequency. What might then be expected from the structure in this case ?

No matter what the basic genes look like and how often crossing over occurs between them, these properties should be reflected in the basic sequences of the variable parts. For demonstration see Fig. 10. Most markedly it should be re-

6*

flected in the N- and C-terminal ends of the variable parts. Any grouping based on sequence homology in the N-terminal end of the variable part should not be valid for its C-terminal end, when crossing over has occurred somewhere between these end points. When crossing over has happened frequently enough, there should be a number of proteins which do not fit into the same grouping at both end points. This should also be expressed in the primary structure of the variable part. With the symbols used in Fig. 3 and 4 we should expect that individual specific exchanges, as distinguished from the basic sequence marked by black boxes, should increase towards the C-terminal end of the variable part when the sequence homology in the N-terminal end has served as a basis for the grouping of the

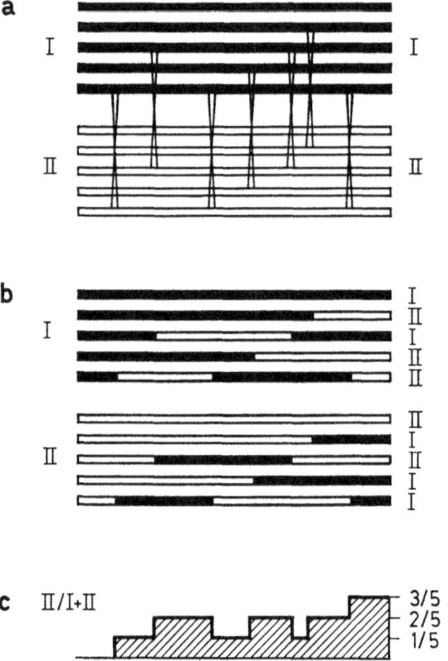

Fig. 10a—c. Consequences of hypothetical crossing-over between V-genes of different subgroups; a 7 assumed crossing-overs between genes of group I and group II, demonstrated on 5 hypothetical gene pairs; b Products of crossing-over would be genes with "blocks" of genetic material either deriving from group I or group II; c Disturbance of group specific sequences as result of crossing-overs, when the proteins of the upper 5 hypothetical recombination products are compared, expressed as sequences from group II/sequences from group I and group II. According to the recombination hypotheses the group specific sequences should be increasingly disturbed towards the C-terminal end (right) of the variable part, when the N-terminal end (left) is taken as reference point.

proteins. This is, however, not the case (Hilschmann *et al.*, 1968). Individual specific exchanges are distributed equally all over the variable parts; no gradient can be observed near the C-terminal end. The groups are constant throughout the entire variable part. This is particularly evident for the λ-chains of group IV which have as distict and remote markers their N-terminal amino acid and the deletions in position 28 and 95/96 (Ponstingl *et al.*, 1968; Langer *et al.*, 1968). These markers have not been observed in a protein of any group other than group IV. Only the C-terminal 10 or so amino acids of the variable parts of the $\varkappa$-chains show

an increased deviation from their group specific sequences (Hilschmann, 1967a).
Even another grouping could be perceived in this region of the molecule. This is so
far the only indication that a recombination process might have occurred. The
accumulation of individual specific exchanges is, however, limited to that part of
the molecule where also the multiple germ line models postulate recombination
between the variable and the constant part.

This constancy of group specific sequences certainly excludes the master and
scrambler gene model which assumes recombination between only two basic genes
(Smithies, 1967). It also excludes models assuming recombination between a
larger number of basic genes, when recombination between genes responsible for
different groups are involved (Hilschmann, 1967b). But even models which
restrict recombination to genes within one group are highly unlikely, since there
is no evidence, in the structure of the variable parts, which could be interpreted as
favoring such an hypothesis.

As clearly can be seen in the N-terminal 20 residues of the $\varkappa$-chains, for which
the most data are available, most differences between the individual chains are
caused by single amino acid replacements. There are no blocks of exchanged
amino acids which could be interpreted as linked groups. Also the nature of the
exchanged amino acids is such that one is not able to designate from which basic
amino acid sequence the particular exchanged residue could be a recombination
product. This might also be impossible to do when the number of recombining
genes is very large, since in this case, the somatic recombination models and multiple germ line models would be structurally indistinguishable. The somatic recombination models would therefore offer no real advantages since the number of
different V-genes which have to be inherited is most likely in the same order of
magnitude as that of the multiple germ line models.

As already mentioned, in the multiple germ line models the number of V-genes
is as large as the number of the variable parts. There is as yet no reasonable
estimation for the maximal number of variants. Only the minimal number can be
estimated from the data already available. There are data for at least 25 different
L-chains of the $\varkappa$-type, some of them only in fragments, but large enough to show
that none of these proteins is identical in structure. From this it has been calculated
with reasonable probability, that the number of different variants must be at least
250 (Cohen and Milstein, 1967). Considering not only the number of investigated
proteins but also the extent of amino acid exchanges which exist between different
variants, the number of variants is most likely much higher. It would not be
surprising if one would have to deal with hundreds or thousands of homologous,
but different genes for the variable parts of one chain type in one chromosome.

The question arose whether so many genes can be carried in one haploid
chromosome set. According to its DNA content (Muller, 1958) a human sperm
cell contains 4×10^9 nucleotide pairs or 0.67×10^9 triplets per single DNA-
strand. If only 0.1% of these DNA would carry the information for immunoglobulin structure 6×10^3 different variable parts for both the L- and the H-
chains would be possible, assuming that the variable parts of both the L- and the
H-chains consist of 110 amino acid residues. Provided the variable parts of both
the L- and the H-chains contribute to the combining site and can combine un-
restrictedly, which is not the case, (Mannik, 1967), $(3 \times 10^3)^2$ or 10^7 different

immunoglobulin structures could result, a figure which is comparable to that calculated from other data (Jerne, 1955).

One might ask whether precedents exist in nature for such a large number of equal or almost equal duplicated genes. There are increasing observations, mainly concerning the DNA of higher organisms, that this is indeed the case. Hybridization experiments show that 30 to 40% of the DNA of higher organism, in contrast to DNA from viruses and bacteria, consist of hundreds of repeating genes (Britten and Kohne, 1968). The length of these repeating genes was cautiously estimated to be 400 to 500 nucleotide pairs. Serially repeating genes are well known for ribosomal (Attardi *et al.*, 1965) and mitochondrial (Borst *et al.*, 1966) DNA, but have also been postulated for other structural genes (Britten and Kohne).

On the other hand recent investigations with the haemoglobins (Schroeder *et al.*, 1968; Huisman *et al.*, 1968), indicate that also for these classical proteins the one gene—one protein dogma in a strict sense is not valid any more. For instance, the γ-chain of human haemoglobin is not determined by just one, but obviously by 4 genes, out of which 3 determine proteins with identical sequences. This was concluded from the investigation of microheterogeneities which formerly were interpreted as ambiguities. More exact genetic analysis has shown that these are not due to translational mistakes, but rather to singular mutations in serially duplicated genes.

Serially repeated genes are therefore no curiosity, they seem to be the rule for higher organisms. The difference between the haemoglobins or the enzymes and the variable parts of the immunoglobulins seems not to be of qualitative, but more of quantitative nature, although their enourmous multiplicity is remarkable.

It can be imagined that with the enzymes the multiplicity was lost during evolution, because these proteins have accepted a restricted and constant responsibility in metabolism. The same selection mechanism might have had the opposite effect on the immunoglobulin genes. The perpetually changing demands which the immune system has to face might have preserved this multiplicity of genes in order to guarantee that antibodies are produced against every possible antigen, even against those which do not occur in nature. The prerequisite for this multipotency is that this variability in structure is produced by a random process, as is true in case of evolution. The antigen selects the "fitting" antibody from a broad spectrum of different structures which are already present. It has a selective, no instructive character.

References

Appella, E., and D. Ein: Two types of lambda polypeptide chains in human immunoglobulins based on an amino acid substitution at position 190. Proc. nat. Acad. Sci. (Wash.) 57, 1449 (1967).

Attardi, G. P., P. C. Huang, and S. Kabat: Recognition of ribosomal RNA sites in DNA. 1. Analysis of the *E. coli* system. Proc. nat. Acad. Sci. (Wash.) 53, 1490 (1965).

Baglioni, C.: The fusion of two peptide chains in hemoglobin Lepore and its interpretation as a genetic deletion. Proc. nat. Acad. Sci. (Wash.) 48, 1880 (1962).

— Homologies in the position of cysteine residues of K and L-type chains of human immunoglobulins. Biochem. biophys. Res. Commun. 26, 82 (1967).

—, L. Alescio-Zonta, D. Cioli, and A. Carbonara: Allelic antigenic factor Inv(a) of the light chains of human immunoglobulins: chemical basis. Science 152, 1519 (1966).

Becker, M. J., and A. Rich: Polyribosomes of tissues producing antibodies. Nature (Lond.) 212, 142 (1966).

Borst, P., G. Ruttenberg, and A. M. Kroon: Mitochondrial DNA. II Sedimentation analysis and electron microscopy of mitochondrial DNA from chick liver. Biochim. biophys. Acta (Amst.) 149, 156 (1967).

Braunitzer, G.: Die Primärstruktur der Eiweißstoffe. Naturwissenschaften 54, 407 (1967).

—, K. Hilse, V. Rudloff, and N. Hilschmann: The hemoglobins. Advanc. Protein Chem. 19, 1 (1964).

Britten, R. J., and D. E. Kohne: Repeated sequences in DNA. Science 161, 529 (1968).

Cebra, J. J., J. E. Colberg, and S. Dray: Rabbit lymphoid cells differentiated with respect to α-, γ-, and μ-heavy polypeptide chains and to allotypic markers AA1 and AA2. J. exp. Med. 123, 547 (1966).

Cohen, S., and C. Milstein: Structure and biological properties of immunoglobulins. Advanc. Immunol. 7, 1 (1967).

Cunningham, B. A., P. D. Gottlieb, W. H. Konigsberg, and G. M. Edelman: The covalent structure of a human γG-immunoglobulin. V. Partial amino acid sequence of the light chain. Biochemistry 7, 1983 (1968).

Hill, R. L., R. Delaney, R. E. Fellows, Jr., and H. E. Lebovitz: The evolutionary origins of the immunoglobulins. Proc. nat. Acad. Sci. (Wash.) 56, 1762 (1966).

Dreyer, W. J., and J. C. Bennett: The molecular basis of antibody formation: a paradox. Proc. nat. Acad. Sci. (Wash.) 54, 864 (1965).

—, W. R. Gray, and L. Hood: The genetic, molecular and cellular basis of antibody formation: some facts and a unifying hypothesis. Cold Spr. Harb. Symp. quant. Biol. 32, 353 (1967).

Edelman, G. M., and J. A. Gally: The nature of Bence-Jones proteins. J. exp. Med. 116, 207 (1962).

— — A model for the 7s antibody molecule. Proc. nat. Acad. Sci. (Wash.) 51, 846 (1964).

— — Somatic recombination of duplicated genes: an hypothesis on the origin of antibody diversity. Proc. nat. Acad. Sci. (Wash.) 57, 353 (1967).

Ein, D.: Nonallelic behaviour of the Oz groups in human lambda immunoglobulin chains. Proc. nat. Acad. Sci. (Wash.) 60, 982 (1968).

—, and J. L. Fahey: Two types of lambda polypeptide chains in human immunoglobulins. Science 156, 947 (1967).

Fleischman, J. B., R. R. Porter, and E. M. Press: The arrangement of the peptide chains in γ-globulin. Biochem. J. 88, 220 (1963).

Frangione, B., and C. Milstein: Disulphide bridges of immunoglobulin G1 heavy chains. Nature (Lond.) 216, 939 (1967).

Good, R. A., and B. W. Papermaster: Ontogeny and phylogeny of adaptive immunity. Advanc. Immunol. 4, 1 (1964).

Gottlieb, P. D., B. A. Cunningham, M. J. Waxdal, W. H. Konigsberg, and G. M. Edelman: Variable regions of heavy and light polypeptide chains of the same γG-immunoglobulin molecule. Proc. nat. Acad. Sci. (Wash.) 61, 168 (1968).

Gray, W. R., W. J. Dreyer, and L. Hood: Mechanism of antibody synthesis: size differences among $\varkappa$-chains. Science 155, 465 (1967).

Green, I., P. Vassalli, and B. Benacerraf: Cellular localization of anti-DNP-PLL and anti-conveyor albumin antibodies in genetic nonresponder guinea pigs immunized with DNP-PLL albumin complexes. J. exp. Med. 125, 527 (1967a).

— —, V. Nussenzweig, and B. Benacerraf: Specificity of the antibodies produced by single cells following immunization with antigens bearing two types of antigenic determinants. J. exp. Med. 125, 511 (1967b).

Haber, E.: Recovery of antigenic specificity after denaturation and complete reduction of disulfide bridges in a papain fragment of antibody. Proc. nat. Acad. Sci. (Wash.) 52, 1099 (1964).

Hilschmann, N.: The chemical structure of immunoglobulins. Proc. 11th Congr. int. Soc. Blood Transf., Sydney 1966, No. 29, Part 2, 501. Basel/New York: Karger 1968.

— Die chemische Struktur von zwei Bence-Jones-Proteinen (Roy und Cum.) vom $\varkappa$-Typ. Hoppe-Seylers Z. physiol. Chem. 348, 1077 (1967a).

— Zum Mechanismus der Antikörperbildung. Hoppe-Seylers Z. physiol. Chem. 348, 1291 (1967b).

Hilschmann, N.: Die vollständige Aminosäuresequenz des Bence-Jones Proteins Cum (*ϰ*-Typ). Hoppe-Seylers Z. physiol. Chem. **348**, 1718 (1967 c).

—, and L. C. Craig: Amino acid sequence studies with Bence-Jones proteins. Proc. nat. Acad. Sci. (Wash.) **53**, 1403 (1965).

—, H. U. Barnikol, M. Hess, B. Langer, H. Ponstingl, M. Steinmetz-Kayne, L. Suter, and S. Watanabe: Structural studies on immunoglobulins and their genetic implications for antibody formation. Proc. 5th FEBS-Meeting, Prague 1968. London: Academic Press Inc. (in press).

Hood, L., W. R. Gray, B. G. Sanders, and W. J. Dreyer: Light chain evolution. Cold Spr. Harb. Symp. quant. Biol. **32**, 133 (1967).

Huisman, T. H. J., G. Brandt, and J. B. Wilson: The structure of goat hemoglobins. II. Structural studies of the α-chains of the hemoglobins A and B. J. biol. Chem. **243**, 3675 (1968).

Jerne, N. K.: The natural-selection theory of antibody formation. Proc. nat. Acad. Sci. (Wash.) **41**, 849 (1955).

Kabat, E. A.: Kabat and Meyer's Experimental Immunochemistry, 2nd. ed. Springfield (Ill.): Thomas 1961.

Koshland, M. E., and F. M. Engelberger: Differences in the amino acid composition of two purified antibodies from the same rabbit. Proc. nat. Acad. Sci. (Wash.) **50**, 61 (1963).

Kunkel, H. G.: Myeloma proteins and antibodies. Harvey Lect. **59**, 219 (1965).

Langer. B., M. Steinmetz-Kayne u. N. Hilschmann: Die vollständige Aminosäuresequenz des Bence-Jones Proteins New (*λ*-Typ). Subgruppen im variablen Teil bei Immunglobulin-L-Ketten vom *λ*-Typ. Hoppe-Seylers Z. physiol. Chem. **349**, 945 (1968).

Mannik, M.: Variability in the specific interactions of H- and L-chains of γG-globulins. Biochemistry **6**, 134 (1967).

Marchalonis, J. J., and G. M. Edelman: Antibodies in the primary immune response of the Sea Lamprey, Petromyzon Marinus. J. exp. Med. **127**, 891 (1968).

Martensson, L.: Genes and immunoglobulins. Vox Sang. (Basel) **11**, 521 (1966).

Milstein, C.: Interchain disulphide bridge in Bence-Jones proteins and in γ-globulin B chains. Nature (Lond.) **205**, 1172 (1965).

— Variations in the amino-acid sequence near the disulphide bridges of immunoglobulin *ϰ*-chains. Nature (Lond.) **209**, 370 (1966 a).

— Chemical structure of light chains. Proc. roy. Soc. B **166**, 138 (1966 b).

— Immunoglobulin *ϰ*-chains. Comparative sequences in selected streches of Bence-Jones proteins. Biochem. J. **101**, 352 (1966 c).

—, J. B. Clegg, and J. M. Jarvis: C-terminal half of immunoglobulin *λ*-chains. Nature (Lond.) **214**, 270 (1967 a).

— Linked groups of residues in immunoglobulin *ϰ*-chains. Nature (Lond.) **216**, 330 (1967 b).

— Studies on the variability of immunoglobulin sequence. Cold Spr. Harb. Symp. quant. Biol. **32**, 31 (1967 c).

— Variations in the C-terminal half of immunoglobulin *λ*-chains. Biochem. J. **104**, 28 c (1967 d).

Muller, H. J.: The gene material as the initiator and the organizing basis of life. Heritage from Mendel, R. A. Bring, and E. D. Styles, Eds., Madison, The University of Wisconsin Press, 1967.

Natvig, J. B., H. G. Kunkel, and T. Gedde-Dahl Jr.: Genetic studies of the heavy chain subgroups of γG globulin. Recombination between the closely linked cistrons. Nobel Symp. 3, Gamma Globulins, J. Killander, Ed. Stockholm: Almqvist and Wiksell 1967.

Niall, H. D., and P. Edman: Two structurally distinct classes of *ϰ*-chains in human immunoglobulins. Nature (Lond.) **216**, 262 (1967).

Pauling, L.: A theory of the structure and process of formation of antibodies. J. Amer. chem. Soc. **62**, 2643 (1940).

Pernis, B.: Relationships between the heterogeneity of immunoglobulins and the differentiation of plasma cells. Cold Spr. Harb. Symp. quant. Biol. **32**, 333 (1967).

—, G. Chiappino, A. S. Kelus, and P. G. H. Gell: Cellular localization of immunoglobulins with different allotypic specificities in rabbit lymphoid tissues. J. exp. Med. **122**, 853 (1965).

Pollara, B., A. Suran, G. Finstad, and R. A. Good: N-terminal amino acid sequences of immunoglobulin chains in polyodon spathula. Proc. nat. Acad. Sci. (Wash.) 59, 1307 (1968).

Ponstingl, H., M. Hess und N. Hilschmann: Die vollständige Aminosäuresequenz des Bence-Jones-Proteins Kern. Eine neue Untergruppe der Immunglobulin-L-Ketten vom λ-Typ. Hoppe-Seylers Z. physiol. Chem. 349, 867 (1968).

— —, B. Langer, M. Steinmetz-Kayne und N. Hilschmann: Über einen Aminosäureaustausch im konstanten Teil eines Bence-Jones Proteins vom λ-Typ. Hoppe-Seylers Z. physiol. Chem. 348, 1213 (1967).

Porter, R. R.: The hydrolysis of rabbit γ-globulin and antibodies with crystalline papain. Biochem. J. 73, 119 (1959).

Press, E. M., and P. J. Piggot: The chemical structure of the heavy chain of human immunoglobulin G. Cold Spr. Harb. Symp. quant. Biol. 32, 45 (1967).

Putnam, F. W., T. Shinoda, K. Titani, and M. Wikler: Immunoglobulin structure: Variation in amino acid sequence and length of human lambda light chains. Science 157, 1050 (1967).

Rudloff, V., M. Zellenik u. G. Braunitzer: Zur Phylogenie des Hämoglobinmoleküls. Untersuchungen am Hämoglobin des Flußneunauges (Lampetra fluviatilis). Hoppe-Seylers Z. physiol. Chem. 344, 284 (1966).

Shapiro, A. L., M. D. Scharff, J. V. Maizel, and J. V. Uhr: Polyribosomal synthesis and assembly of the H and L chains of γ-globulin. Proc. nat. Acad. Sci. (Wash.) 56, 216 (1966).

Singer, S. J., and N. O. Thorpe: On the location and structure of the active sites of antibody molecules. Proc. nat. Acad. Sci. (Wash.) 60, 1371 (1968).

Smithies, O.: Antibody variability. Science 157, 267 (1967).

Suran, A. A., and B. W. Papermaster: N-terminal sequences of heavy and light chains of leopard shark immunoglobulins: Evolutionary implications. Proc. nat. Acad. Sci. (Wash.) 58, 1619 (1967).

Suter, L., H. U. Barnikol, S. Watanabe, and N. Hilschmann: Hoppe-Sylers Z. physiol. Chem. 350, 275 (1969).

Schroeder, W. A., T. H. J. Huisman, J. R. Shelton, J. B. Shelton, E. F. Kleihauer, A. M. Dozy, and B. Robberson: Evidence for multiple structural genes for the γ-chain of human fetal hemoglobin. Proc. nat. Acad. Sci. (Wash.) 60, 537 (1968).

Steinberg, A. G.: Progress in the study of genetically determined human gamma globulin types (the Gm and Inv groups). Progress in medical genetics, Vol. II. New York-London: Grune and Stratton 1962.

Titani, K., E. Whitley, and F. W. Putnam: Immunoglobulin structure: Variation in the sequence of Bence-Jones proteins. Science 152, 1513 (1966).

Valentine, R. C., and N. M. Greene: Electron microscopy of an antibody-hapten complex. J. molec. Biol. 27, 615 (1967).

Waldenström, J.: Studies on conditions associated with disturbed gamma globulin formation (gammopathies). Harvey Lect. 56, 211 (1961).

Whitehouse, H. L. K.: Crossover model of antibody variability. Nature (Lond.) 215, 371 (1967).

Whitney, Ch. L., and Ch. Tanford: Recovery of specific activity after complete unfolding and reduction of an antibody fragment. Proc. nat. Acad. Sci. (Wash.) 53, 524 (1965).

Williamson, A. R., and B. A. Askonas: Biosynthesis of immunoglobulins: The separate classes of polyribosomes synthesizing heavy and light chains. J. molec. Biol. 23, 201 (1967).

Dr. N. Hilschmann
Max-Planck-Institut für experimentelle
Medizin, Abteilung Chemie,
Arbeitsgruppe Immunochemie,
34 Göttingen, Hermann-Rein-Straße 3

Discussion

WELLENSIEK (Mainz): How do you explain that in the constant part of the L-chain an exchange is found only very rarely? Can any major change in this constant part no longer be compatible with the structure of an antibody molecule?

HILSCHMANN (Göttingen): I must point out that the constant part has to be designated as "constant" because there is no possibility for comparison, it is only present once. Otherwise, each species has a different constant part.

GRUNDMANN (Wuppertal): Can this so-called constant part be based on a different eu-chromatisation or hetero-chromatisation? I am not thinking of the simplified scheme according to which every hetero-chromatin is genetically afunctional. Several hetero-chromatic intensities exist which, depending on circumstances, may indicate different genetic activities.

HILSCHMANN (Göttingen): Today we know that very many genetic areas in the chromosome are afunctional. On the other hand we know from hybridisation experiments with DNA that especially in the higher animals DNA is invested for serial doublication. Today, we also know, that the one-gene-one-protein correlation is not factual. For the gamma-chain for example at least 4 genes are necessary according to more recent investigations by Schröder et al. [Proc. nat. Acad. Sci. (Wash.) 60, 537 (1968)]. Other proteins too are probably not conditioned by one gene, but by quite a number of genes.

DE WECK (Berne): If the differences have emerged in phylogeny then the spectrum must be essentially smaller in lower animals.

HILSCHMANN (Göttingen): The heterogenicity of the antibodies has certainly increased during phylogenesis. We know for example that IgD is a relatively recent acquisition. It has never been found in lower animals. We also know that of the H-chains the μ-chain occurred first. Important is that the classes increase and not the heterogenicity within the classes.

Bayer-Symposium I, 91—98 (1969)

The Significance of the Carrier Effect for the Induction of Antibodies

K. Rajewsky

With 1 Figure

Introduction

When an immunogen is injected into a higher organism, antibodies reacting specifically with that immunogen are produced. Since a vast number of antibody specificities exist, and since cogent evidence indicates that antibody specificity is determined by the primary structure of the antibody polypeptide chains, the question has to be asked of how antigen induces the structural genes coding for the "right" antibodies, and only these, to initiate protein synthesis.

Upon immunization with an antigen, only a small proportion of the population of immunocompetent cells present in the organism starts to multiply and to produce specific antibodies. Strong evidence supports the idea that for any given antigen a specific subpopulation of immunocompetent cells exists, which is antigen-sensitive, i.e. which can be stimulated by that antigen to produce specific antibodies. If a given immunocompetent cell has the capacity to produce antibodies of just one or very few specificities, the problem of antibody induction is reduced to the question of how antigen specifically stimulates those cells that are able to produce an antibody fitting to that antigen. The simplest way of specific stimulation would be the presence of specific receptors for antigen on the surface of the immuno-competent cells. Since these receptors must have the same range of specificities as the specific product of the cells, e.g. the antibodies, it is straightforward to believe that the postulated receptors for antigen on the cell surface are antibody, — that antibody, that a given cell is capable to produce. This in fact is just a restatement of Jerne's original idea (Jerne, 1960) that antigen recognition must occur via specific antibodies. Though direct evidence for cellular immunoglobulin receptors of the type described here is lacking, there is strong evidence favouring this view (Mitchison, 1969 b).

The induction process would be based, then, on combination of a given antigenic determinant with a specific receptor on a specific immunocompetent cell. We are going to describe in this article recent experiments which point to a more complex mechanism of antibody induction.

The Carrier Effect: Cooperation of Antigenic Determinants

We will discuss here the evidence showing that the induction of specific antibodies by an antigen requires the recognition of more than one determinant of the antigen. This implies that immunogenic substances must possess at least two antigenic determinants.

The work of Landsteiner (1947) has established that in order to be immunogenic, simple chemical compounds have to be coupled to a macromolecular carrier. Substances that are unable to induce an immune response by themselves, but which can be recognized by antibody, were designated as haptens. What is the role of the carrier in rendering a hapten immunogenic ?

It has long been known that there is some specificity associated with the role of the carrier: An animal primed with hapten on carrier A responds poorly or not at all to a secondary injection of the hapten on carrier B, whereas injection of the hapten on carrier A leads to a good secondary response. Since antigenic determinants are frequently composed of the hapten and some of the adjacent carrier surface, this finding does not a priori need an elaborate explanation. Recent studies indicate, however, that the role of the carrier cannot be fully understood on the basis of a "local environment hypothesis" (see Mitchison, 1967). Hapten-carrier systems have been described where hapten and carrier are macromolecules of similar size. As shown by Benacerraf and his coworkers (Benacerraf, *et al.*, 1967), DNP-polylysine (DNP-PLL; molecular weight approximately 60,000) is non-immunogenic in a certain strain of guinea pigs. The same guinea pigs respond, however, to immunization with DNP-PLL complexed with foreign serum albumin with the formation of large amounts of antibodies to serum albumin *and* to the DNP determinant. The five lactic dehydrogenase (LDH) isozymes are tetrameric molecules composed of two types of subunits (A and B) in all possible combinations (for review see Kaplan, 1964). It was found (Rajewsky *et al.*, 1967; Rajewsky and Rottländer, 1967; Armerding and Rajewsky, 1969) that a certain line of rabbits was unable to fully respond to the B_4 enzyme, whereas a normal response occurred upon immunization with the A_4 enzyme. If the animals were immunized with the $B_2 A_2$ hybrid, however, similar amounts of anti-A *and* anti-B antibodies were formed. In both systems, antibodies to the haptenic macromolecule did not show any detectable reaction with the carrier.

The role of the carrier was specific in both systems: DNP-PLL complexed with guinea pig serum albumin proved to be non-immunogenic. And porcine haptenic B-subunits hybridized with (carrier) A-subunits from rabbit were unable to induce a secondary anti-B response in rabbits primed with the porcine $A_2 B_2$ hybrid. Perhaps most striking, it could be shown in both systems that induction of tolerance to the carrier led to a reduced response to carrier *and* hapten upon immunization with the hapten carrier complex. Quantitatively, the reduction of the response was similar in this situation for anti-hapten and anti-carrier antibodies, as demonstrated in the LDH system (Fig. 1).

Thus, in both the LDH and the DNP-PLL-BSA system, it appears unlikely that the carrier only completes the antigenic determinants of the hapten. Instead, antigenic determinants of the hapten and those of the carrier seem to cooperate in some way in the induction of the immune response to the hapten carrier complex. Mitchison, who has clearly stated this idea of cooperating antigenic determinants, came to the same conclusion in his conventional hapten carrier system. He showed, that for the induction of the secondary response, the hapten could be separated from the carrier by a spacer group without abolishing the carrier effect (Mitchison, 1967). Further evidence supporting the cooperation concept came from the work of Schierman and McBride (1967) in their system of chicken isoantigens. Recent studies on the mechanism of the carrier effect (Rajewsky *et al.*, 1969) again strongly suggest cooperation between the haptenic determinant and determinants of the carrier molecule. It was shown that a hapten-specific secondary response to a hapten-carrier complex is obtained in animals primed with the carrier and the hapten separately (i.e. with the uncoupled carrier and the hapten on a second, unrelated carrier). Table 1 shows the experimental design and the result of one of the experiments relevant here. Again Mitchison (1969a) has done similar studies in his transfer system in mice. It should be mentioned that the clear-cut result obtained corresponds very well to earlier findings in the LDH-system (Rajewsky and Rottländer, 1967). Animals primed with the carrier subunits responded to an injection of the hybrid enzyme with the production of antibodies directed to carrier

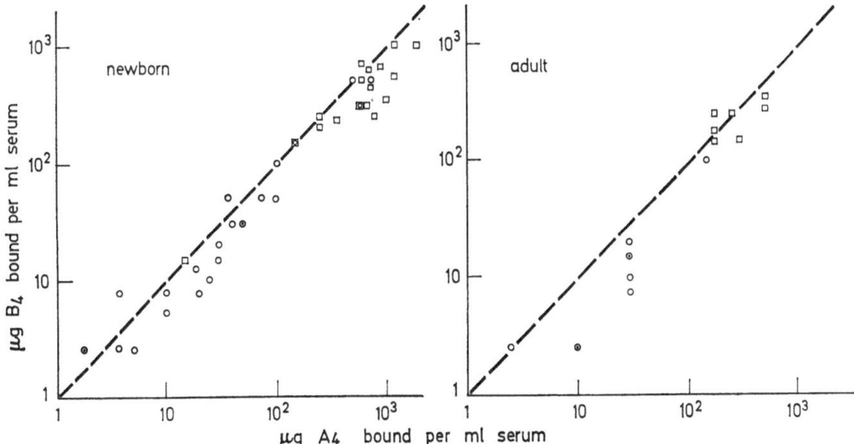

Fig. 1. Induction of tolerance to porcine LDH-III ($A_2 B_2$) in newborn (left) and adult (right) rabbits by injection of LDH-V (A_4). Newborn animals were given 1 to 10 mg LDH-V (A_4) on the day of birth. Adult animals were injected intravenously with a total of 100 mg LDH-V (A_4) within 3 days before immunization. Tolerant (circles) and control animals (squares) were immunized with the $A_2 B_2$ hybrid according to a standard procedure, at the age of 10 to 12 weeks. Secondary anti-B titers are plotted versus secondary anti-A titers. Each point represents the response of a single rabbit. Taken from Rajewsky *et al.*, 1967, and Rajewsky and Rottländer, 1967, with modifications

and haptenic subunits. Since the animals had not been primed with the haptenic subunits before, less anti-hapten antibody than anti-carrier antibody was formed. These experiments suggest that cooperation also occurs in the induction of the primary immune response.

Evidently, the results described in this section are incompatible with the "local environment hypothesis." It seems clear that the function of the carrier in the induction of the immune response has to be assigned to its antigenic determinants. How does cooperation between the haptenic determinant and the determinants of the carrier molecule occur? The carrier effect suggests an interaction of antigen with at least two specific, antibody-like receptors. Whereas we have reason to believe that one of these receptors is produced by and localized on the antigen sensitive cell, origin and localization of the cooperating receptor are unclear. Cooperation could occur between receptors of the same type, situated either on the same or on different cell populations. The cooperating receptor could also be represented, however, by some sort of conventional antibody.

Let us reconstruct the experimental situation described above. Animals primed with hapten and carrier produce anti-hapten and anti-carrier antibodies during the primary response. The carrier effect found in secondary stimulation could be brought about by this antibody production. Circulating anti-carrier antibody could combine with the hapten carrier complex to form an immunogenic compound (Terres and Wolins, 1961; Morrison and Terres, 1966). Cytophilic anti-carrier antibody, adsorbed to certain cell membranes, could trap the hapten-carrier complex and expose it efficiently to the target cells.

Our experiments and the experiments of Mitchison argue against the idea that circulating anti-carrier antibodies are responsible for the carrier effect. Passive

Table 1. *Carrier specificity in the secondary response: Pretreatment with secondary carrier*

No. of rabbits	1. injection[a]	2. injection[b]	$T_2 - T_1$[c] (log$_2$ dilution)	standard error[d]
8	sulf$_{19}$-BSA[e]; HGG[f]	sulf$_{19}$-BSA; HGG	3.3	0.6
6	sulf$_{23}$-HGG	sulf$_{23}$-HGG	2.0	0.3
7	sulf$_{19}$-BSA	sulf$_{23}$-HGG	0.4	0.3
8	sulf$_{19}$-BSA; HGG[g]	sulf$_{23}$-HGG	3.4	0.4

[a] 1 mg of each antigen in Freund's complete adjuvant injected in footpad.

[b] 1 mg of each antigen injected intravenously, 4 weeks after primary injection.

[c] Mean primary (T_1; determined 1 day before 2. injection) and secondary (T_2; determined 7 days after 2. injection) anti-sulfanilic acid (sulf) hemagglutination titers.

[d] Normal distribution of log$_2$ titer differences not proven.

[e] Sulfanilic acid coupled to bovine serum albumin.

[f] Human γ globulin.

[g] HGG could be injected in other foot and even 2 weeks later than sulf$_{19}$-BSA, without changing the result. This eliminates the possibility of in vivo transfer of sulf groups from BSA to HGG. For experimental details and complete results see Rajewsky et al., 1969.

infusion of anti-carrier antibody into animals primed with the hapten on another carrier did not prepare the animals to respond to a secondary injection of the hapten-carrier complex. Our data do not strictly exclude, however, the participation of cytophilic anti-carrier antibody in that part of the induction process, which is characterized by the carrier effect. In any case, we feel inclined to link the finding of cooperating antigenic determinants to the concept of two cooperating cell-bound receptors, probably two cell types, in the induction of the immune response. In the next section, we will briefly discuss direct evidence, which points to the cooperation of two cell types in antibody induction.

Thymus Dependency of the Immune Response: Cooperation of two Cell Types

It is well established that the thymus is of fundamental importance for the immune reactivity of an animal (see Miller and Osoba, 1967). One aspect of the role of the thymus has come clearly into focus by the recent work of Mitchell and

Miller (1968 a). In these experiments, strong evidence was provided for the existence of two types of lymphoid cells cooperating in the induction of the immune response to sheep red blood cells (SRC). While both cell types originate in the bone marrow, one of them exerts its function only after having passed through the thymus. The two cell types, which were designated as bone marrow-derived and thymus-derived lymphocytes, have been studied extensively by several groups of workers (Davies *et al.*, 1966, 1967; Claman *et al.*, 1966; Miller and Mitchell, 1967, 1968; Mitchell and Miller, 1968 a, b). We are not going to deal with the many other reports in the literature (see Rajewsky *et al.*, 1969) that all point to cell cooperating taking place in the induction of antibodies and that may in part be related to the work referred to in this section.

Of special relevance for the argument presented here were the findings that the ancestors of the antibody forming cells exclusively belong to the bone marrow-derived cell population (Mitchell and Miller, 1968 a; Miller and Mitchell, 1968 a), and that the thymus-derived cells seem to be antigen-specific. This was derived mainly from tolerance experiments which in two independent systems led to the conclusion that tolerance was localized in the thymus-derived cells (Taylor, 1969; Miller and Mitchell, 1968). Further evidence is needed, however, to confirm this point and to establish, whether bone marrow-derived cells can also be made tolerant under suitable conditions. Since the possibility to render a cell tolerant to an antigen is a strong argument for the specificity of the cell, such studies would answer the question of whether thymus-derived *and* bone marrow-derived cells are antigen-specific, or only the former ones. It will be discussed below, why we tend to believe that *both* cell types might be antigen-specific.

Thymus-Derived and Bone Marrow-Derived Cells Linked together by Antigen: A Mechanism for Antibody Induction

If the concepts of cooperating antigenic determinants and of cooperating cells in the induction of antibodies can be generalized, a mechanism for antibody induction can be pictured which accounts for both lines of evidence (Mitchison, 1969 a; Rajewsky *et al.*, 1969).

According to this hypothesis, activation of the precursors of the antibody producing cells, which are bone marrow-derived, requires their interaction with thymus-derived helper cells[1]. This interaction is thought to be antigen-dependent in that the two cells are linked together by antigen. The linkage is brought about by the binding of antigenic determinants present on the antigen to specific immunoglobulin receptors on the surfaces of the two cells. It is obvious that this type of cell interaction requires the presence of at least two antigenic determinants on an immunogenic molecule, and that these determinants need not be identical.

As pointed out above, there is reason to believe that one of the two types of receptors postulated here is localized on the surface of those cells by which it is produced. For the other type of receptor, we have to decide whether it is a receptor of the same kind or some sort of cytophilic antibody, which is randomly adsorbed to the membranes of the second type of cell. If just one of the two interacting cells

---

[1] The identity of helper cells and thymus-derived cells has not yet been formaly proven in hapten-carrier cooperation. Although thymus-derived cells are probably the most common helper cells, other cell types may also be able to function as helpers.

were precommitted to the synthesis of antibodies of a single specificity we would have to assign this precommitment to the thymus-derived cell since this cell can be specifically paralyzed. This would almost necessarily imply an information transfer from thymus-derived to bone marrow-derived cell, since the latter cell is the ancestor of those cells that produce specific antibody. A number of arguments will be discussed below which make us think that the receptors present on the thymus-derived cells might have a limited spectrum of specificities as compared with the spectrum of specificities present on conventional antibody. For this reason and because of simplicity we assume that both types of cells are precommitted to a single antibody specificity[2].

We do not know at present, why cell interaction is needed in the induction of the immune response. Do the helper cells just serve as an antigen concentrating device (Mitchison, 1969 a)? Are they needed to trigger proliferation of the precursors of the antibody forming cells? In any case, the helper cells must play an important rôle in the regulation of the immune response. One possibility is that the thymus-derived cell receptors are selected for certain specificities, and in this way limit the immune reactivity of the animal.

In fact, the cooperation hypothesis accounts for a number of immunological phenomena especially if we attribute to the thymus-derived cells a certain class of immunoglobulin, which does not allow for as many different specific combining sites as do the immunoglobulins produced by the marrow-derived cells. This would mean that for any given antigen, only certain surface structures possess "carrier property" (Rajewsky et al., 1967) i.e. can be recognized by certain clones of thymus-derived cells and thus mediate the immune response to the whole spectrum of antigenic determinants present on that antigen. In this way an explanation can be offered for the finding in certain of our hapten-carrier experiments (Rajewsky et al., 1969), that the haptenic groups present on the carrier did not cooperate efficiently with each other, whereas carrier determinants were strongly cooperative. In other systems, cooperation of haptenic groups seems to be more clearly detectable (Steiner and Eisen, 1967; Paul et al., 1967).

On the basis of the hypothesis, it can be easily understood that frequently substances that prove to be immunogenic in certain strains of laboratory animals, function as haptens in others. Examples for this, LDH in rabbits and DNP-PLL in guinea pigs, have already been mentioned (for further literature see World Health Organization, Techn. Rep., 1968). Though the antibody response to the respective antigens is heterogeneous in responder animals, relatively simple Mendelian genetics are found in some of these systems, responsiveness being dominant over non-responsiveness. One can imagine that in the non-responder animals, the thymus-derived cells do not possess an immunoglobulin receptor that recognizes any of the determinants of the substance to which the animal is unre-

---

[2] The mechanism of antibody induction proposed requires the interaction of two types of presumably rare cells. Preliminary calculations, done by Prof. J. Hajdu from the Institute for Theoretical Physics, University of Köln, have shown (unpublished) that the frequency of such cell interactions could be easily high enough to account for a normal immune response, if it is assumed that $10^3 - 10^4$ specific cells of each type are present in the spleen of a normal mouse and that the mobility of these cells corresponds to the one observed by Drs. W. Ax and H. Fischer, Freiburg, (personal communication) in organ culture.

sponsive. As predicted by the hypothesis, non-responder animals are fully responsive to the haptenic substance if it is coupled to an immunogenic carrier.

Finally, the assumption of immunoglobulin receptors with a limited range of specificities on the thymus-derived cells has interesting consequences for the phenomenon of immunological tolerance, since tolerance seems to be more easily inducible in these than in the bone-marrow-derived cells. One would have to assume that the specificity of tolerance need not necessarily be identical with antibody specificity, since it would reflect the specificity of the receptors on thymus-derived cells rather than the specificity of conventional antibody. Cross-tolerance of serologically non-crossreacting substances has indeed been found (Austin and Nossal, 1966). Furthermore, for the induction of tolerance only those determinants of an antigen would be needed that possess "carrier property." This has been verified in both the LDH- and the DNP-PLL-BSA system (see above). It can be imaged that this finding will be important for clinical immunology and especially for the transplantation problem.

It should be mentioned that in several systems tolerance has been found to be determinant-specific. In the terms of the cooperation hypothesis this would mean that bone marrow-derived cells can also be paralyzed under certain conditions. The two types of immunological tolerance that can be distinguished by their specificity (see Rajewsky et al., 1967) could thus be localized in different cell populations. This could also hold for low and high dose paralysis (Mitchison, 1964).

Many of the arguments presented in this article have been developed in a continous discussion with Prof. N. K. Jerne, Paul Ehrlich-Institut, Frankfurt am Main. This does not mean that he aggrees with all of them. The author is also grateful for discussion to Dr. N. A. Mitchison, National Institute for Medical Research, Mill Hill, London, who has so much contributed to this field of research. The experimental work has been done together with R. Kappis, B. Müller, S. Nase, G. Peltre, E. Rottländer and V. Schirrmacher and was supported by the Deutsche Forschungsgemeinschaft and the Stiftung Volkswagenwerk.

Summary

The induction of antibody formation seems to require the cooperation of antigenic determinants of the immunogen and the cooperation of two cell types. Cell interaction could be brought about by antigen linking the two cells together specifically. The possibility is discussed that one of the two cell types carries on its surface immunoglobulin receptors of a special class with a restricted spectrum of specificities.

References

Armerding, D., and K. Rajewsky. In: Proceedings of the XVIIth Colloquium Protides of the Biological Fluids, Brugge 1969 (H. Peeters, Ed.). Oxford, Pergamon Press (in press).
Austin, C., and G. J. V. Nossal: Aust. J. exp. Biol. med. Sci. 44, 341 (1966).
Benacerraf, B., I. Green, and W. E. Paul: Cold Spr. Harb. Symp. quant. Biol. 32, 569 (1967).
Claman, H. N., E. A. Chaperon, and R. F. Triplett: Proc. Soc. exp. Biol. (N. Y.) 122, 1167 (1966).
Davies, A. J. S., E. Leuchars, V. Wallis, and P. C. Koller: Transplantation 4, 438 (1966).
— — —, R. Marchant, and E. V. Elliott: Transplantation 5, 222 (1967).
Jerne, N. K.: Ann. Rev. Microbiol. 14, 341 (1960).
Kaplan, N. O.: Brookhaven Symp. Biol. 17, 131 (1964).
Landsteiner, K.: The specificity of serological reactions. Washington: Howard University Press 1947.

Miller, J. F. A. P., and G. F. Mitchell: Nature (Lond.) **216**, 659 (1967).
— — J. exp. Med. **128**, 801 (1968).
—, and D. Osoba: Physiol Rev. **47**, 437 (1967).
Mitchell, G. F., and J. F. A. P. Miller: Proc. nat. Acad. Sci. (Wash.) **59**, 296 (1968a).
— — J. exp. Med. **128**, 821 (1968b).
Mitchison, N. A.: Proc. Royal Soc. B **161**, 275 (1964).
— Cold Spr. Harb. Symp. quant. Biol. **32**, 431 (1967).
— In: Immunological Tolerance (Landy, M., and W. Braun, Ed.). New York: Academic
    Press, 1969 a.
— In: Handbook of General Pathology, Suppl. Vol. Immunology, Chapter **IV** A, New York:
    Springer (in press, b).
Morrison, S. L., and G. Terres: J. Immunol. **96**, 901 (1966).
Paul, W. E., G. W. Siskind, B. Benacerraf, and Z. Ovary: J. Immunol **99**, 760 (1967).
Rajewsky, K., and E. Rottländer: Cold Spr. Harb. Symp. quant. Biol. **32**, 547 (1967).
— —, G. Peltre, and B. Müller: J. exp. Med. **126**, 581 (1967).
—, V. Schirrmacher, S. Nase, and N. K. Jerne: J. Exp. Med. **129**, 1131 (1969).
Schiermann, L. W., and R. A. McBride: Science **156**, 658 (1967).
Steiner, L. A., and H. N. Eisen: J. exp. Med. **126**, 1185 (1967).
Taylor, R. B.: Transplantation Reviews I, 114 (1969).
Terres, G., and W. Wolins: J. Immunol. **86**, 361 (1961).
World Health Organization, 1968. Technical Report No. 402.

Prof. Dr. K. Rajewsky
Institut für Genetik der Universität,
5 Köln-Lindenthal, Weyertal 121

Discussion

DE WECK (Berne): Do you think you need on the same molecule two antigenic determinants of different structures or of the same structure ? If you take the case of an animal which is immunised with its own protein to which you added one determinant, for example, by conjugation in vivo, you will have one determinant structure added, but this nevertheless induces antibody formation. On the other hand you know that a synthetic oligopeptide antigen having one single determinant on the molecule is immunogenic.

RAJEWSKY (Cologne): I think this is an important point. According to the hypothesis, at least two determinants must be present on an immunogenic molecule. These determinants may or may not be identical. To my knowledge, there is no example of an immunogen possessing only one antigenic determinant.

HILSCHMANN (Göttingen): In your model, Dr. Rajewsky, two cells are present, an assistant cell and the other one which produces the antibodies. You say that the assistant cell is mono-specific. Usually the antibody producing cells are called monospecific, are they not ?

RAJEWSKY (Cologne): Until now we have not been able to decide whether both the assistant cell and the precursor of the antibody forming cell or only one of them is monospecific. The finding that tolerance can be induced in the population of thymus derived cells can be most easily explained by the assumption that these cells are monspecific.

HAUROWITZ (Bloomington): If a carrier protein is coupled with a large amount of hapten, e.g. diazotized arsanilic acid, it loses its antigenicity. The reasons for this phenomenon are not clear. Most probably, substitution with an excess of hapten leads to a loss of susceptibility of the antigen to 'processing' by proteolytic enzymes. This view is supported by the fact that antibodies have been produced by the administration of haptens such as acetyltyrosine azophenylarsonate which can undergo transpeptidation.

FISCHER (Freiburg): I would like to know precisely what function the assistant cell has and whether of necessity it must be specific. A second question: Could it be that the induction of antibody formation requires several differentiating steps and cellular divisions, while sensitization and the development of a relatively crude antibody fragment on the cell membrane can take place without so many steps? Thus, we may be concerned with a problem of cell-differentiation.

RAJEWSKY (Cologne): In the sense of the hypothesis put forward the assistant cell must, of course, be specific. It binds antigen specifically as does the precursor of the antibody forming cell. The interaction of the two cell types is thus specifically brought about by the bridging antigen molecule.

ROITT (London): I want to give some evidence that there are antigen sensitive cells in two lymphocyte populations. Firstly the work of Taylor [Nature (Lond.) **220**, 611 (1968)] using a thymus-bone marrow combination, which on injection into an irradiated mouse with sheep red cells gives an antibody response, has shown that with thymus from a tolerant animal there is suppression of the immune response in the recipient. Secondly Dr. Playfair [Immunology **15**, 815 (1968)] in our department has been studying a similar system where he takes the mouse strains A and B and uses FI hybrid AB as the recipient for thymus and foetal liver cells from either A or B in different combinations. He finds that there is a strain difference: one produces a very good response to the sheep red cells, the other produces a very poor response. Then he took thymus from the FI hybrids and foetal liver cells from either A or B. If B is the strain which gave a very good response to sheep red cells, then the foetal liver cells together with the thymus from the hybrid gave a good response. The foetal liver cells from the poorer responding animals gave a poorer response in the hybrid. Dr. Playfair has subsequently shown that when tolerance is induced by injection of sheep cells plus cyclophosphamide, it is the bone marrow rather than the thymus cell population which is specifically unresponsive. Thus both bone narrow and thymus cells can be shown separately to contain antigen sensitive cells.

WESTPHAL (Freiburg): If diffusion processes or migration of cells are necessary then they may be dependent upon temperature, and one might use such a system to find out whether something like that really happens.

WALFORD (Los Angeles): There is evidence for a two stage process based upon the effect of temperature on the antibody response. If you immunise turtles at 6 °C and maintain same, you get no response at all or you may get a response many weeks or months later. If you immunize the turtles at 6 °C and a few weeks later raise the temperature, a prompt response is seen. They can recognize the antigen at the lower temperature, but a higher temperature is required for an actual antibody response.

7*

DEICHER (Hannover): How do you explain by your hypothesis the difference between low-dose tolerance on the one hand and the absence of antigen on the other.

RAJEWSKY (Cologne): Small doses of antigen may induce paralysis without bringing about a significant number of cell interactions.

Bayer-Symposium I, 101—111 (1969)

The Effect of Cytostatic Agents on Nucleic Acid and Protein Synthesis and on Immunological and Non-Immunological Inflammation

H. Begemann

With 7 Figures

The indication for the use of cytostatic substances has been expanded significantly by the knowledge that almost without exception cytostatic agents exert an immunosuppressive effect. At present, the clinical importance of this property is nearly equal to their actual cytostatic effects. The frequency in the use made of cytostatic agents is in noticeable contrast to our limited knowledge of their mode of action. On account of this the choice of the respective agent, the time of its administration, the combination possibilities of various substances which act in a similar manner is largely left to coincidence or to the experience of the individual physician.

After having studied the proliferation dynamics of human lymph nodes under normal and pathological conditions (publication Theml *et al.*, 1967) for a prolonged period of time it was obvious that the action of substances with a cytostatic effect also had to be examined. This idea was particularly obvious since it is generally assumed that a major part of the cytostatic agents effect the formation of nucleic acids by various biochemical pathways.

Also for these experiments, which were performed in association with Trepel, Stockhusen and Rastetter we used short periods of 1 h of incubation of particles of human lymph nodes. This method is similar to that which was suggested by Johnson *et al.* for other organs. Immediately after surgery the excised lymph nodes were prepared. The tissue particles which were used had a mean size of 1 mm³. This method (details of which have been reported by us elsewhere) enabled us to imitate in vivo conditions due to rapid processing and the choice of culture medium. It was possible to confirm this by previously performed simultaneous autoradiographic experiments in vivo and in vitro. To the customary culture media (7 parts TC-medium according to Morgan, Morton and Parker 3 parts patient serum with ³H-thymidine or ³H-cytidine or ³H-leucine) we now added the cytostatic substances which were to be examined. In this manner we tested ibenzmethyzin (Natulan), nitrogen mustard, actinomycin C (Sanamycin), vinblastine (Velbe) and prednisolone. We tested these agents in concentrations (dose I), which corresponded to a mean to high single human dose and in a second preparation which contained a tenfold concentration (dose II). We used the following individual levels:

Methylhydrazine:	0.01 mg/ml	(dose I corresponds to the clinical administration of 6.5 mg/kg)
	0.1 mg/ml	(dose II)

Nitrogen mustard:	0.0001 mg/ml	(dose I corresponds to the administration of a clinical dose of 0.06 mg/kg)
	0.001 mg/ml	(dose II)
Actinomycin C:	0.005 µg/ml	(dose I corresponds to the clinical administration of 3.5 µg/kg)
	0.05 µg/ml	(dose II)
Vinblastine:	0.0004 mg/ml	(dose I corresponds to the clinical administration of 0.24 mg/kg)
	0.004 mg/ml	(dose II)
Prednisolone:	0.001 mg/ml	(dose I corresponds to the clinical administration of 0.7 mg/kg)
	0.01 mg/ml	(dose II).

In addition to this, an even higher concentration of 1.0 mg/ml of prednisolone was used.

Lymph node tissue from 10 patients with hyperplasia of the lymph nodes, 9 patients with lymphogranulomatoses, 5 patients with reticulosarcomas and 5 patients with lymphadenoses served as a start. By comparing the synthesis-indices of the various lymph nodes with and without the effect of cytostatic agents it was possible to determine the effect of each of the studied substances on the DNA, RNA and protein syntheses.

Interpretation of our results must take into consideration the fact that the method used offers various advantages to the clinician, but that on the other hand it only permits limited conclusions regarding the inhibition of the individual phases of the cell cycle. Thus we cover the phase of DNA-synthesis, of RNA and protein syntheses, whereas the postmitotic and premitotic resting phase as well as mitosis itself can only be studied in vivo or in tissue cultures.

We shall select only a few of the results of our experiments which are of interest in connection with today's symposium:

Even under the action of the various cytostatic agents the 'markation pattern' of the lymph nodes remains unchanged. Now as before, the three large basophil cell types, the large lymphatic reticulum cell, the basophil round-cell and the plasmoblast are the carriers of DNA-synthesis and thus of the proliferation of the lymphatic tissue. The more differentiated reticulum cell and the lymphoblast also participates in the DNA-synthesis, but to a considerably smaller extent. The

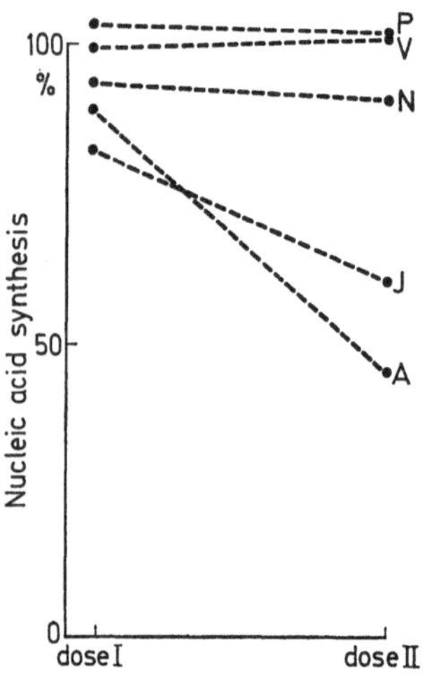

Fig. 1. The effect of cytostatic agents of nucleic acid. Mean effect of the normal dose (dose I) and of tenfold the normal dose (dose II) of various substances on the synthesis of nucleic acids of all lymphomas on which two concentrations of one substance were tested. For prednisolone (P), vinblastine (V), nitrogen mustard (N) and ibenzmethyzin (J) the effect on the DNA synthesis is given; for actinomycin (A) the effect on the RNA-synthesis is also given

effect of cytostatic agents decreases the markation index and the number of granules with ^{3}H-thymidine as well as with ^{3}H-cytidine or uridine labelling. In this context it is assumed that the number of cells which synthetize DNA and

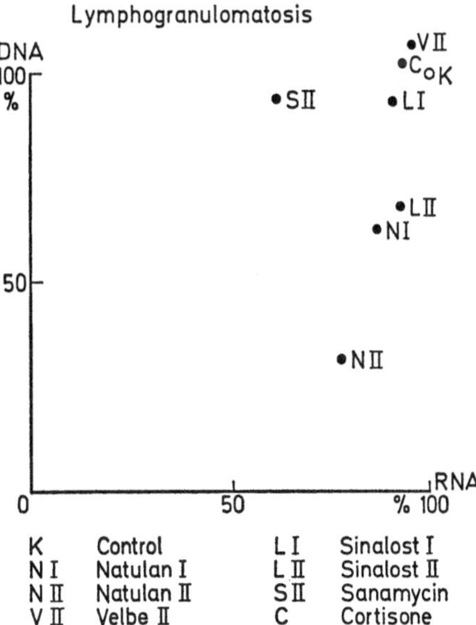

Fig. 2. Mean effect of the stated drug on the DNA and RNA syntheses of 9 cases with lymphogranulomatosis. The comparative value without cytostatic agents is set at 100%

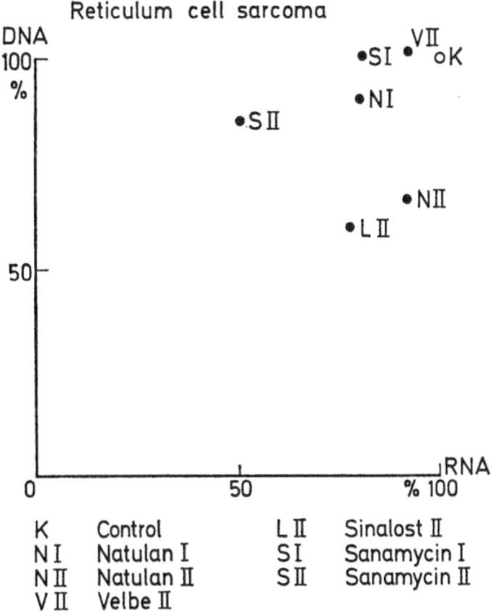

Fig. 3. Mean effect of the stated drug on the DNA and RNA syntheses of 4 cases with reticulum cell sarcoma

RNA becomes smaller and that ther ate of synthesis is also decreased (see Figs. 1—5).

The individual cytostatic agents have a very different effect on DNA, RNA and protein synthesis. Ibenzmethyzin and nitrogen mustard produce quite pronounced inhibition of DNA-synthesis (up to 60% of the starting value). These substances exert a significantly smaller effect on the RNA-synthesis. Actinomycin C almost selectively inhibits the RNA-synthesis (up to 50% of the starting value),

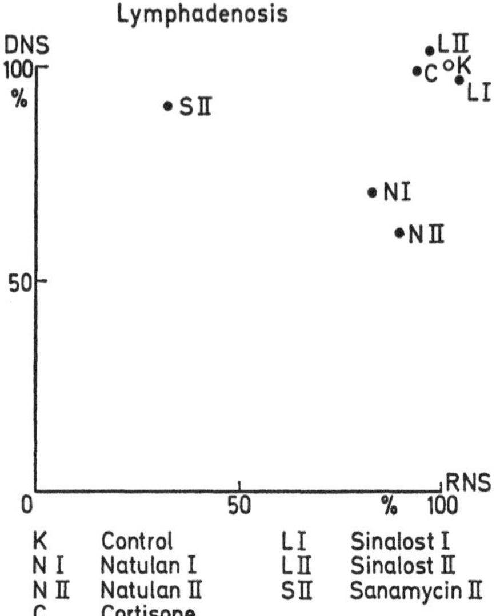

Fig. 4. Mean effect of the stated drugs on the DNA and RNA syntheses of 4 cases with lymphadenosis

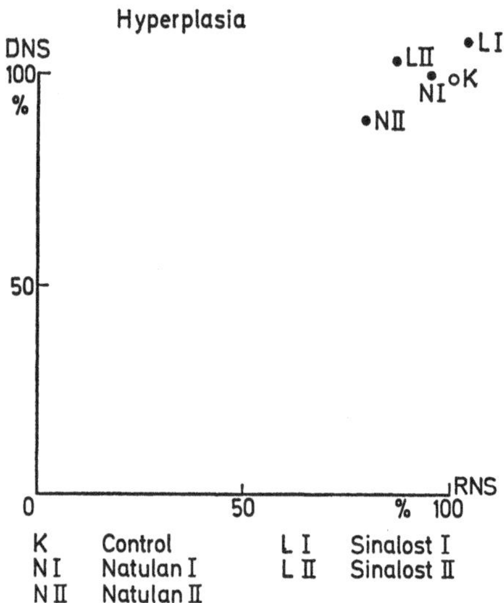

Fig. 5. Mean effect of the stated drugs on the DNA and RNA syntheses of 9 cases with hyperplasias of the lymph nodes

whereas the synthesis of DNA and protein are not affected by this substance. The synthesis of protein is, most of all, inhibited by ibenzmethyzin (up to 40% of the starting value). Vinblastine does not show a recognizable action on the synthesis of nucleic acids nor of proteins. This finding is in good agreement with other experimental results according to which vinblastine has a selective inhibitory effect in the metaphase of mitosis (Boggs *et al.*, Bruchovsky *et al.*). In clinical doses and in 10 to 100-fold increased concentrations prednisolone does not have a definite effect on the synthesis of nucleic acid. Only a 1000-fold concentration produced a definite reduction of the DNA-synthesis by 53 to 90%. In contrast to ibenzmethyzin and nitrogen mustard, prednisolone primarily affected the speed of synthesis and only to a lesser extent did it affect the percentage of cells involved with synthesis. We do not have any exact knowledge regarding the action of cortisone on patients with hemoblastoses. The known lymphoclastic effect of this drug-group is probably due to an action on the postmitotic resting phase and this has also been assumed by Trowell and Nowell.

The inhibition of the synthesis of nucleic acid—if present at all—is not strictly dosage-dependent. An inhibition value is achieved by a certain concentration (dose I) which frequently can only be insignificantly increased by increasing the dosage. This was particularly obvious with nitrogen mustard, whereas actinomycin C and ibenzmethyzin in the concentrations used by us showed that the effect was definitely dosage-dependent. On account of their potential major clinical importance these findings absolutely require additional checking and control.

The observation that the inhibition of the synthesis of nucleic acid depends on the type of disease of the lymph nodes under examination is of particular interest and importance. Lymphogranulomatous tissues were inhibited most, reticulum cell sarcomas and lymphadenomas were inhibited to a somewhat lesser degree, whereas reactive hyperplasias were hardly affected. Since we have shown in previous experiments (Theml *et al.*, 1967) that the DNA-markation-index of lymphogranulomatoses, reticulum cell sarcomas and lymphosarcomas is definitely lower than that of reactive lymph node hyperplasias and that thus the generation time of the individual cells with the fore-mentioned diseases must be prolonged, the usual interpretation according to which cytostatic agents are stated to exert their therapeutic action by affecting cell division, is no longer justified. Regarding this point we are unable to agree with Bruce *et al.* in the acceptance of their findings. It is rather to be assumed that the cells of malignant lymphomas, as far as significant vital functions (amongst others cell maturation and cell proliferation) are concerned, are inferior to normally functioning, adequately stimulated cells and that they thus are more susceptible to the action of cytotoxic substances.

From the clinical use of cytostatic agents, the following question arises amongst others: How do the cellular defence mechanisms of the organism react to the effects of cytostatic agents? We attempted to clarify this question through animal experiments (Trepel, Schick and Begemann). These experiments were carried out with male guinea-pigs of mixed races. Their weight ranged from 400 to 700 gm. Five weeks after intracutaneous immunization with 0.1 ml of double-concentrated BCG-vaccine the intensity of the tuberculin reaction was determined with an intracutaneous injection of 0.1 ml of tuberculin GT (concentration 10^2), (first test). Subsequently, groups of 10 animals each received daily intraperitoneal injections of the cytostatic agents Endoxan (cyclophosphamide), Natulan (ibenzmethyzin), TEM (trimethylenmelamine), Sanamycin (actinomycin C), Velbe (vincaleucoblastin), Proresid (podophyllinic acid glycoside), Methotrexate (amethopterin), Puri-Nethol (6-mercaptopurin) and the antiphlogistic agents

Decortin H (prednisolone) and Butazolidine (phenylbutazone) for 10 days. The selected dosage (Table 1) generally was already within the toxic range (weight loss of 0 to 20%, a mortality of 0 to 10% within the first 11 days). A control group received 1 ml of NaCl solution i.o. per day. After treatment for 5 days a second tuberculin test was performed, after treatment of 10 days a third tuberculin test and after recovery had occurred after 23 to 28 days a fourth tuberculin test was carried out. The tuberculin reactions were read after 24 h and the thickness of the infiltration as well as the surface area of the erythema were measured.

A skin-window (Rebuck and Crowley) was constructed in two animals from every group, as well as in all 10 control animals after termination of treatment for

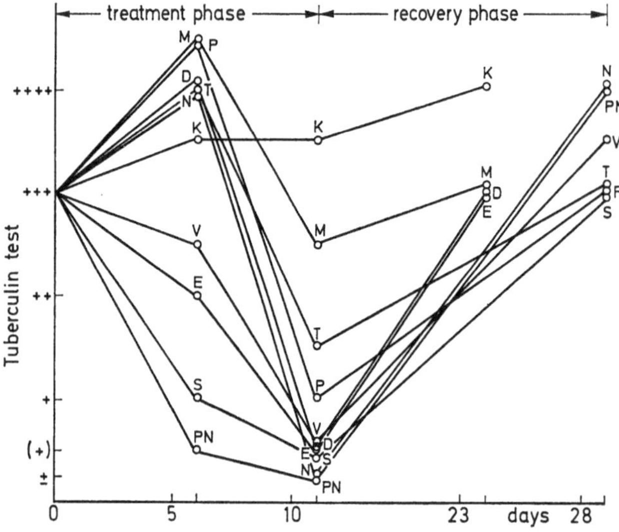

Fig. 6. Mean effect of the various drugs on the tuberculin reaction during treatment, immediately after treatment and during the recovery phase. M = Methotrexate, P = Proresid, D = Decortin H, T = TEM, N = Natulan, K = control, V = Velbe, E = Endoxan, S = Sanamycin, PN = Puri-Nethol. The values for Butazolidine are identical to the values for Endoxan

10 days. In this context attention was paid to temporal coincidence with the third tuberculin test. In addition to this, groups of 4 additional animals were treated for 24 h with high doses of the following drugs which were subdivided into four individual doses (intensive therapy): Endoxan (4 × 7.5 mg/kg), Natulan (4 × 20 mg/kg), Puri-Nethol (4 × 25 mg/kg), Decortin H (4 × 4 mg/kg) and Butazolidine (4 × 20 mg/kg). A skin-window was constructed at the start of intensive treatment. After 24 h all skin-windows were removed from the subcutaneous tissues of the animals, they were stained according to May-Grünwald-Giemsa and they were evaluated. The density of the cells in the inflammatory exudate was evaluated and the ratio of mononuclear macrophages to granulocytes was determined by counting.

The changes of the tuberculin reactions during and immediately after treatment as well as during the recovery phase are compiled in Fig. 6. Whereas the control value during and after treatment with NaCl increases or remains unchanged, Puri-Nethol, Sanamycin, Endoxan, Butazolidine and Velbe already produce a decrease of the tuberculin reactions after 5 to 6 days and Methotrexate, Proresid, Natulan, TEM and Decortin still produce a transient increase but subsequent to this, after treatment for 10 days, they produce a mild to severe decrease of the tuberculin reaction. In comparison to the starting value and the control value, the smallest decrease (produced by Methotrexate) is insignificant but it, nevertheless, becomes definite by comparing it to the result of the 5th to 6th day. Obviously the reduction of the tuberculin test was not dependent on the degree of

Table 1. *The effect of treatment for 10 days with 8 cytostatic agents and 2 antiphlogistic agents on the white cell count, the reaction of the skin-window and on the tuberculin reaction. The treated animal groups are arranged according to the absolute leukocyte numbers after treatment*

	Leukocytes		Skin-window			Tuberculin test
	Absolute	Relative to the starting value %	Cellular exudate	Makro-phagen	Granulo-cytes	
Controls 1 ml NaCl	17800	99	+++	45:55		+++
Sanamycin 13 γ/kg	29800	151	++	55:45		(+)
Decortin-H 10 mg/kg	24100	93	++++	55:45		(+)
Methotrexat 2 mg/kg	15100	91	++(+)	50:50		++(+)
Butazolidine 50 mg/kg	14300	76	+++	60:40		(+)
Velbe 18 γ/kg	12400	114	+++	55:45		+
Proresid 100 mg/kg	10500	60	++(+)	25:75		+
Natulan 40 mg/kg	6000	30	++	30:70		±
Puri-Nethol 70 mg/kg	4000	25	+	5:95		±
Endoxan 15 mg/kg	3100	22	++	15:85		(+)
TEM 0,3 mg/kg	2000	18	(+)	5:95		++

toxicity of a drug: with the dosage levels used, Endoxan and Decortin did not have a general toxic effect but they did diminish the tuberculin reaction more than the very toxic TEM. During the recovery phase the tuberculin reaction regularly shows an increase once again, frequently in excess of the starting value.

After treatment for 10 days the cellular inflammatory exudate in the skin-window was not significantly changed by the antiphlogistic agents Decortin and Butazolidine and by Sanamycin, Methotrexate and Velbe (Table 1). Proresid and (increasing in this order) Natulan, Endoxan, Puri-Nethol and TEM not only effected a definite to extreme decrease of the total cellular exudate but also of the percentage of macrophages. In Table 1 the result of the skin-window is compared

to that of the tuberculin test 1 day after the 10 day treatment period. It is noticeable that, with the exception of Methotrexate and of TEM, the tuberculin reaction
was suppressed more than the skin-window reaction.

As opposed to longterm treatment for 10 days, the exudate of the skin-window
was not affected during intensive treatment for 24 h with the cytostatic agents
Endoxan, Natulan, Puri-Nethol. In contrast to this, it was decreased by the antiphlogistic agents Decortin and Butazolidine without a change of the ratio of
macrophages to granulocytes (Fig. 7).

With the exception of Proresid, the more or less pronounced immunosuppressive action of the tested substances is known (Schwartz and Andre, Trepel

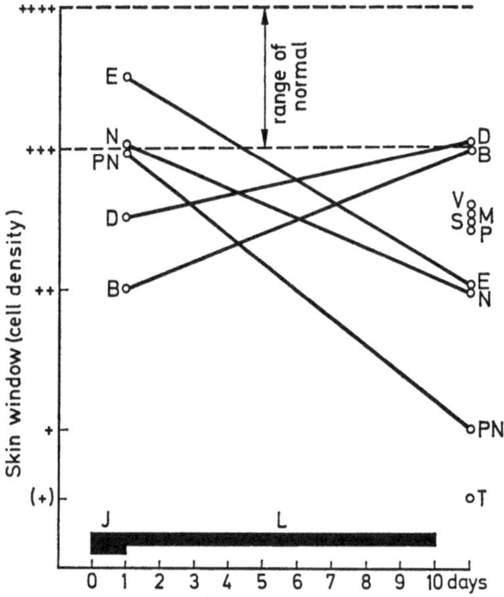

Fig. 7. Mean effect of various drugs on the cellular inflammatory exudate in the skin-window:
left, during intensive treatment for 1 day (1) and right, after longterm treatment for 10 days
(L). Designations: See Fig. 6. The joining lines do not indicate an aimed change between the
measured values, they are only intended to connect the various test phases of the same drug

et al.). However, it had to be determined whether the suppression of the immune
reaction of allergies of the delayed type is due to elimination of the specific
immunological defence or whether it is due to suppression of the non-specific
inflammatory reaction. The available findings indicate that immunosuppressive
substances suppress the specific immunological inflammatory infiltrate to a
larger extent than the non-specific cellular infiltrate. The importance of these
results is discussed elsewhere (Trepel *et al.*). Hitherto only the cytostatic agent 6-
mercaptopurine and Amethopterin were known to suppress the non-specific inflammatory reaction (Hersh *et al.*; Page *et al.*). These findings could be confirmed
with the 6-mercaptopurine. With the dosage levels used by us Amethopterin,
vincaleucoblastine and actinomycin C only produce a minimal decrease of the
cellular exudate, whereas podophyllinic acid glycoside, cyclophosphamide,
ibenzmethyzin and triethylenmelamine produced a pronounced decrease of the
cellular exudate.

A comparison of the findings during intensive treatment and after longterm treatment is characteristic regarding the antiphlogistic action of the cytostatic agents, as well as that of the antiphlogistic agents themselves. With shortterm treatment only, the antiphlogistic agents decrease the cellular inflammatory exudate and the interrelationship of the cellular elements remains unchanged. The cytostatic agents remain ineffective, obviously because they do not have primary antiphlogistic properties. Prolonged pre-treatment with cytostatic agents apparently decreases the prerequisites for a normal inflammatory reaction since, with such pre-treatment, a frequently extremely decreased exudation of inflammatory cells—particularly of macrophages—results. Thus, the cytostatic agents must be regarded as indirect, secondary, antiphlogistic agents. Pre-treatment with the classical antiphlogistic agents does not result in an anti-inflammatory effect since obviously the antiphlogistic effect of these agents is related to their presence.

In summary it can be observed that the non-specific as well as the immunologically specific inflammatory reaction is decreased by prolonged treatment with cytostatic agents. This means that two of the possible defense mechanisms of the host against the tumor are interfered with by cytostatic agents. Testing of various cytostatic agents in vitro in tumor tissue prior to the start of treatment would be desirable, since the cytostatic agents definitely restrict the defense mechanisms of the body and usually do not necessarily restrict tumour growth. Permanent treatment of a patient with cytostatic agents is probably only acceptable if the tumour cells are definitely more sensitive than the normal cells, thus enabling one to get by with low maintenance doses which do not strongly depress the endogenous defence mechanisms of the organism. In patients with less sensitive tumors, which require higher, toxic maintenance doses, the cytostatic agents would damage "friend and foe" alike and thus no advantage would be gained. In such cases massive treatment at intervals would theoretically be more promising since, as has been shown by our tests, the effects of a few cytostatic agents on the tumour cell occur immediately, whereas the detrimental effects on the defences of the host only take place later and—where single administration is concerned—probably occur in a much attenuated manner.

The pronounced anti-inflammatory effect of cytostatic agents is also of importance where the success evaluation of treatment through cytostatic agents against solid tumors is concerned. For example, during treatment with cytostatic agents, tumour metastasis may simply become smaller by regression of the peritumoral inflammatory infiltrates without the occurrence of a genuine carcinostatic effect.

Summary

At present, the spectrum of application of cytostatic substances is being expanded well beyond mere tumour therapy.

We have experimentally studied three potential uses for cytostatic agents:

1. Inhibition of tumour cells.
2. Inhibition of immunological inflammation.
3. Inhibition of non-specific inflammation.

On 1. The uptake of ³H-thymidine and of ³H-uridine into lymph node cells after in vitro incubation for 1 h with ibenzmethyzin, nitrogen mustard, actinomycin C, vincaleublastine and prednisolone was determined in 29 pathological or irritated human lymph nodes (9 lymphogranulomatoses, 5 reticulum cell sarcomas, 5 lymphadenoses and 10 hyperplasias). Ibenzmethyzin reduced the DNA-synthesis and, to a lesser extent, the RNA-synthesis in 8 out of 9 cases with lymphogranulomatosis and in approximately one half of the cases with reticulum cell sarcomas and with lymphadenosis. Nitrogen mustard decreased the DNA-synthesis in approximately one third of the lymph node tumors. In all of the examined cases actinomycin C reduced the RNA-synthesis. Vincaleucoblastine which is a mitotic toxin, did not affect the synthesis of the nucleic acids. In contrast to lymph node tumors these substances did not have a definite action on thymidine and uridine uptake rate in cases with lymph node hyperplasias. Prednisolone depresses the DNA and RNA synthesis only in extremely high concentrations.

On 2. Groups of 10 guinea-pigs each which had been immunized with BCG, received daily doses of Natulan, cyclophosphamide, triethylenmelamine, actinomycin C, 6-mercaptopurine, Amethopterin, vincaleucoblastine, podophyllinic acid glycoside, prednisolone or phenylbutazone intraperitonealy for 10 days after the tuberculin test had become positive. After treatment for 5 days the intensity of the tuberculin reaction usually was not as yet significantly changed, however, after treatment for 10 days, with one exception (Amethopterin), it was definitely decreased.

On 3. The inhibition of the inflammatory reaction of a specific immunological process such as the tuberculin reaction is not parallel to inhibition of the non-specific reaction with all of the ten tested substances: After the conclusion of a 10 day treatment period, the cellular infiltrate of a non-specific inflammatory reaction (skin-window) was only reduced by: 6-mercaptopurine, triethylenmelamine, ibenzmethyzin and cyclophosphamide. As has been shown by stringent tests, these cytostatic agents do not have the primary antiphlogistic effect of prednisolone and phenylbutazone. Rather, their anti-inflammatory action only manifests itself during a prolonged treatment due to a decrease of the inflammatory cells.

References

Boggs, D. R., J. W. Athens, O. P. Haab, P. A. Cancilla, S. O. Raab, G. E. Cartwright, and M. W. Wintrobe: Leukokinetic studies. VII. Morphology of the bone marow and blood of dogs given vinblastine sulfate. Blood **23**, 53 (1964).

Bruce, W. R., B. E. Meeker, and F. A. Valeriote: Comparison of the sensitivity of normal hematopoietic and transplanted Lymphoma colony-forming cells to chemotherapeutic agents administred in-vivo. J. nat. Cancer Inst. **37**, 233 (1966).

Bruchovsky, N., A. A. Owen, A. J. Becker, and J. E. Till: Effects of vinblastine on the proliferative capacity of L-cells and their progress through the division cycle. Cancer Res. **25**, 1232 (1965).

Hersh, E. M., V. G. Wong, and E. J. Freireich: Inhibition of the local inflammatory response in man by antimetabolites. Blood **27**, 38 (1966).

Johnson, H. A., and V. P. Bond: A method of labeling tissues with tritiated thymidine in vitro and its use in comparing rates of cellproliferation in duct epithelium, fibroadenoma and carcinoma of human heart. Cancer (Philad.) 14, 639 (1961).

Morgan, J. F., H. J. Morton, and R. C. Parker: Nutrition of animal cells in tissue culture. Proc. Soc. exp. Biol. (N. Y.) **73**, 1 (1950).

Nowell, P. C.: Inhibition of human leucocyte mitosis by prednisolone in vitro. Cancer Res. **21**, 1518 (1961).

Page, A. R., R. M. Condie, and R. A. Good: Effect of 6-mercaptopurine on inflammation. Amer. J. Path. **40**, 519 (1962).

Rebuck, J. W., and J. H. Crowley: A method of studying leukocytic functions. Ann. N. Y. Acad. Sci. **59**, 757 (1955).

Schwartz, R., and J. Andre: The chemical suppression of immunity. In: Grabar, P., and P. Miescher: Mechanism of cell and tissue damage produced by immune reactions, p. 385. II. Internat. Sympos. Immunpath., Basel (Schweiz)-Stuttgart 1965.

Theml, H., F. Trepel, J. Rastetter u. H. Begemann: DNS- und RNS-Synthese in benignen und malignen Lymphomen. Klin. Wschr. **45**, 609 (1967).

Trepel, F., P. Schick u. H. Begemann: Morphologische und funktionelle Veränderungen im Blutzellsystem des Meerschweinchens mit zytostatischen Substanzen, Prednisolon und Phenylbutazon. III. Veränderungen einer immunologischen und einer unspezifischen Entzündungsreaktion. Z. ges. exp. Med. **149**, 25 (1968).

—, G. Stockhusen, J. Rastetter u. H. Begemann: Zytostatikawirkung auf die Nukleinsäure- und Proteinsynthese von benignen und malignen Lymphomen. Chemotherapia (Basel) **12**, 182 (1967).

Trowell, O. A.: The action of cortisone on lymphocytes in vitro. J. Physiol. (Lond.) **119**, 274 (1953).

Prof. Dr. H. Begemann
I. Medizinische Abteilung des Städtischen
Krankenhauses München-Schwabing,
8 München 23, Kölner Platz 1

Discussion

LAUENSTEIN (Wuppertal): Does the skin window method enable to distinguish definitely between anti-inflammatory effect and immunosuppressive effect ? Clinically, in the individual case it is very difficult to differentiate the so-called immuno-suppressive action of cytostatics from the anti-inflammatory action.

GRUNDMANN (Wuppertal): In the examination of the inflammatory exudate by the skin window method, lymphocytes appear rather late. If differences between the cytological composition in the skin window and the tuberculin reaction exist, one has to consider that the tuberculin reaction is the typical delayed reaction, i.e. a lymphocyte transferred reaction.

BEGEMANN (Munich): With regard to all these questions we must compare immunological and non-immunological inflammations. In non-immunological inflammation, e.g. in a traumatic inflammation, lymphocytes certainly play no role initially. In the immunological inflammation on the other hand very few lymphocytes, about 5% of the cells, suffice to set the mechanism in motion as studies by Prendergast have shown. This small number may not become noticeable in the skin window method.

WESTPHAL (Freiburg): Does any inflammation take place independent of immunology ? When you use the skin window method you always apply a local trauma and then the release of immunologically active substance is possible.

BEGEMANN (Munich): This would then be a local auto-immune disease — a new interpretation of inflammation in injuries.

HARTMANN (Hannover): To the definition of an immuno-suppressive agent: —
In my opinion we cannot at present speak of any drug as an immuno-suppressive.
Of no substance do we have definite proof that the mechanisms belonging to a
genuine immune reaction are disturbed, i.e. the uptake of antigen, the recognition
of antigen, the induction of the antigen-antibody reaction, etc. The only thing
that has been proved is that something before or after this chain is inhibited; but
the drug makes no specific attack. This is also true of the immuno-suppression by
prednisone, if its lymphoclastic effect is considered to be the essential action.
Lymphoclasia is no definition of immuno-suppression.

DEICHER (Hannover): The reported investigations are clinically very important since we must attempt to achieve effective immuno-suppression without
severe side reactions. A combination of several drugs with different mechanisms
of action might bring better clinical results with less undesirable effects then
higher doses of a single agent. Besides organ transplantation, such regimen are
being tried e.g. in rheumatoid arthritis (Deicher, H., u. R. Fricke: Zur Behandlung
der rheumatoiden Arthritis mit Cytostatika. Z. Rheumaforsch., in press) or lupus
erythematodes visceralis (Miescher, P.: Vortrag Dtsch. Ges. inn. Med., Wiesbaden
1968, in press).

WARNATZ: Do the results seen in the in vitro system for testing cytostatics
agree with the clinical success ?

BEGEMANN (Munich): In preliminary studies on rats good concord has been
found between in vitro results concerning DNA and RNA synthesis and the
in vivo effects. We have also clinically compared the results and in the majority
of cases found good agreement.

HAMMER (Freiburg): It is known that cytostatics can also have an adjuvant
effect. How may this be explainable ?

FISCHER (Freiburg): Membrane damage releases the so-called endogenous
adjuvants. This may explain the adjuvant actions of surface active substances
which are of a very diverse chemical nature. A recent example is vitamin A-
alcohol [Dresser, W.: Nature (Lond.) **217,** 527 (1968)].

Bayer-Symposium I, 113—120 (1969)

Studies on the Cytotoxicity of Lymphocytes

H. Fischer, W. Ax, H. Malchow, and I. Zeiss

With 14 Figures

The higher organisms are equipped with two different systems for immunological defence. One system is characterized by the production of humoral antibodies, the other by the appearence of specifically sensitized lymphocytes, which are capable of direct interaction with the antigen. If the antigen happens to be attached to a cell, this interaction may lead to the destruction of the antigen carrying cell.

The cytotoxic activity of specifically sensitized lymphocytes is of great biological significance. It is a major manifestation of immune reactions of the cellular type which include such important phenomena as tumour control, autoimmune diseases and allograft rejection. In spite of its obvious importance the actual mechanism of cell destruction by sensitized lymphocytes has not yet been elucidated.

In choosing a suitable model for the analysis of lymphocyte cytotoxicity, the following considerations have to be taken into account:

Lymphocyte cytotoxicity can be induced in two ways: firstly by specific immunological sensitization in vivo or in vitro (Rosenau, 1963; Wilson, 1965; Ginsburg, 1965); secondly by nonspecific activation, for instance, by mitogens such as PHA, Streptolysin S and staphylococcus filtrate (SF) (Möller, Perlman et al., 1965; Hirschhorn et al., 1964; Ling, 1968).

The question thus arises whether specifically and non-specifically induced cytotoxicity are identical or essentially different processes.

The process is an interaction of two cells, and its criterion is the destruction of the target cell. Different types of target cells are known to vary in their susceptibility to lymphocyte attack (Perlman et al., 1968; Holm, 1967a; Brunner). The variation probably depends on special qualities of the membranes of the different types of cells. Thus the study of target cell membranes will be a crucial step in the analysis of the whole phenomenon.

Experimental

The answer to the first consideration will be of great biological interest (see above), but will also be extremely important for technical reasons: even optimal specific stimulation will activate but a small fraction of the total lymphocyte population to cytotoxicity; by contrast, non-specific stimulation may yield up to 80% of cytotoxic lymphocytes (Ling, 1968). A preponderance of cytotoxic cells of this order will be required for valid biochemical analyses.

In a pilot study the question of identity or diversity of specific and non-specific cytotoxicity was approached by a comparison of lymphocyte behaviour

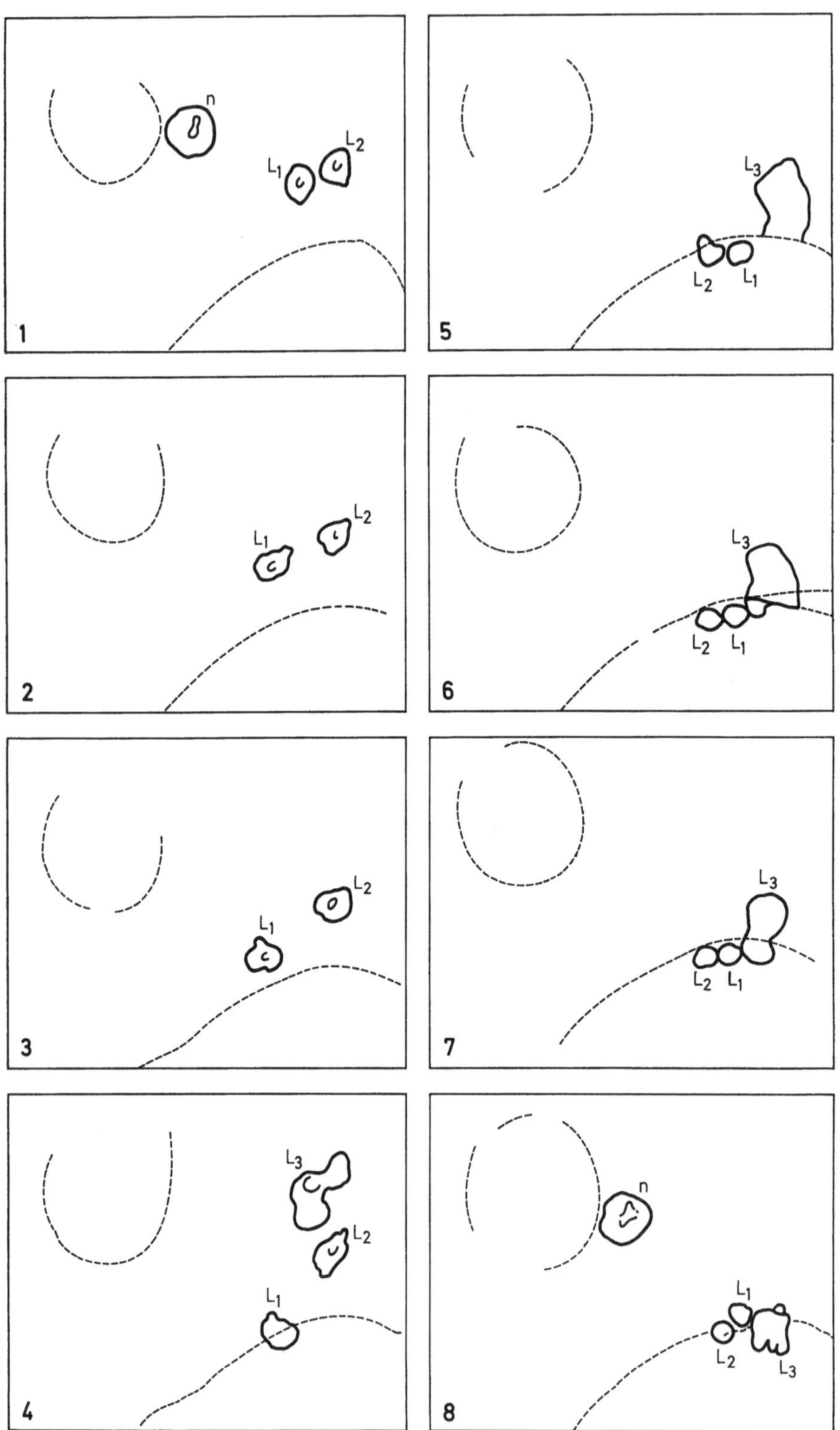

Figs. 1—8: Legends see page 116

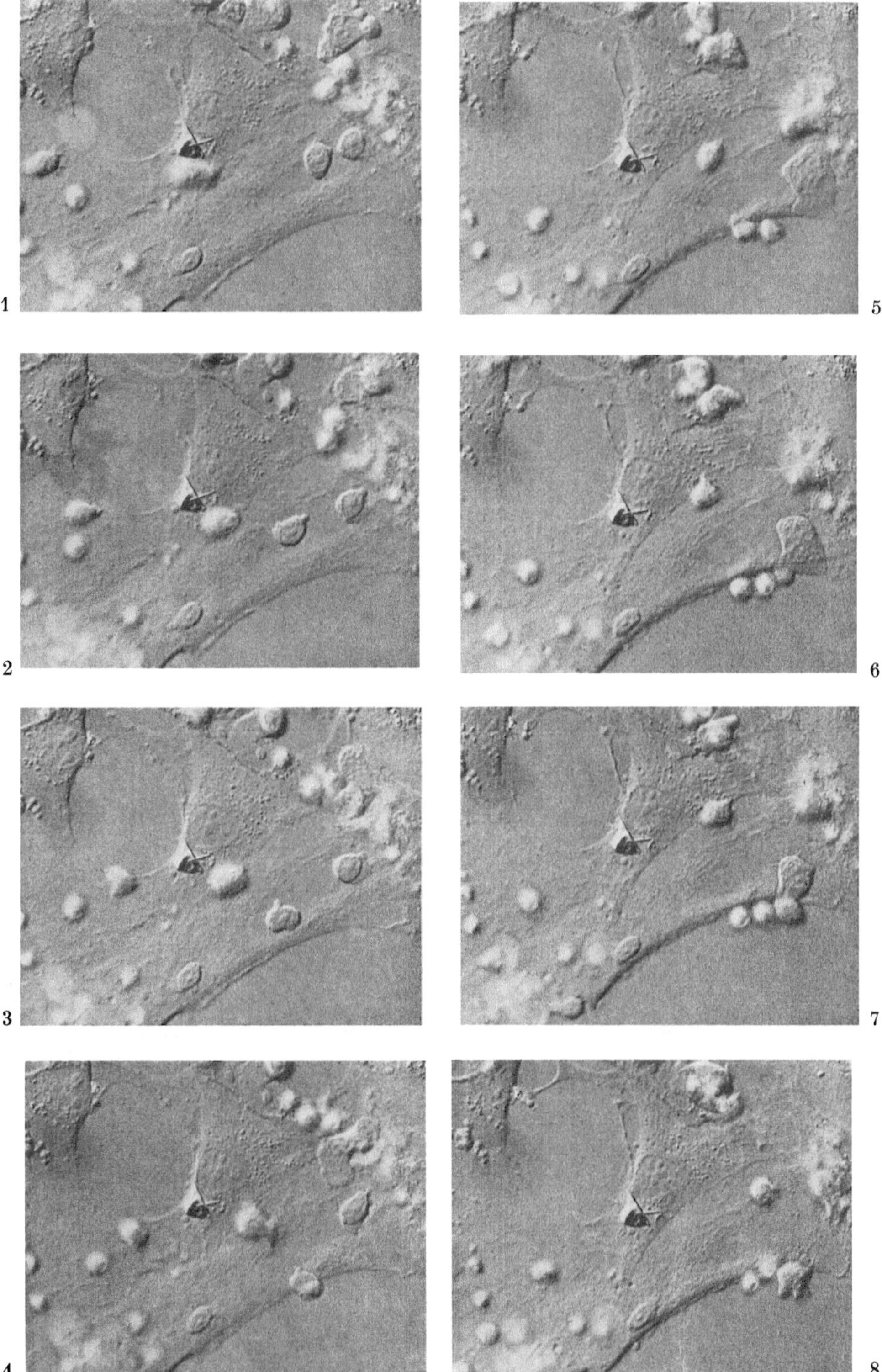

Figs. 1—8

8*

in the process of target cell destruction in vitro. The observations were made by time lapse cinematography (Ax *et al.*, 1968). The specific type of cytotoxicity was represented by Ginsburg's system (Ginsburg), the non-specific one by the system of Möller (Möller, 1965). Ginsburg uses lymphocytes which have been sensitized on heterogeneic fibroblast monolayers, i.e. by primary sensitization in vitro. The experimental system of Möller requires the addition of Phytohaemagglutinin for lymphocyte activation. The main features of the two systems are compared in the table.

Common to both types of reaction was the striking motility of the lymphocytes during their prolonged and close contact with the target cells. The sequence of photographs on Figs. 1—8 is but a poor illustration of the processes which are most impressively documented by cinematography. The pictures were taken with interference-phase contrast equippment according to Nomarski. This technique made it possible to distinguish clearly whether lymphocytes moved inside on, or underneath the target cells. There was no doubt that emperipolesis—if it occurred —was an extremely rare event and certainly of no significance for target cell destruction. This again emphasizes the role of the outer membrane as the actual target of the attacking lymphocytes. In summary it can be stated that locomotion of the lymphocytes on the outer membranes of the target cells seems to be an essential feature in both types of lymphocyte cytotoxicity.

Motility of in vivo sensitized allogeneic rat lymphocytes on rat target cell monolayer, (DA and Lewis).

Figs. 1—3: 2 Lymphocytes (L_1, L_2) crawling underneath fibroblast, i.e. between monolayer and coverslip, n = nucleus of fibroblast; dotted line = outline of fibroblast

Fig. 4. Lymphocyte L_1 is leaving the area underneath the fibroblast; part of the lymphocyte is still "squeezed" between target cell and coverslip. A third lymphocyte (L_3) can be seen underneath the fibroblast

Fig. 5. Lymphocytes L_1, L_2 have left the fibroblast area and can now be seen in spherical shape on the coverslip. Lymphocyte L_3 is reaching the edge of the target cell

Figs. 6—8: Lymphocyte L_3 leaves the space between target cell and supporting coverslip. Time intervals: Fig. 1—4: 2 min; Fig. 5—8: 6 min. All pictures are shots from time lapse cinematography using an interference contrast system (Nomarski-Zeiss), scale 600:1

Action of rat lymphocytes (DA) on rat target cell monolayer (Lewis). Lymphocytes had been sensitized in vivo. After transfer into tissue culture they start to destroy target cells. The control is showing the action of lymphocytes on a syngeneic monolayer

Fig. 9. Day 1 after transfer — mobile lymphocytes (DA rat) on target monolayer (Lewis); dark lymphoid cells are in contact with target fibroblasts i.e. on and underneath the latter

Fig. 10. Day 3 after transfer — large lymphoid cells attack fibroblasts

Fig. 11. Day 3 after transfer—same field as in 10. Target fibroblast undergoes lysis. Aggressor lymphocytes can be seen in the area where the target cell cytoplasm is scattered

Fig. 12. Day 3 after transfer—almost complete destruction of the target monolayer; shrinking fibroblast cytoplasm, remaining fibres, and aggregated lymphocytes

Figs. 13 and 14. Day 3 in vitro—control; same time as 10 and 12; lymphoid cells interacting with syngeneic monolayer cells. Formation of small lymphocyte aggregates, no destruction. All pictures are taken from 35 mm time lapse cinematography; phase contrast, scale 400 to 600:1 approx.

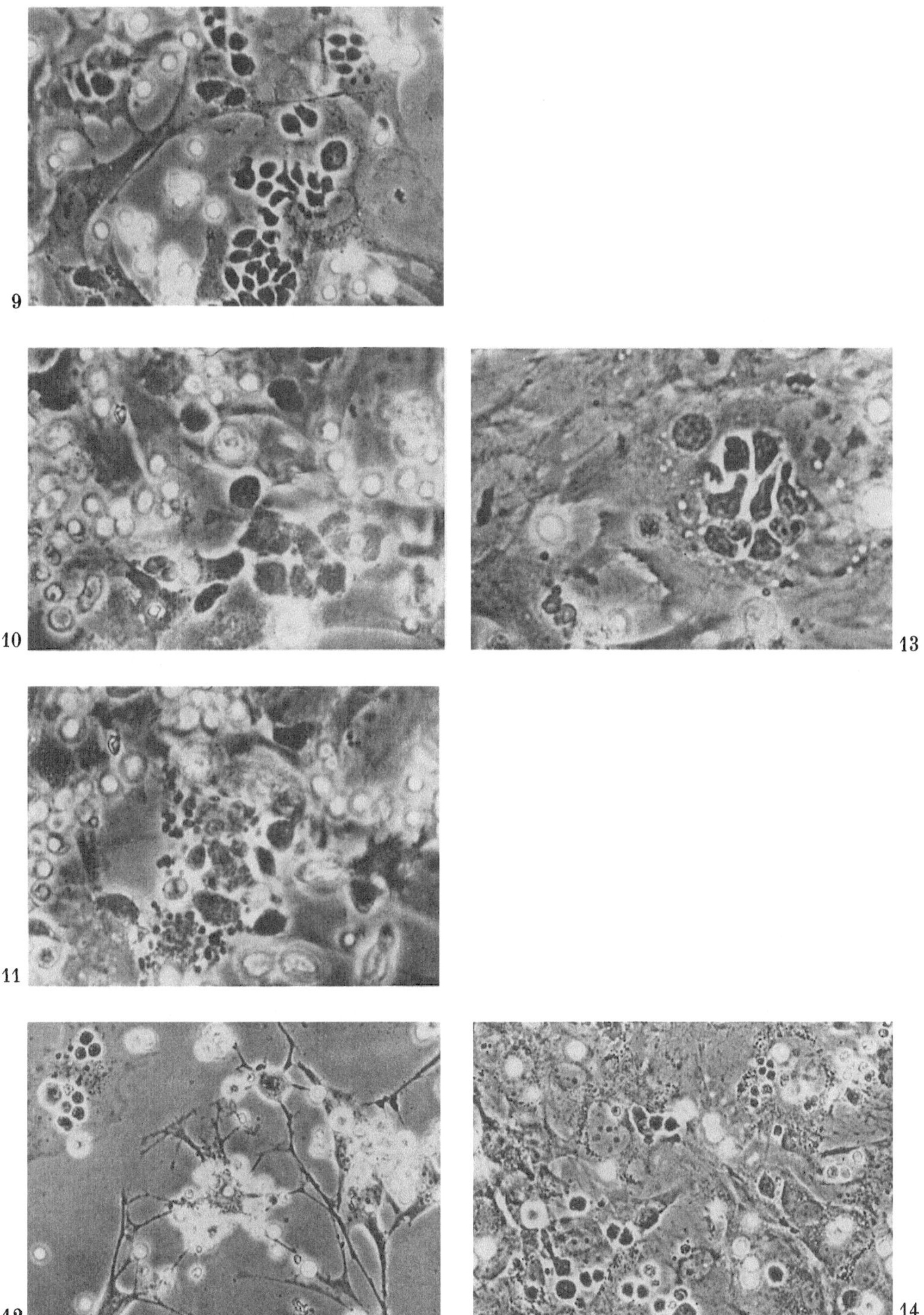

Figs. 9—14

Table. *Comparison of immunologically and PHA induced cytotoxicity*

Test system	Ginsburg	Möller
Similarities in cell behaviour		
Lymphocyte perambulation	Fast	Fast
Hand mirror shape of	Yes	Yes
Lymphocytes	(Pronounced)	(Not very pronounced)
Emperipolesis	No	No
Differences in cell behaviour		
Target cell death within	5 days	48 h
Transformation of lymphocytes	Yes	No
Lymphocyte mitoses	Mitotic wave	None
Lymphocytes develop uropod	Yes	No

The differences between the two systems mainly consisted in the earlier onset of cytotoxicity after nonspecific (PHA-mediated) stimulation. In this case target cell destruction was evident within 48 h. It thus seems that transformation of lymphocytes, development of the "uropod," and lymphocyte mitoses did not occur in this system simply for lack of time. However, these three changes were typical of specific sensitization. Taken in conjunction, the differences and the common features suggest that lymphocyte transformation and mitosis were not essential steps in the development of cytotoxicity. They may rather have been the expression of the cell proliferation and differentiation which ensues after specific sensitisation, and results in increased numbers of specifically cytotoxic lymphocytes.

Three additional observations seem worth mentioning:

1. In the initial stages of lymphocyte attack, lymphocytes moved freely from one target cell to another. It is thus possible that one lymphocyte is responsible for the death of more than one target cell.

2. Dead target cells and fragments of killed cells were regularly surrounded by a cluster of highly active lymphocytes. There was little to suggest that "anaphylactic death" of lymphocytes occurred (compare Figs. 9—14).

3. Retraction of the protoplasmic processes was the first sign of target cell damage The increasingly spherical, partially detached cells seemed particularly ready to divide. Mitoses were frequently seen, many of them remained incomplete. The increased mitotic activity of target cells under lymphocyte attack may be the in vitro analogon of the host cell proliferation in the graft versus host reaction in vivo.

Thus, the mitotic stimulation of target cells which precedes cell death seems an important stage which should not be neglected by biochemical analysis.

Speculations and Working Hypotheses

As pointed out above, thus far no biochemical mechanism has been proposed to explain lymphocyte cytotoxicity. Relevant information has come from inhibitor studies by Holm (Holm *et al.*, 1967 c; Holm, 1967 b) and Brunner. There is general agreement, that

1. only *living* lymphocytes are cytotoxic,

2. the energy generating metabolism (oxydative phosphorylation) must be intact,

3. RNA and DNA synthesis are not essential. The role of protein synthesis is still controversial.

Our current work on the membrane metabolism in lymphocyte cytotoxicity benefits from our previous studies on the phospholipid metabolism of membranes of irritated *macrophages*. In macrophages irritation and damage results in an increased degradation of diacylphospholipids and an accumulation of intermediary lysocompounds (Munder *et al.*, 1966).

An increase in the lipid turn-over has been demonstrated in *lymphocytes* soon after stimulation (Kay, 1968; Fisher, 1968). It may well be that during increased phospholipid turnover imbalances occur and lead to strictly localized accumulations of intermediates such as lysophospholipids and free fatty acids. These substances are highly surface active and cytotoxic. It may therefore be speculated that the activation of phospholipase A or alternatively the inhibition of lysophospholipase or acyltransferase, (which are both processes resulting in an accumulation of lysophospholipids) may be the decisive steps in cytotoxicity. These events may occur in certain localized areas of the membranes of either participant: lymphocyte or target cell. Investigations on the membrane metabolism of target cells and lymphocytes are in progress.

Acknowledgement

We thank Mister Heunert, Institut für Wissenschaftlichen Film, Göttingen, for expert help in cinematographic work. Part of the work was supported by grants from the Deutsche Forschungsgemeinschaft.

References

Ax, W., H. Malchow, I. Zeiss, and H. Fischer: The behaviour of lymphocytes in the process of target cell destruction in vitro. Exp. Cell Res. **53**, 108 (1968).

Brunner, K. T.: Personal communication. Swiss Institute for Experimental Cancer Research, Lausanne, Schweiz, Bugnon 21.

— Personal communication.

Fisher, D. B., and G. C. Mueller: An early alteration in the phospholipid metabolism of lymphocytes by phytohaemagglutinin. Proc. nat. Acad. Sci. (Wash.) **60**, 1396 (1968).

Ginsburg, H., and L. Sachs: Destruction of mouse and rat embryo cells in tissue culture by lymph node cells from unsensitized rats. J. cell. comp. Physiol. **66**, 199 (1965).

Hirschhorn, K., R. R. Schreibman, S. Verbo, and R. H. Gruskin: The action of streptolysin S on peripheral lymphocytes of normal subjects and patients with acute rheumatic fever. Proc. nat. Acad. Sci. (Wash.) **52**, 1151 (1964).

Holm, G.: The in vitro cytotoxicity of human lymphocytes; comparison with other cells. Exp. Cell Res. **48**, 327 (1967a).

— The in vitro cytotoxicity of human lymphocytes: the effect of metabolic inhibitors. Exp. Cell Res. **48**, 334 (1967b).

—, P. Perlmann, and B. Johansson: Impaired phytohaemagglutinin-induced cytotoxicity in vitro of lymphocytes from patients with Hodgkin's disease or chronic leukemia. Clin. exp. Immunol. **2**, 351 (1967c).

Kay, J. E.: Phytohaemagglutinin: An early effect on lymphocyte lipid metabolism. Nature (Lond.) **219**, 172 (1968).

Ling, N. R.: In: Lymphocyte stimulation, p. 152. Amsterdam: North-Holland Publ. Co. 1968.

Möller, E.: Contact-induced cytotoxicity by lymphoid cells containing foreign isoantigens. Science **147**, 873 (1965).

Munder, P. G., M. Modolell, E. Ferber u. H. Fischer: Phospholipide in quarzgeschädigten Makrophagen. Biochem. Z. **344**, 310 (1966).

Perlmann, P., H. Perlmann, and G. Holm: Cytotoxic action of stimulated lymphocytes on allogenic and autologous erythrocytes. Science **160**, 306 (1968).

Rosenau, W.: In: Interaction of lymphoid cells with target cells in tissue culture. Cell bound antibodies, p. 75—80. (Amos, B., H. Koprowski, Eds.). Philadelphia: Wistar Institute Press 1963.

Wilson, D. B.: Quantitative studies on the behaviour of sensitized lymphocytes in vitro. J. exp. Med. **122**, 143 (1965).

Prof. Dr. H. Fischer
Max-Planck-Institut für Immunbiologie,
78 Freiburg-Zähringen, Stübeweg 51

Discussion

WELLENSIEK (Mainz): Have you carried out histochemical examinations concerning different enzyme activities in your lymphocytes ? It may be possible that lymphocytes which actively attack target-cells show enzymatic activities which are different from those of sensitized lymphocytes which are not in contact with their homologous antigen.

FISCHER (Freiburg): So far we have not carried out such investigations. Unfortunately we do not know any method which could reliably indicate changes of the phospholipids of the cell membrane.

GRUNDMANN (Wuppertal): The film we have seen makes the function of the lymphocytes particularly clear. Can you add more details about the mitoses of the lymphocytes ?

FISCHER (Freiburg): In the system of H. Ginsburg [Immunology 14, 621 (1968)] the mass of mitoses occur about the fifth day. However, the mitoses proceed very rapidly and therefore very often go unoticed in the film.

WARNATZ (Erlangen): Does the stimulation of lymphocytes specifically depend on the antigen or does a stimulated lymphocyte attack every kind of cell ?

FISCHER (Freiburg): From our movie it is evident that **specifically** stimulated lymphocytes are characterized by a very pronounced tail, the so-called "uropod". It is by this part of the cell that intimate contact with the antigenic target cell is established. **Non-specifically** stimulated lymphocytes seem to be more labile and more sticky than controls. It may very well be, that this stickyness, besides other factors, renders them cytotoxic.

WESTPHAL (Freiburg): At present we are testing various models of synthetic phosphatides, employing the system Dr. Fischer has shown. This filming method is an especially favourable screening test. The fact that the acylating system is very important for the fate of the cell may also deserve special mention.

FISCHER (Freiburg): In fact, we have found that aged cells have a decreased capacity to metabolize lysophosphatides, because the activities of acyltransferase and of lysophospholipase are considerably lower in aged erythrocytes. One might speculate whether this impairment renders aged erythrocytes more susceptible to the lytic action of the lysolecithin produced by the macrophages which line the sinuses of the RES. [Ferber, Munder, Kohlschütter and Fischer: Europ. J. Biochem. 5, 395 (1968)].

Bock: Have corresponding examinations already been carried out on bank blood of different storing ages ? I would suggest such examinations. Since the experiments of Waller, Löhr, Schlegel et al. we know much about the differences in metabolism and behaviour of ageing erythrocytes.

Fischer (Freiburg): Comparative analyses of erythrocytes stored in acid citric dextrose medium (ACD) have shown, that "ageing in vitro" at 4 °C has no effect on the activities of those two enzymes.

Macher (Freiburg): In the film, it could be seen that the still living "target cells" were vividly searched by lymphocytes. However, when the target cells had died the lymphocytes were firmly attached to them and did not move any longer. Have these lymphocytes perished with the target cells ?

Fischer (Freiburg): "Allergic death" of agressing lymphocytes is a relatively rare event. Most of the lymphocytes which are attached to a dead target cell are still active and alive. One single lymphocyte may very well kill several target cells.

Popper (New York): Is Freund's adjuvant also bound to phospholipases ?

Fischer (Freiburg): Complete as well as incomplete Freund's adjuvant leads to an increased formation of lysolecithin in cultures of macrophages.

Fischer (Hamburg): In a tuberculin test following the passive transfer of lymphocytes from animals sensitised with tuberculin, it is seen that only a very small percentage — perhaps 5% — of the specifically stimulated lymphocytes are found at the reaction site. How do the other, i.e. the larger number of lymphocytes behave ?

Oettgen (New York): In this respect the migration-inhibition factor is again of interest. The supernatant of a culture of lymphocytes from sensitized animals in presence of antigen not only inhibits macrophage migration but also stimulates lymphocytes to undergo transformation.

Schwick (Marburg): Do fairly exact ideas of the mechanism of the stimulation of lymphocytes by PHA exist ? Some findings indicate that alpha-2-macroglobulin is present on or contained in the lymphocytes. This has been shown with the aid of fluorescent serological methods [Burtin, P., S. von Kleist, W. Rapp, F. Loisillier, A. Bonatti, and P. Grabar: In: Immunopathology, IVth International Symposium, Monte Carlo 1965. Basel-Stuttgart: Schwabe & Co. (Publishers)]. It is also known that alpha-2-macroglobulin is precipitated with phytohaemagglutinin, similar to an antigen-antibody reaction. [Bo Gahne: Hereditas 51, 375 (1964)].

Bayer-Symposium I, 122—129 (1969)

Contact Sensitivity and Immunological Tolerance as Competitors in Sensitization to Simple Chemical Compounds

Egon Macher

With 6 Figures

Data will be presented which indicate that during the induction period of contact sensitivity two immunologic processes are occurring independently which in principle act antagonistically, one leading to a state of specific immunological tolerance, the other one to contact sensitivity. It will be shown that the tolerogenic stimulus derives from a fraction of the injected chemical which escapes from the site early, whereas the allergenic fraction is retained at the site for many hours or even days. From these findings, sensitization to simple chemical compounds can be interpreted as a process, in which the cellular immunological apparatus of the organism is stimulated at different sites simultaneously by different chemical products which compete with one another, thus on balance defining the final degree of hypersensitivity. The outcome probably reflects genetic differences between animals in their readiness for sensitization as well.

The experiments were undertaken under the following conditions:

(i) The allergenic chemicals (picryl chloride [PCl]: 1-chloro-2,4,6-trinitro-benzene; dinitrochlorobenzene [DNCB]: 1-chloro-2,4-dinitrobenzene) were administered on day 0 by a single intradermal injection into one ear of Rockefeller University albino guinea pigs.

(ii) The dose used for active sensitization was intended to approach the minimal sensitizing dose in order to avoid excess hapten which could flood the organism and deviate attention from sites significant for sensitization. The doses actually chosen were 0.25 µg of PCl, i.e. approximately 1×10^{-9} M, and 5 µg of DNCB, i.e. approximately 25×10^{-9} M.

(iii) For determination of contact sensitivity a single contact test was performed on day 14 (one drop of a 1% solution of the chemical in olive oil applied on a freshly clipped site of the back). The reactions were read blindly at 24 h and 48 h and graded quantitatively [4].

(iv) Non-responders upon primary contact testing as well as weak responders were subjected to secondary treatments of 10 to 12 daily intradermal injections of 2.5 µg of PCl or DNCB respectively, made *seriatim* along the flanks. Many experimental animals were sensitized simultaneously to the unrelated allergen o-chlorobenzoyl-chloride, the chemical being administered by daily injections of 5 µg doses on the other flank.

(v) Final contact tests made with the two unrelated chemicals in parallel, determined the sensitivity attained by the secondary sensitizing courses.

In order to determine the fate of the chemical allergens during the induction period of contact sensitivity, carbon[14]-labelled PCl or DNCB were applied as stated above (i), (ii), with a specific activity of 2 mc/mM or 4.86 mc/mM, respectively. The injected ears were excised after each of these chemicals had been allowed to escape from the site of deposition for varying times ranging from $^1/_2$ min following the injection up through 10 weeks. The tissues taken were immediately frozen in liquid nitrogen, and subsequently divided into segments which were combusted to $C^{14} O_2$ and H_2O within scintillation vials according to Gupta [1—3], the radioactivity being determined by liquid scintillation counting. Efficiency, accuracy and reproducibility of the method were high, as detailed elsewhere [4].

The injected chemicals indeed disseminated from the site of deposition with great rapidity (Fig. 1), though at different rates, thus reflecting their unequal chemical reaction constants. At 3 h following the injection, 50% of the injected

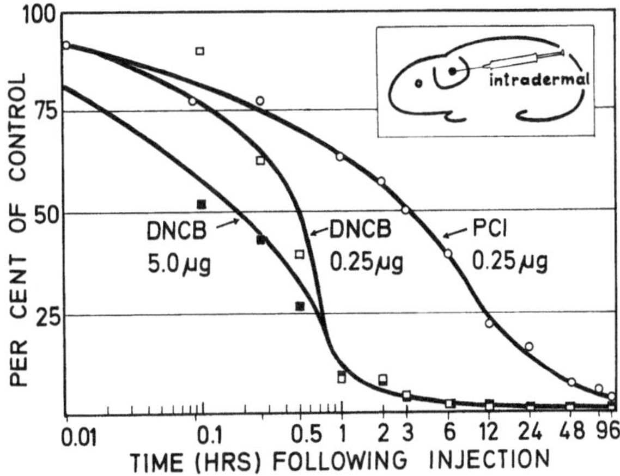

Fig. 1. Comparative escape of C^{14}-labelled chemicals from an intradermal ear site. Data are plotted against time, as percent of the values of 10 control ears excised before injection

PCl had disappeared; at 12 h about 25%, at 4 days only 3% were left at the site. DNCB escaped more rapidly. About 90% were gone after 1 h regardless of whether 0.25 µg or 5 µg had been injected. (The smaller DNCB dose had proved ineffective in sensitization, whereas the higher dose induced hypersensitivity of a degree comparable with that secured by the PCl dose.)

The measurements obtained at various times also suggest that the chemical allergens leave the site in three phases or stages (Fig. 2). The first phase of rapid escape commenced immediately after the injection and ceased about 12 h later. When the body pH is taken into account with regard to the capability of the chemical allergens to unite with proteins by covalent bonds, the first large proportion to leave probably represents free chemical still uncoupled.

Thereafter, the rate of dispersal slowed down considerably, apparently in connection with increasing dominance of the coupling reaction. The second phase material constituted a local depot which remained traceable for about 4 or 5 days despite slow leakage. No such depot was found to have formed, when a non-sensitizing amount had been injected such as 0.25 µg of DNCB (Fig. 2). This finding is highly suggestive for the second phase material as representing the allergenic fraction. More evidence in favour of this interpretation will be given below.

Finally, a small fraction was found to be retained at the site for several weeks escaping at a very slow rate. It probably represents insoluble coupling products which might share the fate of local tissue components such as fibres or cells. With delayed hypersensitivity then already being established, the significance of this fraction is unknown.

Unexpectedly, the principal pathway for escape proved to be the local ear veins. Blood samples taken from the central ear vein or the retroauricular vein during the early phase of escape, regularly carried radioactivity. Excretion through the kidneys, at least in part, in the form of decomposition products, was ascertained as early as 3 to 4 h after the injection.

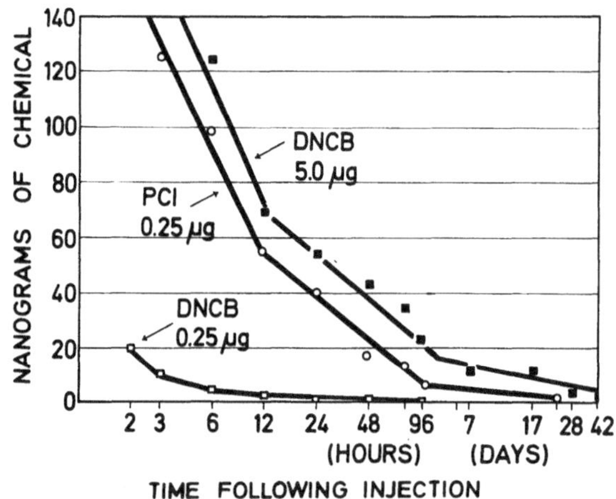

Fig. 2. Chemical actually retained in intradermal ear site. The data of Fig. 1 are replotted on the basis of absolute amounts of chemical remaining in the tissue at different times

In contrast, the regional lymph nodes contained either no radioactivity or only bare traces. Lymph fluid collected for several hours directly from the cervical duct by cannulation was also free of radioactivity. Lymph nodes remained non-radioactive throughout the observation period for several weeks. In particular, no radioactivity could be detected to accumulate in the regional nodes during the second phase of escape in which leakage of coupling products of high molecular weight is taken to occur.

Contralateral lymph nodes, mesenteric lymph nodes, spleen and thymus were found to be non-radioactive at any time during the observation period.

The concept of consecutive release of chemical substances in more than one form from the injection site was challenged by a simple experimental design of spaced excisions of the injected ears [5]. The excisions were intended to differentiate between immunologic effects of the portion of the chemical already flowed off and the fraction retained at the site. If, for example, the local depot which formed at about 12 h following the injection and remained at the site for about 4 days were essential for sensitization, then early removal of the ear prior to the formation of the depot would have to cancel sensitization completely. This was actually found to be true. When the injected ear including the residual chemical was surgically removed at 12 h (or earlier), practically every animal escaped sensitization as revealed by contact testing on day 14 (Fig. 3, top row). Extension of the time interval between deposition of allergen and excision of site to 24 h and 48 h led to gradual increase in the rate of sensitization (Fig. 3).

This indicates clearly that the local depot does play an essential role in sensitization, that it is put into effectiveness about 12 h after the intradermal injection and that it provides "immunologic information" which is picked up therefrom progressively. Furthermore, it seems necessary to conclude that the large fraction of the allergen which escapes from the site early (75% of PCl, 99% of DNCB within 12 h) is irrelevant for sensitization.

Nevertheless, this portion of the chemical shown to travel presumably uncoupled *via* the blood stream was found to be immunologically active, though in a

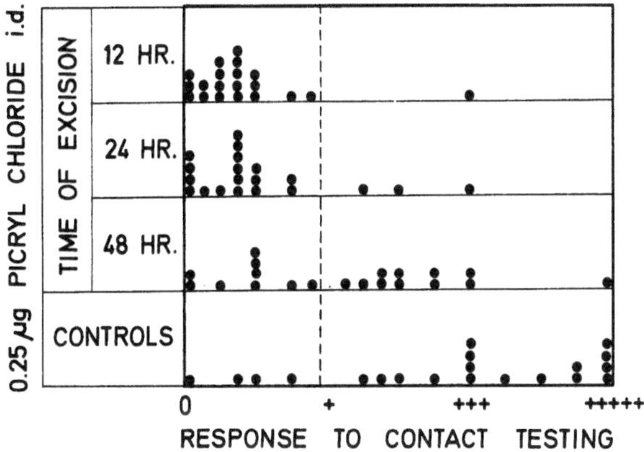

Fig. 3. Contact sensitivity following excision of site. Surgical excision of the ear including the site was practiced at 12 h, 24 h, and 48 h. Animals are indicated in closed circles. Abscissa shows responses to contact tests 2 weeks later, graded from 0 to $+++++$. The vertical dashed line divides the experimental groups into non-responders (on the left) and responders (on the right)

different direction. When those animals which remained unsensitized owing to the early excision of the ear (Fig. 4, closed circles) were subsequently subjected to a series of daily intradermal injections of PCl, the average sensitivity attained (Fig. 4, open circles) was much lower than that of a control group of normal animals not pretreated. Analysis of individuals shows that the early escaping fraction rendered about 50% of the animals unresponsive in subsequent attempts to sensitize them. However, sensitization to the unrelated chemical o-chlorobenzoyl chloride was not restrained, which proves that the state of tolerance attained was immunologically specific.

Animals found unresponsive were taken at random for spot-checks on antibody production. They were test-bled after the secondary sensitizing treatments and the sera were examined for hapten-specific circulating antibody by passive cutaneous

126　　　　　　　　　　　　　　　　　　E. Macher

anaphylaxis. Generally, no evidence of antibody production was found in tolerant animals or antibody could be detected only in traces, whereas positive controls exhibited distinct antibody levels.

The tolerogenic effect of site excision following application of sensitizing doses could be mimicked by intradermal injection of non-sensitizing doses without subsequent excision. Here it is necessary to recall the pattern of escape of labelled allergen from an ear site, when the dose applied was inefficient in sensitization, i.e., 0.25 µg of DNCB (Fig. 2). At 12 h following the injection no more than 3 nanograms of the 250 nanograms initially injected were left at the site. In contrast, doses capable of securing mild but definite sensitivity were locally represented at 12 h by at least 50 nanograms of the originally free chemical now presumably being coupled.

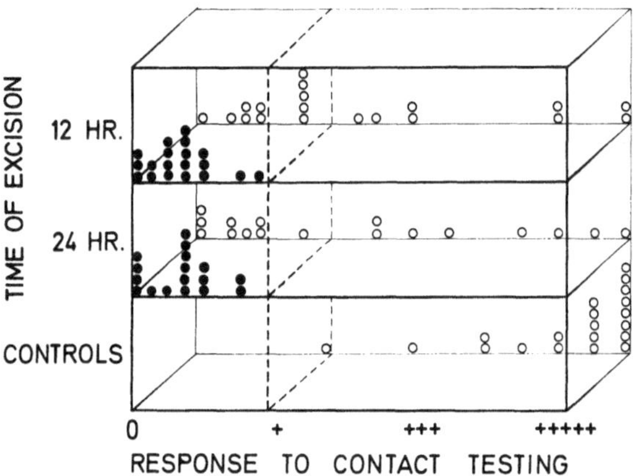

Fig. 4. Tolerogenic effect of excision of site. Non-responders of Fig. 3 are replotted in the near plane. The far plane (animals indicated in open circles) shows the responses of the same animals, and of newly introduced controls, following 10 daily intradermal injections of 2.5 µg PCl

Indeed, animals which had been injected intradermally with this non-sensitizing dose of DNCB (Fig. 5, top row, closed circles) and had subsequently received a series of intradermal injections for active sensitization (Fig. 5, top row, open circles) were found to be specifically tolerant to DNCB to the extent of about 50%.

Since it had been found that about 90% of the intradermally injected DNCB leaves the skin within 1 h (Fig. 2), the effect of injecting this amount of DNCB (0.22 µg) directly into the jugular vein was examined. None of the animals was sensitized by this injection, giving negative contact test reactions (Fig. 5, middle row, closed circles), but subsequent attempts to sensitize the animals by means of daily intradermal injections of DNCB showed that about 50% were unresponsive (Fig. 5, middle row, open circles), quite in contrast with positive controls not pretreated (Fig. 5, bottom row). This provides further evidence that the tolerogen, in fact, travels *via* the blood. Its later localization, however, could not be traced given the specific radioactivity available under the conditions used. In this respect, it might be interesting to record that the thymus was always free of detectable radioactivity. Therefore, no selective accumulation of the escaping allergen or of coupling products formed later could have occurred in the thymus.

Any amount present exceeding about one nanogram of the chemical initially injected would have been detectable with the method used.

The tolerogenic effect of non-sensitizing doses could be elicited with the use of PCl as well. When a single intradermal injection of 0.0125 µg of PCl was applied,

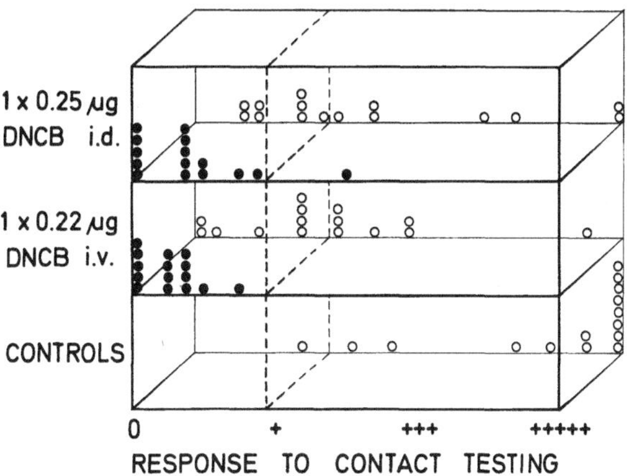

Fig. 5. Tolerogenic effect of chemical escaping from ear site. Near and far plane have significance as in Fig. 4. The near plane (closed circles) indicates responses to contact testing 2 weeks after injection of DNCB in non-sensitizing doses: intradermally in the top row, intravenously in the middle row. The far plane (open circles) shows sensitivities of the same animals, and of newly introduced controls (bottom row) following 10 daily intradermal injections of 2.5 µg DNCB

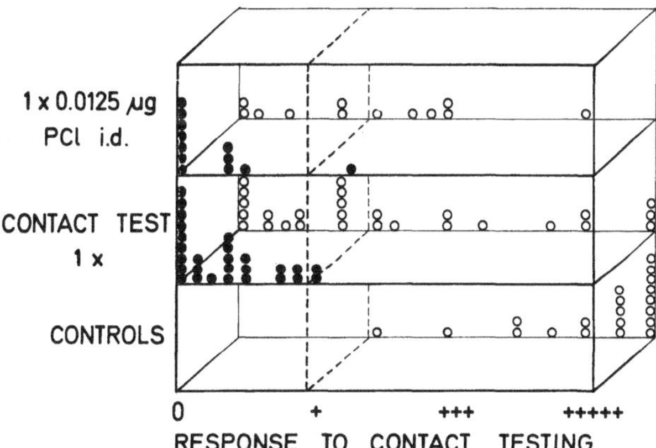

Fig. 6. Tolerogenic effect of non-sensitizing doses. Near and far plane have significance as in Fig. 4. Top row shows response to contact test of animals injected with a non-sensitizing dose of PCl, middle row shows reactions of normal animals (toxicity controls) following a single contact test of 0.02 ml of 1% PCl in olive oil. The far plane (open circles) shows the distribution of sensitivities of the same animals, and of newly introduced controls, following 12 daily intradermal injections of 2.5 µg PCl

only one of twelve animals treated gave a positive but weak response to contact testing on day 14 (Fig. 6, top row, closed circles). Subsequent rigorous sensitization by daily injections and a final contact test revealed that 50% were specifically tolerant (Fig. 6, top row, open circles).

Similar findings were made with animals which served as "toxicity controls" in the course of several previous experiments. They had been given a single contact test of 1% PCl in olive oil for evaluation of possible toxicity of the test solution on normal animals, thus providing a baseline for contact reactions on sensitized animals (Fig. 6, middle row, closed circles). This "treatment" imposed a similar restraint on susceptibility of contact sensitivity as did intradermal injection of non-sensitizing doses. Again, about 50% of the animals which had received the single contact test were found to be specifically tolerant (Fig. 6, middle row, open circles).

The object intended here is not a new method of inducing immunological tolerance to simple chemical compounds. Superior methods exist, although it can be reasoned that careful timing of repeated applications might increase the rate of tolerance, since even a single application was so often effective which in itself is surprising. The findings rather point to a situation in which emission of tolerogenic stimuli is an inevitable part of sensitization to simple chemicals.

Tolerance appears to dominate, when the initial contact with the free chemical does not favour the formation of an effective allergen due to non-sensitizing routes or an unfavourable chemical structure or too low a dosage. Under marginal conditions, that is to say, with the use of doses approaching the minimal sensitizing amount, the individual will embark on one path or the other leading either to tolerance or to sensitivity. Genetic differences among the animals seem to determine the status to be attained as the rate and route of dispersal of the chemical from the site of deposition were actually alike in both tolerant and sensitized animals. With somewhat higher doses applied, the rate of tolerance decreases. But even with methods of sensitization known to establish high degrees of contact sensitivity, single animals will escape from sensitization (Fig. 4: $^1/_{20}$; Fig. 5: $^1/_{15}$). Such animals have often been found to fail to respond only to the one sensitizing agent in question.

When sensitization results, tolerance may be regarded to be either depressed or hidden. The latter view seems acceptable in animals which display only low levels of sensitivity (Figs. 4, 5, 6). Tolerance induction must have entered into the process of sensitization modifying the acquisition of delayed hypersensitivity. Thus, partial tolerance lies behind the appearance of low levels of sensitivity.

From the findings reported here, it seems reasonable to conclude that sensitization toward chemical allergens naturally involves two immunologic processes. They are triggered simultaneously by a single application of an allergenic chemical into or onto the skin. A large proportion of the applied chemical will escape presumably uncoupled during the first few hours *via* the blood and act as tolerogen. Under conditions favouring the local fixation of a suitable amount of chemical at the site of deposition, this remaining portion acts as allergen. The two different immunologic stimuli set two processes going which in principle lead into different directions, but on balance define the resultant immunological status.

Acknowledgements

The author wishes to express his sincere thanks to Dr. Merrill W. Chase for his steady interest in this work and for kind advice, and to Dr. G. N. Gupta for many helpful suggestions. The experiments reported here have been performed in Dr. Chase's laboratory at the Rockefeller University, New York. N.Y., USA.

References

1. Gupta, G. N.: A simple in-vial combustion method for assay of hydrogen-3, carbon-14, and sulfur-35 in biological, biochemical, and organic materials. Analyt. Chemistry 38, 1356 (1966).
2. — Simplified solid-state scintillation counting on glass microfiber medium in plastic bag for hydrogen-3, carbon-14, and chlorine-36 in biological and organic materials. Analyt. Chemistry 39, 1911 (1967).
3. — A new approach of combustion in plastic bags for radioassay of H^3, C^{14}, and S^{35} in biological, biochemical, and organic materials. Microchem. J. 13, 4 (1968).
4. Macher, E., and M. W. Chase: Studies on the sensitization of animals with simple chemical compounds. XI. The fate of labeled picryl chloride and dinitrochlorobenzene after sensitizing injections. J. exp. Med. 129, 81 (1969).
5. — — Studies on the sensitization of animals with simple chemical compounds. XII. The influence of excision of allergenic depots on onset of delayed hypersensitivity and tolerance. J. exp. Med. 129, 103 (1969).

Prof. Dr. E. Macher
Hautklinik der Universität
78 Freiburg i. Br., Hauptstraße 7

Discussion

DE WECK (Bern): It seems the reported investigations show for the first time that immunisation with an allergen which conjugates in-vivo leads to low-dose tolerance. We have not so far seen this in our own studies. In work Dr. Frey carried out with us [J. invest. Derm. 42, 41 (1964)] and in unpublished experiments animals were sensitised with dinitrochlorobenzene. If varied doses of dinitrobenzene sulfonate are intravenously given 14 day prior to the sensitisation attempt, a dosage range is observed where the animals do not become sensitized but are primed; within this dosage range they react much more strongly to the sensitisation attempt than the controls. In another dosage range they become sensitised and in yet another one they become tolerant. Thus we found high-dose tolerance but never encountered low-dose tolerance.

HAMMER (Freiburg): When in a parabiosis test the animals have large amounts of circulating allergen in their blood, is it then possible to sensitise also the contact partner ?

MACHER (Freiburg): Such parabiosis experiments were carried out [Kalkhoff: Med. Welt 18, 140 (1944)]. Sensitising the parabiosis partner is readily achieved. But now to Dr. de Weck's remark: The detection of low-dose tolerance depends on the test applied to the phenomenon tolerance. If, for example, the second immunisation is too powerful, a weak degree of tolerance may not be detectable. If the second sensitisation is carried out with Freund's adjuvant the phenomenon may not at all be traceable.

RAJEWSKY (Cologne): I would like to ask whether you really induce tolerance in your experiments ?

MACHER (Freiburg): At least utilising the PCA reaction we have searched for antibodies. In the tolerant groups, either no antibodies are found or the titres are substantially lower than in the control groups, even after 6 weeks. Mainly we are not dealing with complete but with partial tolerance.

RIETHMÜLLER (Tübingen): I would like to refer to the investigations of Russell and Monaco using antilymphocytic globulin [Proc. Transplant. Soc. 1 (1968) (in press)]. During treatment with this globulin, skin was excised on the 4th or 5th day after transplantation, and 20 to 30 days later an equal skin graft was applied. Thereafter, a very long lasting tolerance persisted for 200 to 300 days across the H-2 locus. These experiments certainly approach Dr. Macher's model in some points.

DE WECK (Berne): Finally I would like to draw attention to the following phenomenon: If sensitised guinea pigs are given a single intravenous injection of 60 to 30 mg/kg neoarsphenamine, then, in dependence on the dose, a temporary inhibition of the immune reaction is observed. If, however, a markedly smaller dose, about 150 gamma/kg, is intradermally injected 6 h after the intravenous injection, the animals remain unresponsive for months. We have unsuccessfully attempted to reproduce these results with dinitrochlorobenzene. Turk and Polak [Clin. exp. Immunol. 3, 245 (1968)] recently found the same phenomenon in hypersensitivity to chronium. If people who are locally sensitised against nitrogen mustard are given the same substance intravenously and then tested within two days they may remain contact-negative for several months. I do not know whether this is real tolerance.

Bayer-Symposium I, 131—137 (1969)

Results of Some Investigations on Lymphocyte Transformation in vitro

H. WARNATZ

With 6 Figures

1. Estimation of the O_2-consumption of lymphocytes stimulated by phytohemagglutinin (PHA) or tuberculin

The activation of DNA- and RNA-metabolism in transforming lymphocytes is accompanied by an increase of the whole metabolism of the cell; especially the activity of the glycolytic and oxydative enzymes is enhanced [1, 2, 4, 5]. Morpholo-

Table 1. *Mean values of transformed lymphocytes in cultures with (P-culture) and without added phytohemagglutinin (N-culture) counted 24 to 96 h after onset of cell culturing*

Hours from start of culture	Average percentage of cells transformed	
	N-cultures %	P-cultures %
24	less than 3.00	less than 3.00
48	4.87	15.67
72	4.82	20.00
96	3.55	19.12

gically a higher number of mitochondria in the lymphocyte corresponds to this findings [1, 2]. In our investigations the O_2-uptake of transformed lymphocytes was measured in daily intervals after addition of the stimulating agent.

The experiments were performed on lymph node lymphocytes of guinea pigs. The lymphocytes were cultured with PHA and the counts of ^{3}H-thymidine labelled cells were determined by autoradiography (Table 1).

The O_2-consumption of 1×10^6 lymph node cells was estimated by a stabilized whole glas platin electrode according to Lübbers [3] in a chamber described by Munder and Fischer [6, 7] (polarizing tension 6.5 mV, movement of the chamber in a shaking water bath of 37 °C). The decrease of the P_{O_2} in the chamber was continuously recorded by a mikrograph Kipp BD2. The time necessary for a P_{O_2} decrease from 128 to 71 mmHg was defined as measuring time. Two representative O_2-uptake curves are drawn in Fig. 1.

The results of our experiments are summarized in Table 2. According to our results a significant increase in the O_2-uptake of the PHA stimulated lymphocytes was observed in comparison with the non stimulated cells. This increased O_2-

9*

uptake could be demonstrated as soon as 24 h after onset of cell culture and precedes the increase of the DNA metabolism.

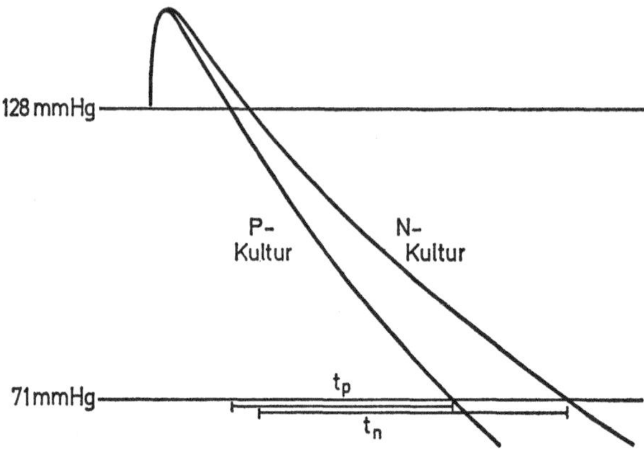

Fig. 1. Curves of the O_2-uptake of lymphocytes cultured with (P-culture) and without added
phytohemagglutinin (N-culture). The distances t_p or t_n, respectively, are the measuring times
in which the P_{O_2} decreased from 128 to 71 mm Hg

Table 2. *Mean values of the measuring times and standard deviations
estimated in lymphocyte cultures 24 to 96 h after onset of culturing.
Measuring times for P-cultures in bold figures differ significantly from
those of the N-cultures (p = 0.05)*

Hours from start of culture	No. of cultures	Mean measuring times	
		N-cultures	P-cultures
24	21	20.73 ± 7.74	**15.38 ± 6.73**
48	24	19.31 ± 7.45	**15.44 ± 8.48**
72	18	18.20 ± 5.57	**15.60 ± 5.36**
96	14	17.65 ± 5.35	19.91 ± 7.63

Table 3. *Mean values of cultures of 14 tuberculin negative and
14 tuberculin sensitive animals with added tuberculin related to
the measuring times of the cultures of the same animals without
added tuberculin, the latter were set as 100%. The measuring time
was defined as the time necessary for the P_{O_2} decrease from 128
to 71 mm Hg. Long measuring times indicate a small, short
measuring times a high O_2-consumption*

Hours of cell culture	Measuring times of cultures with added tuberculin in % of those without added tuberculin	
	Lymphocytes of tuberculin negative animals	Lymphocytes of tuberculin sensitive animals
24	88.75 ± 4.45	97.19 ± 3.93
48	88.36 ± 3.56	93.95 ± 2.23
72	97.57 ± 3.89	87.50 ± 4.16
96	98.14 ± 5.92	89.86 ± 2.90

Similar results were obtained in lymphocyte cultures of tuberculin sensitive animals when tuberculin was added to the culture medium [11]. The results of these experiments are given in Table 3.

2. Transformation of lymphocytes stimulated by antilymphocyte sera (ALS)

ALS have a cytotoxic and a mitogenic activity on lymphocytes [8—10]. We studied the correlation between the dose of ALS and the counts of ^{3}H-thymidine labelled cells in lymphocyte cultures evaluated by autoradiography. We were

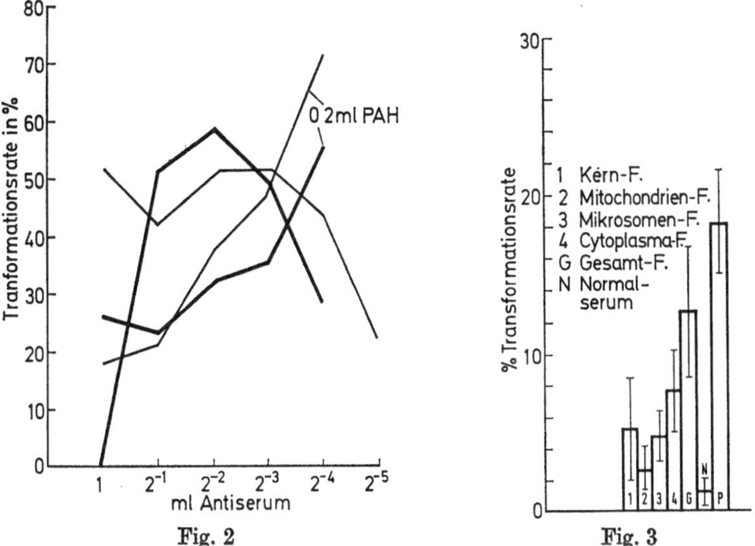

Fig. 2   Fig. 3

Fig. 2. Transformation rate of lymphocytes obtained from 10 different persons which were cultured with dilutions of a horse-antilymphocyte-serum; the lymphocytes were cultured with 0.5 ml guinea pig complement or without added complement, respectively. In the PHA marked cultures dilutions of the antilymphocyte serum and 0.2 ml phytohemagglutinin were added to the lymphocyte cultures

Fig. 3. Mean values and standard deviations of labelled cells in lymphocyte cultures of normal rats after addition of the antisera against the different lymphocyte fractions

kindly supplied with the ALS by Dr. R. Pichelmayr, München. Furthermore we investigated the effect of complement on the transformation of lymphocytes in cultures. The results obtained in lymphocyte cultures with different dilutions of the ALS with and without added complement are summarized in Fig. 2.

Lymphocytes cultured without complement showed an equal transformation rate from 500 to 125 µl of ALS. By further reducing the quantity of ALS the blast cell counts decreased in the same manner in the experiments with and in those without complement. The cytotoxic effect of complement only could be demonstrated in cultures with high concentrations of ALS. However, it was uneffective when the ALS was diluted. In the case of high concentration of ALS phytohemagglutinin caused a depression of the blast cell formation; this effect was absent in higher dilutions of the ALS.

In experiments with rats it should be investigated if ALS produced by sensitization with lymphocyte fractions have a different effect on the lymphocyte transformation in comparison with an antiserum against the whole lymphocyte extract. It should be demonstrated whether the lymphocyte transformation test (LLT) is a suitable method for the standardization of an ALS and if the results of the LTT are comparable with those of the usual techniques for the evaluation of ALS, especially the cytotoxic reaction and the immune depressive effect.

The antisera were produced by long time immunization of rabbits with fractions of lymphocytes which were obtained by differential centrifugation of homogenized lymph node lymphocytes of rats in hypertonic sucrose solution. The fractions were proved for impurities by microscopical examination and enzyme

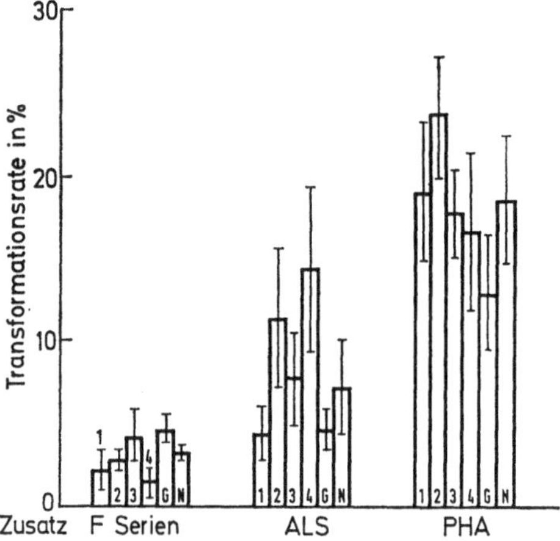

Fig. 4. Mean transformation rates of lymphocytes cultured with antisera against different lymphocyte fractions. The lymphocytes were obtained from animals which were pretreated with the ALS against the different lymphocyte fractions over a period of 3 weeks. 1 = rats pretreated with antiserum against nuclear fraction; 2 = rats pretreated with antiserum against mitochondrial fraction; 3 = rats pretreated with antiserum against microsomal fraction; 4 = rats pretreated with antiserum against cytoplasmic fraction; G = rats pretreated with antiserum against whole lymphocyte extract; N = rats pretreated with normal rabbit serum

techniques; no intact cells were detected in the nuclear fraction. A slight malate dehydrogenase activity, however, was demonstrated in the nuclear as well as in the microsomal fraction.

Lymphocytes of the rat were cultured with the antisera against the different lymphocyte fractions; the transformation rate was evaluated by the ^{3}H-thymidine uptake in autoradiographic experiments.

The results of the LTT are summarized in Fig. 3. Lymphocytes of normal rats showed an increase in blast cell formation. The transforming capacity of the anti-cytoplasmic antiserum was the most conspicuous, but it did not exceed that of the antiserum against the whole lymphocyte extract.

Lymphocyte cultures of the animals which were pretreated with the anti-lymphocyte serum showed no enhanced transformation rate, when the ALS was added to the cultures (s. Fig. 4). This result was the same in the antisera against the different lymphocyte fractions. The transformation of lymphocytes, however, could be stimulated by a ALS against the whole lymphocyte extract. In these experiments, too, a depression of the transformation rate could be observed in cultures from animals injected with the different ALSs when 0.2 ml of phytohemagglutinin was added to the culture medium.

For the characterization of the antisera the results of other methods for the evaluation of ALS are reported. After intravenous injection of the antisera a decrease of the peripheral lymphocyte could be observed in the rats which is

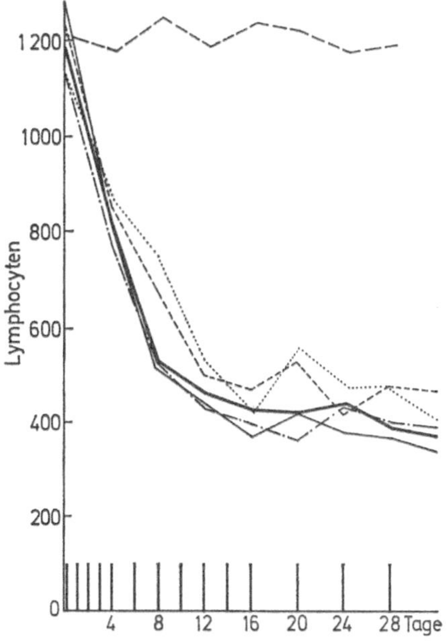

Fig. 5. Decrease of the peripheral lymphocytes in the rats after intravenous injection of antisera against different lymphocyte fractions. The columns give the time schedule of the i.v. injection of 0.5 ml antiserum. ——————— Rats injected with antiserum against the whole lymphocyte fraction; ——————— rats injected with antiserum against the nuclear fraction; —————— rats injected with antiserum against the mitochondrial fraction; —·—·—·— rats injected with antiserum against the microsomal fraction; ---------------- rats injected with antiserum against the cytoplasmic fraction; ————— rats injected with normal rabbit serum

demonstrated in the following Fig. 5. The most effective depression of the peripheral lymphocyte counts was observed after injection of the antisera against the nuclear and the microsomal fraction.

The cytotoxic reaction was performed with lymphocytes obtained from the thoracic duct of normal rats. The results of the cytotoxic are summarized in Fig. 6. In these experiments, too, the antisera against the nuclear and the microsomal fraction showed the highest cytotoxic activity.

Finally the immune depressive effect of the antisera was determined by grafting skin from Sprague-Dawley rats to the Wistar rats which were treated with the antisera against the different lymphocyte fractions. The survival time of the homologous skin was prolonged from 10.8 days in untreated rats to 17.3 days

in animals treated with 0.5 ml antiserum against the whole lymphocyte fraction
in intervals of 2 days. From the antisera against lymphocyte fractions the antimicrosomal and the antinuclear antisera were most effective (survival of skin
grafts 16.2 or 15.3 days, respectively).

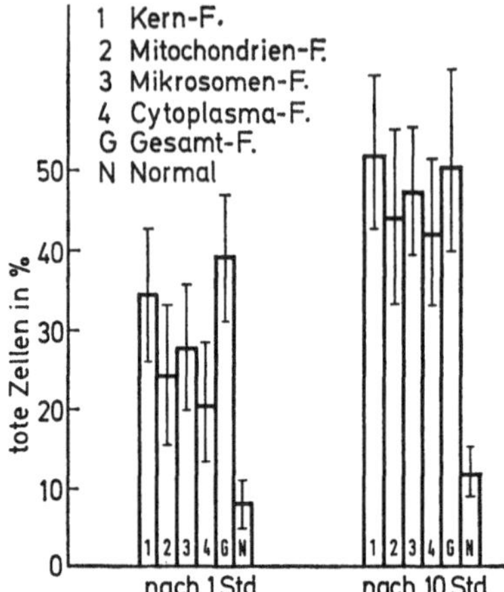

Fig. 6. Results of the cytotoxic reaction. The columns represent the percentage of dead cells
after addition of 1:32 diluted antisera against the different lymphocyte fractions to lymphocytes obtained from the thoracic duct of untreated rats

It is concluded from these results that no correlation exists between the cytotoxic activity of ALS which was the strongest in the antinuclear and the antimicrosomal antisera and the mitogenic capacity. Here the anticytoplasmic antiserum was the most effective.

3. The transformation of lymphocytes of thymectomized mice

The importance of thymectomy for the transformation of lymphocytes was
investigated in experimental studies. Mice of the inbred strain C57Bl were neonatally thymectomized. After 6 weeks the animals were sacrificed and lympho-

Table 4. *Counts of labelled cells in percent in lymphocyte cultures
of thymectomized mice, of non-thymectomized mice of the same age
and of adult mice after stimulation with phytohemagglutinin*

	Without PHA	With PHA
Thymectomized mice	3.2 ± 1.92	5.7 ± 0.84
Non-thymectomized mice	3.7 ± 0.96	8.8 ± 1.07
Adults	6.9 ± 1.18	22.6 ± 16.17

cytes of the lymph nodes and the spleen cultured for 3 days with and without
phytohemagglutinin. In comparison cultures of lymphocytes obtained from non-
thymectomized mice of the same age and those of adult mice were performed.
0.1 ml of phytohemagglutinin M was added to the cultures as stimulating agent
and the counts of cells labelled with ^{3}H-thymidine were determined by autoradiography. The results are summarized in Table 4.

A depressive effect on the transformation rate was observed in the cultures of thymectomized mice. The counts of labelled cells in the non thymectomized mice also were lower than the counts in lymphocyte cultures of the adult mice. It must be considered, however, that other cell types, for instance reticulum cells, may impair the results in the cultures of thymectomized mice.

References

1. Elves, M. W.: The in vitro transformation of lymphocytes. In: Hayhoe's Current research in leukaemia. Cambridge: University Press 1965. — The Lymphocytes. London: Lloyd-Luke 1966.
2. Fischer, R., u. A. Gropp: Zytologische und zytochemische Untersuchungen an normalen und leukämischen in vitro gezüchteten Blutzellen. Klin. Wschr. 42, 111 (1964).
3. Gleichmann, U., u. D. W. Lübbers: Die Messung des Sauerstoffdruckes in Gasen und Flüssigkeiten mit der Platinelektrode unter besonderer Berücksichtigung der Messung im Blut. Pflügers Arch. ges. Physiol. 271, 431 (1960).
4. Gropp, A., u. R. Fischer: Untersuchungen zur Phytohämagglutinin-stimulierten Umwandlung von menschlichen Blutlymphozyten zu blastenartigen Zellen. Virchows Arch. path. Anat. 338, 64 (1964).
5. Hedeskov, C. J., and V. Esman: Respiration and Glycolysis of normal human lymphocytes. Blood 28, 163 (1966).
6. Munder, P. G., u. H. Fischer: Über die polarographische Bestimmung des Sauerstoffverbrauchs von Leukozyten und Makrophagen und dessen Beeinflussung durch silikogene Stäube. Silikose-Forsch. 5, 21 (1963).
7. —, u. M. Modelell: Fortlaufende registrierende Bestimmung der Zellatmung durch elektrochemische Sauerstoffmessung. Z. analyt. Chem. 212, 177 (1965).
8. Sell, S.: Studies on rabbit lymphocytes in vitro. VII. The induction of blast transformation with the F(ab)^2 and Fab fragments of sheep antibody to rabbit IgG. J. Immunol. 98, 786 (1967).
9. —, and P. G. H. Gell: Studies on rabbit lymphocytes in vitro. IV. Blast transformation of the lymphocytes from newborn rabbits induced by antiallotype serum to a paternal IgG allotype not present in the serum of the lymphocyte donors. J. exp. Med. 122, 923 (1965).
10. — — Studies on rabbit lymphocytes in vitro. I. Stimulation of blast transformation with an antiallotype serum. J. exp. Med. 122, 423 (1965).
11. Warnatz, H., and F. Scheiffarth: The influence of tuberculin on the O_2-requirement of lymphocyte cultures of tuberculin sensitized animals. Int. Arch. Allergy 32, 463 (1967).

Priv.-Doz. Dr. H. Warnatz
Abteilung für klinische Immunologie
des Universitäts-Krankenhauses
Erlangen-Nürnberg,
852 Erlangen, Krankenhausstraße 12

Bayer-Symposium I, 138—143 (1969)

In vitro Stimulation of Lymphoid Cells
by Antilymphocytic Globulins[1]

GERT RIETHMÜLLER, DORIS RIETHMÜLLER, PETER RIEBER, and HANS STEIN

With 3 Figures

The in vitro irritability of lymphoid cells expressed as their proneness to respond to a great number of foreign macromolecules with blastoid transformation and subsequent mitosis seems to be related to their basic immunologic function: the recognition of antigens or foreigness and the production of specific antibody.

At present we do not know how the primary signal for cell division is mediated from the lymphocyte's surface to the cytoplasm or to the nucleus. An immunoglobulin is implied as a specific receptor site on the lymphocyte during an ordinary primary immune response when antigen provides the proliferative stimulus. In vitro, however, the release of the signal for proliferation does not seem to occur only through a reaction with an immunoglobulin receptor, since many mitogenic substances stimulate through trigger sites other than immunoglobulins. Antilymphocytic antibodies for instance induce blastoid transformation also after absorption with immunoglobulins of the lymphocyte donor.

Experiments with peptic fragments of antilymphocytic antibodies have shown that only divalent fragments [F (ab') 2] transform lymphoid cells, whereas univalent fragments are inactive [4, 9]. Heterologous univalent antibody fragments against IgG, however, retained the transformatory activity of the intact or divalent antibody [6]. It is not certain at the moment if this difference between anti-IgG antibodies and antilymphocytic antibodies reflects a difference in the generation of the signal for cell division. As a first approach to this problem we have studied the transformation of lymphocytes by different antibodies of various species and of different biological classes. We wanted to know if the Fc part of the immunoglobulin was important in triggering off the proliferation. Uhr has shown that the affinity for cell membranes of the Fc part of the immunoglobulin is increased by binding with an antigen [7]. Another question to be answered was whether an antigen-antibody reaction occurring on the lymphocyte's surface would necessarily lead to proliferation of the cell. The answer to this question could shed some light on the cellular mechanism of tolerance induction.

As an introduction to the experimental system a short description of used methods shall be given.

Rabbits were immunized with A/NMRI mouse thymocytes in complete Freund's adjuvant as outlined by Nagaya and Sieker [1]. The rabbits were bled at various times after the third intravenous booster and after later multiple booster injections.

---

[1] Supported by the Deutsche Forschungsgemeinschaft.

Guinea pigs of a partially inbred strain (Isabel), obtained from Dr. Timm, Bundesforschungsanstalt für Virusforschung, Tübingen were immunized by two different procedures: One group received 1×10^8 mouse thymus cells in complete Freund's adjuvant, the other group was immunized with mouse thymus cells suspended in normal saline by subcutaneous injections.

Ducks of a single litter of a Württemberg village were immunized by mouse thymus cells suspended in complete Freund's adjuvant 10^9 cells per animal at the first injection, followed by three intravenous booster injections with 10^8 thymus cells at intervals of 10 days.

Immunoglobulin preparation: The sera were inactivated at 56 °C and absorbed three times with mouse erythrocytes. Immunoglobulins were used either as crude ammonium sulfate precipitates or after purification on DEAE-cellulose. Guinea pig immunoglobulins were further fractionated as outlined by Oettgen and

Table 1. *In vitro and in vivo effects of duck anti-mouse lymphocyte serum*
Effect of duck-ALS on skin-transplant survival: C57/Bl/6J on A/NMRI

Cytotoxic titer of duck-ALS against mouse-thymus cells:

1:160 (with fresh duck serum as complement source)
1:10   (with guinea pig complement)
Lymphocyte agglutinating titer: 1:320 to 1:640

Treatment	No. of animals	Median survival time (days)
0.5 ml normal duck serum on days —2.0, +2, +5 i.p.	14	10.7 ± 2
0.5 ml duck ALS on days —2.0, +2, +5	16	10.9 ± 2

Benacerraf into γ_1 and γ_2 globulins on DEAE-cellulose. Two separate peaks were eluted, the second containing γ_1 globulins was rechromatographed on DEAE cellulose [3].

Lymphocyte culture: Mouse lymphocyte cultures were set up using lymph node cells or thymus cells. The lymphnodes were gently dissected with a pair of curved scissors and suspended in modified Eagle's medium fortified with 10% fetal calf serum. The cells were washed by centrifugation at 800 rpm for 10 min and pre-incubated for 12 to 18 h. After this period the cells not adhering to glass were divided into aliquots of 1.5 ml containing 1.5×10^6 cells/ml. All cultures were maintained at a humid atmosphere of 5% CO_2 in air.

Uridine-14C or thymidine-14C uptake of cells was taken as parameter of transformation of cells. Uridine labelling was performed during a 1 h pulse, thymidine uptake was measured after 6 h incubation. Cold TCA-precipitable material was collected on millipore filters and radioactivity was counted in a liquid scintillation counter. Cultures were set up as duplicates and all experiments were designed as dosis-effect reactions.

As summarized in Table 1 antilymphocytic serum prepared in ducks against mouse thymuscells proved to be ineffective with respect to delaying allogeneic skin graft rejection. Unanue and Dixon had shown that avian immunoglobulins do not fix mammalian complement to a measurable degree [8]. We ascribed the failure to get an immunosuppressive effect in vivo with duck ALS to its inactivity to bind mouse complement [5]. It was of interest to study the transformatory activity of duck ALS in vitro. In spite of its high agglutinating power (1:640) duck ALS did not induce blastoid transformation at various concentrations tested (Fig. 1). Competition studies revealed that preincubation of the lymphoid cells with duck ALS at a concentration of 1:10 did not inhibit a subsequent response of these cells to phytohaemagglutinin or to rabbit antilymphocytic globulins (Fig. 2). Thus agglutination of lymphoid cells by antibodies does not provide the necessary stimulus for proliferation. As a further conclusion we postulated that an antigen-antibody reaction on the lymphocyte's surface is by itself not sufficient to trigger

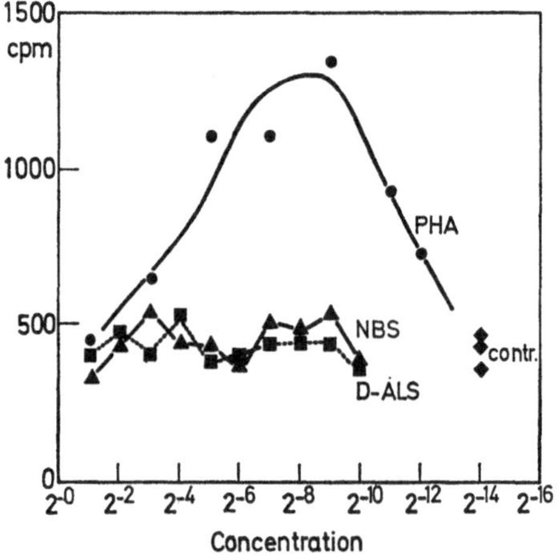

Fig. 1. Stimulation of mouse lymph node cells by: NDS ▲————▲ normal duck serum, D-ALS ■————■ duck anti-mouse antilymphocytic serum, PHA ●———— ● phytohaemagglutinin P (Difco). Abscissa: 0.1 ml antiserum dilution in Eagle's modified medium was added for 12 to 18 h prior to uridine pulse. Ordinate: Uridine-^{14}C- incorporated per culture

off the events leading to cell division. From the competition experiments it may be concluded that duck antilymphocytic antibodies react with surface antigens which are not not involved in the early steps of initiation of the mitotic response.

To study the role of the Fc part of the antilymphocytic globulins more closely we compared the chromatographically purified γ_1 and γ_2 fractions of guinea pig anti-mouse lymphocyte globulins with respect to immunosuppressive activity in vivo and induction of blastoid transformation in vitro.

Guinea pig γ_1 and γ_2 fractions are well characterized by different biological activities due to structural differences in the Fc part of the heavy chain. The γ_2-7s globulins readily bind complement but do not give a positive passive cutaneous anaphylaxis reaction. In contrast, γ_1 globulins do not activate complement but are highly active when tested with the PCA reaction [2]. As shown by Nussenzweig and Benacerraf [2] the amount of γ_1 and of γ_2 synthesized after antigenic stimulation is greatly influenced by the mode immunization. The use of complete Freund's adjuvant enhances formation of γ_2 antibodies, whereas γ_1

production is greater when the antigen is incorporated in incomplete Freund's adjuvant or suspended in saline only. We have immunized two groups of guinea pigs each comprising 15 animals with mouse thymus cells. One group was injected with the cells incorporated in complete Freund's adjuvant, the other group received the thymus cells supsended in saline.

Agglutination titers of the sera ranged from 1:128 to 1:512 in both groups, cytotoxic titers against thymocytes were about 1:64 to 1:128 in the first group, and 1:16 to 1:32 in the second group immunized without complete Freund's adjuvant.

After pooling the sera and after fractionation on DEAE-cellulose the γ_2 and γ_1 fractions were concentrated by ultrafiltration and brought to the same agglutina-

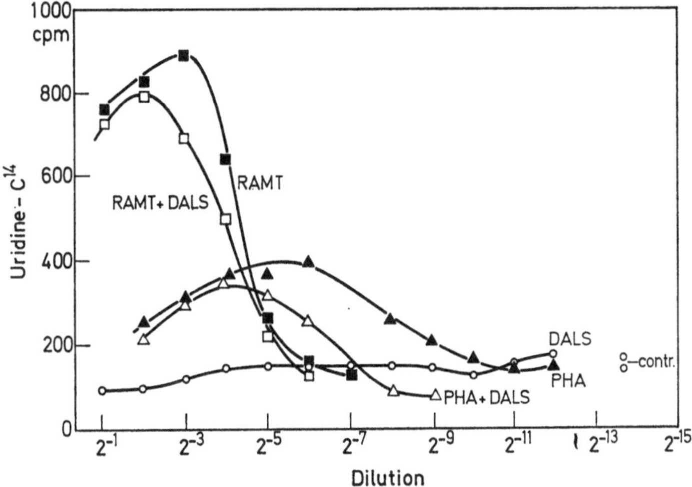

Fig. 2. Effect of duck ALS on subsequent response of mouse lymph-node cells to PHA and rabbit ALG: RAMT ■————■ rabbit anti-mouse lymphocytic globulin; RAMT + DALS □————□ preincubation of cells with duck ALS 1:10 for 30 min and subsequent incubation with RAMT; DALS O————O duck antilymphocytic serum; PHA + DALS △————△ preincubation of cells with duck ALS 1:10 for 30 min and subsequent incubation with phyto-haemagglutinin. Abscissa: Antisera dilution; Ordinate: Uridine-^{14}C- incorporated per culture

tion titer per unit of volume. Immunosuppressive activity of the two fractions was assayed in a graft-versus-host system by injecting C57/Bl spleen cells into adult C57/Bl × C3H/he F1 hybrids.

Surprisingly, as Table 2 demonstrates, the two globulin fractions tested by preincubation with the cells in vitro at two comparable concentrations were almost equally well effective in suppressing the graft-versus-host syndrome when tested with the Simonsen assay. Unspecific cytotoxicity after the incubation with the globulin fractions was less than 10% as assayed with the trypan blue exclusion test. We are cautious in interpreting these results; a more rigorous test system for detecting difference between the two fractions with respect in vivo immuno-suppressive activity would be an allogeneic skin transplantation system.

As Fig. 3 demonstrates both globulin fractions are effective in transforming lymphoid cells in vitro. When whole guinea pig sera with antilymphocytic activity were tested in vitro the cytotoxic effect was predominant, probably due to the high asparaginase concentration in the guinea pig serum. We have, however, found a few sera of animals immunized with mouse thymus cells in saline which induced a rather high thymidine uptake comparable to stimulation with phytohaemag-

Table 2. *Effect of preincubation of parental spleen cells with guinea pig γ_2 and γ_1 ALS-globulin on the graft versus host reaction in mice* [100×10^6 C57/*BL* spleen cells into (C57/*BL* × C3H) F_1 *adult hybrids*]

Cells preincubated in 199 medium with	Total (g)	Spleen (mg)	Kidney $\frac{R+L}{2}$ (mg)	$\frac{Spleen}{Total}$	$\frac{Spleen}{Kidney}$	Index mean
Normal γ_2-globulin 1:100	27.62	295	218	10.70	1.355	1.509
(11 mg protein/ml)	26.67	344	204	12.90	1.690	11.85
	30.38	358	239	11.80	1.50	
	31.64	334	240	10.55	1.39	
	27.15	363	226	13.30	1.61	
ALS-γ_2-globulin 1:100	27.42	90.0	215	3.28	0.420	0.4205
L.A.-titer 1:256	24.79	75.0	199	3.02	0.376	3.22
	25.86	82.0	206	3.17	0.398	
	22.39	78.0	168	3.48	0.465	
	24.51	77.0	182	3.14	0.423	
ALS-γ_2-globulin 1:500	29.70	323	235	10.86	1.375	1.303
	27.05	280	204	10.35	1.370	10.37
	26.31	272	207	10.34	1.315	
	26.40	301	210	11.85	1.433	
	26.83	250	213	9.33	1.175	
	28.57	271	236	9.50	1.150	
ALS-γ_1-globulin 1:100	25.10	106	189	4.22	0.561	0.815
L.A.-titer 1:256	27.16	171	184	6.31	0.930	5.80
	27.14	176	190	6.50	0.926	
	24.41	160	172	6.56	0.930	
	26.10	141	193	5.40	0.730	
ALS-γ_1-globulin 1:500	25.97	321	203	12.35	1.59	1.478
	29.42	396	213	13.47	1.88	11.38
	31.20	325	239	10.45	1.36	
	26.78	333	215	12.45	1.51	
	27.17	263	224	9.68	1.175	
	27.95	276	204	9.87	1.354	

Trypanblue cytotoxic-test prior and after incubation with globulins and after centrifugation: $\leq 10\%$.

glutinin. As fas as guinea pig anti-mouse lymphocytic γ_1 and γ_2 globulins are concerned we have been unable to detect a true difference in stimulatory activity in vitro.

Comparative studies with anti-IgG antibodies of different biological activities should yield more information on the triggering events leading to cell division. Anti-IgG antibodies can be specifically purified, so that the minimum number of

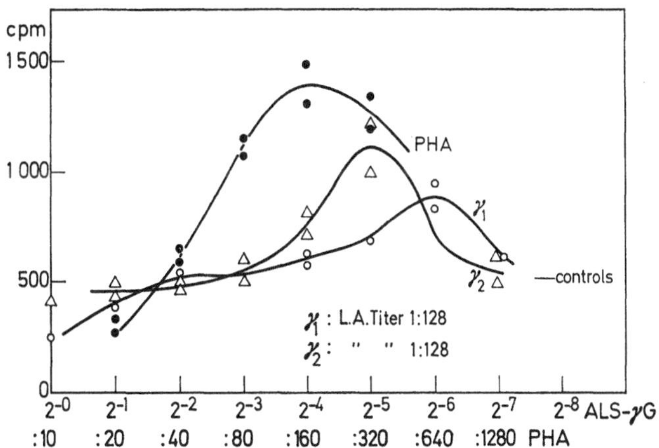

Fig. 3. Stimulation of lymphnode cells by guinea pig γ_1 and γ_2 anti-lymphocytic globulin, 0.1 ml globulin of lymphocyte agglutination titer 1:128 was added to 1.5 ml of culture medium, 1.5 × 10- cells/ml. Abscissa: Dilution of globulin. Ordinate: Uridine-^{14}C incorporated per culture

antibody molecules can be assessed which would be required for transformation. The expert technical assistance of Miss Ilke Piepmeyer is gratefully acknowledged.

References

1. Nagaya, H., and H. O. Sieker: Science **150**, 1181 (1965).
2. Nussenzweig, V., and B. Benacerraf: In: Gammaglobulins. Stockholm: J. Killander 1967. p. 233.
3. Oettgen, H. F., R. A. Binaghi, and B. Benacerraf: Proc. exp. Biol. (N. Y.) **118**, 336 (1965).
4. Riethmüller, G., D. Riethmüller, H. Stein, and P. Hausen: J. Immunol. **100**, 969 (1968).
5. — Lancet 1967 II, 1210.
6. Sell, S.: J. Immunol. **98**, 786 (1967).
7. Uhr, J. W.: Proc. nat. Acad. Sci. (Wash.) **54**, 1599 (1965).
8. Unanue, E. R., and F. J. Dixon: J. exp. Med. **119**, 965 (1964).
9. Woodruff, M. F. A., B. Reid., and K. James: Nature (Lond.) **215**, 591 (1967).

Dr. G. Riethmüller
Medizinische Klinik der Universität,
74 Tübingen, Olfried-Müller-Straße

Discussion

Hammer (Freiburg): I would like to ask Dr. Riethmüller a question about the separation of γ-1-globulin from guinea-pig serum: can γ-1-globulin be more effectively purified by rechromatography on DEAE Sephadex or DEAE cellulose ?

Riethmüller (Tübingen): Dr. Nussenzweig tried this but his γ-1-globulin still contained about 5 to 10% of γ-2 (pers. comm., see also Nussenzweig, V., and B. Benacerraf: In: Gammaglobulins, p. 233. Killander, Ed. Stockholm (1967).

Roitt (London): I would like to say something about the cell type which is transformed by phytohaemaglutinin (PHA). The experiments which Dr. Greaves and I did on thymectomised and bursectomised chickens show quite clearly that in the bursectomised chicken PHA transformation is completely undiminished whereas in the thymectomised chicken the PHA response is completely suppressed. Depending upon the degree of thymectomy you approach closer and closer to zero transformation. Reports by Good and his group are very similar to this. Therefore the first thing we would say is that there is one population in the peripheral blood which is responding to phytohaemaglutinin and it is related to the cell type which is responsible for so-called cell mediated immunological reaction. That covers graft-rejection, graft-versus-host-reaction delayed typ hypersensitivity and presumably the co-operation with other cell types in the response to certain antigens.

RIETHMÜLLER (Tübingen): Do isolated thymus cells respond to PHA? At least according our experiments with mouse thymus cells, we are sure that they can be stimulated [J. Immunol. **100**, 969 (1968)].

ROITT (London): Yes. If you accept that the cell type responding to phytohaemagglutinin is that which is responsible for cell mediated reactions, then we have another relevant observation in the human. We find that anti-human light-chainserum (anti-L) causes significant transformation of lymphocytes. If we take a series of patients who differ in their degree of impairment of delayed hypersensitivity we find that the PHA and anti-L responses are diminished. For example, in sarcoidosis where there is a poor delayed hypersensitivity reaction, the responsiveness to anti-L is similarly diminished. So there is a correlation between PHA and anti-L transformations. This suggests that the cell type responsible for cell mediated reactions has some sort of immunoglobulin on the surface. This cell type which is transformed is the typical PHA looking cell as the morphology under the electron microscope is concerned: there is no rough endoplasmic reticulum but abundant free polyribosomes, and there is no evidence whatsoever for the presence of immunoglobulin **within** this cell. Greaves and I have suggested that Hirschhorn's result — he treated transformed lymphocytes with fluorescent anti-immunoglobulin in sera and showed that the transformed cells were stained — is due to the fact that he used living cells. When living lymphocytes are taken we believe that addition of anti-immunoglobulin induces endocytosis by combination with immunoglobulin on the surface, so leading to uptake of the label. You can do the same thing with a combination of anti-lymphocyte serum and anti-ovalbumin labelled with fluorescein. In fixed cells you cannot see any immunoglobulin by immunofluorescence. I am sure that this evidence implies that there are immunoglobulin markers on the surface of the lymphocytes and recently Greaves, Torrigiani and I have been able to show that the PPD and mixed lymphocyte reactions in culture can be inhibited by anti-L serum.

OETTGEN (New York): Concerning the question of correlation of lymphocyte stimulation with cell mediated or humoral immunity: When the guinea-pigs are immunized with hapten-protein conjugates, lymphocytic stimulation in vitro is carrier specific in the early phase of immunization. If immunization is continued, it appears to become hapten-specific. Thus it seems as though a change takes place in time.

RIETHMÜLLER (Tübingen): I believe that not only reactions of a cell-mediated type are shown to occur in this system but also — as Dutton has shown — humoral reactions. There is no strict correlation in the response between delayed type hypersensitivity and transformation. We can only say that most of all these experiments were done with lymphocytes of donors who showed delayed type reactions.

HAMMER (Freiburg): Does the possibility exist that after pre-treating lymphocytes with duck anti-lymphocyte-serum a subsequent treatment with a guinea-pig anti-lymphocyte-serum still leads to blast formation or would the steric inhibition which possibly results from the treatment with duck anti-lymphocyte-serum prevent any later transformation ?

RIETHMÜLLER (Tübingen): We only carried out experiments with rabbit antibodies after coating the lymphocytes with duck antibodies, and in this case no inhibition occurred, although we are sure that the concentration of 1:10 duck anti-lymphocyte-globulin results in massive cell agglutination.

HAMMER (Freiburg): You find differences between the reactivity of γ-1 and γ-2-globulins. This would really indicate that in one animal γ-1 and γ-2 globulin as antibodies are equipped with different specificities.

RIETHMÜLLER (Tübingen): That I don't know. I only find that in vivo these two γ-globulins with biologically antagonistic actions exist; this is an exciting fact. I am reminded of Humphrey's experiments. After immunizing guinea pigs with sheep erythrocytes, he first incubated these sheep erythrocytes in vitro with the γ-1-globulin fraction, then added the γ-2-globulin fraction together with complement, and the result was that haemolysis was inhibited.

WALFORD (Los Angeles): It is important to specify the exact animal strains used in the experiments. It is for example difficult to produce tolerance neonatal in C57BL mice because their RE system is somewhat more mature at birth than that of other mouse strains.

WESTPHAL (Freiburg): One should not generalize at all. There are many immunological findings which refer to the rabbit only and others which are valid for the human only. It is always more important that we work under standardized experimental conditions.

Bayer-Symposium I, 146—148 (1969)

The in vitro Transformation of Lymphocytes of Premature and Mature Infants[1]

J. OEHME

With 2 Figures

The functions of organs in newborn infants are immature according to Salge [8]. He was speaking of "developing functions," a notion that has prompted a great number of studies. Oftentimes the newborn is thought helpless. From the neurological point of view and that of behavioral research this view has first been vigorously attacked by Peiper [7]. Decisive progress has been made in immunology during recent years, suggesting that the newborn infant is not helpless as regards also his resistance. This does not apply so much to the transplacental transmission of immune antibodies as to the fact that the fetus is able to form antibodies upon stimulation by antigens while still in the uterus. IgM-globulin was thus demonstrated following intrauterine inoculation with syphilis or toxoplasmosis and found to be of diagnostic value as in the case of the FTA-absorption test.

We posed ourselves the question as to whether the cell-bound immunological systems interacting with lymphocytes will respond to stimulation in a mature way at birth. To this end the transformation of lymphocytes by phyto-hemagglutinin (PHA) in the form of the so-called lymphocyte function test appeared to be a suitable approach.

Nowel [4] observed the appearance of large lymphocytes upon the addition of PHA in his analytical studies of chromosomes. In addition, the blast-like cells showed a high mitotic activity. According to Gropp and Fischer [2] this transformation of lymphocytes to lymphoblasts in the PHA-test may be regarded as immunopathological reaction. Thus, we have at our disposal the PHA-test as an in vitro model for immuno-cytological reactions.

We have examined the cellular response of newborns by stimulating both the transformation into lymphoblasts and the mitotic activity with PHA and relating the results to those obtained in adults; these studies were carried out in 20 premature and 5 mature infants. Of the 20 premature infants 11 were immature, including fetuses and infants weighing 650 to 1250 g, and 9 were premature weighing 1251 to 2500 g.

Methods:

Blood for examination was drawn under sterile conditions into a 10 ml-syringe containing 0.8 ml Liquemin, followed by thorough mixing. For sedimentation the syringe was placed with the tip pointing up in the incubator at 37 °C for 1 h. Equal aliquots were then pipetted into Erlenmeyer flasks containing 5 ml tissue culture medium 199 (Difco, USA) and 1000 IU Sodium Penicillin G.

[1] The experimental studies were supported by a grant of the "Deutsche Forschungsgemeinschaft", which is also hereby gratefully acknowledged.

To flask A (sample flask) 0.1 ml phytohemagglutinin (Wellcome, London) was added. No PHA was added to the control flask (flask B). The cultures were subsequently incubated at 37 °C for 72 h. The contents of the flasks were then transferred to centrifuge tubes with conical bottom and centrifuged at 800 rpm (100 g) for 5 min. The sediment was spread on two microslides cleaned with a mixture of ethanol-ether to remove fat, dried, fixed with methanol and stained with May-Grünwald's stain 1:10 and Giemsa's stain 1:25.

This was followed by the evaluation under the light microscope, i.e. 4000 cells were counted and differentiated as lymphocytes, lymphoblasts and mitoses.

Results:

The results disclosed a strikingly high degree of plasticity of the lymphocytes of immature infants (Fig. 1 and 2). The values correspond to the results obtained by stimulating the lymphocytes of adults with PHA. As measured by the PHA

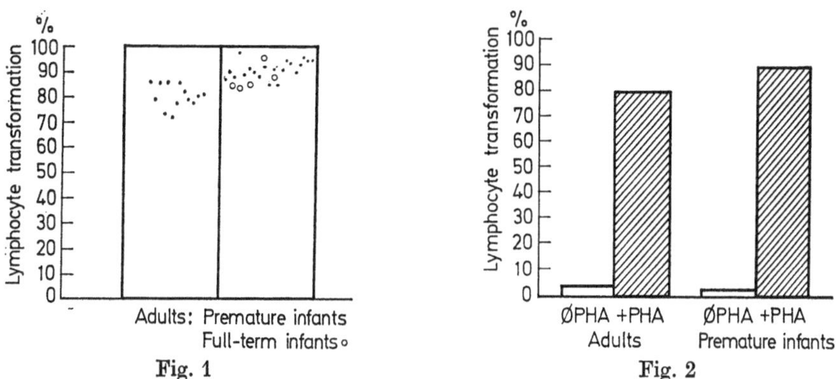

Figs. 1 and 2. Lymphocyte transformation values after stimulation with phytohemagglutinin (PHA and without PHA)

function test of lymphocytes an immature infant of 600 g birth weight has thus matured amazingly early and is not different from infants born at term or from adults in terms of the cell-bound part of the immunological system interacting with lymphocytes.

Discussion:

In mature newborns Lindahl et al. [3] could not detect lymphocytes differing in shape and number from those seen in adults upon stimulation with PHA. We are able to extend this observation by stating that the normal rate of blast formation both in premature and immature infants exceeds 90%. Thus, the values are not different from those of adults possessing an intact immunological defense. According to Brody et al. [1] the strength of the lymphocytic reaction may be regarded as an even better indicator of an intrauterine exposure to bacteria than the production of IgM. In any case, their experimental approach revealed that the mitosis rate of the lymphocyte culture test—cell-free extracts of E. coli were used as antigen—was significantly higher in infants whose mothers had contracted pyelonephritis due to E. coli than in infants born of healthy mothers.

10*

The high rate of transformation of lymphocytes of premature newborns is of significance not only for the general cellular reactivity of the young infant, but also in regard to the question as to the rejection of leukocytes of maternal origin entering the fetal circulation. Depending on the time of the event and their number transmitted transplacentally, the cells will be deposited within an immunologically defenseless organism and turn against the antigen system of the host. This pathogenetic mechanism causes a runt disease to develop, a syndrome characterized by retarded growth, swelling of spleen and lymphnodes, dermatitis, and perioral and perianal excoriations. The pathogenesis requires—as mentioned above—a host that is rendered immunologically defenseless by a "sensibilization through foreign cells" (Oehme [5, 6]). However, unequivocal evidence for the occurrence of runt disease in newborn infants could not be brought about as yet. Therefore, one has to assume that the transmitted, immunologically competent cells—for that there is transplacental transmission of cells in individual cases can no longer be denied—are destroyed within the host organism rather than deposited to multiply. This requires, however, an immunological capacity for defense which we have just shown to exist in premature newborns provided that the transformation of lymphocytes following the stimulation with PHA is indeed indicative of an immunological reaction. Like phagocytosis the cell-bound portion of the immunological system related to lymphocytes is not a developing postnatal function (Salge [8]) but has matured at an early time. This development may be accelerated even before birth by stimulation.

Summary

The widespread notion that the newborn infant is helpless, has already been refuted from several points of view. We have examined the question regarding the maturation of the cell-bound portion of the immunological system related to lymphocytes by means of the PHA-stimulation test. To this end, the transformation of lymphocytes of immature and premature infants (n = 20) and of mature newborns (n = 5) was studied and compared to results obtained in adults. The rate of blast formation was in all cases in excess of 90%; the rate is thus not different from that of adults. The results are discussed also with respect to the origin of runt disease.

References

1. Brody, J. I., F. A. Oski, and E. E. Wallach: Lancet 1968 I, 1396.
2. Gropp, A., u. R. Fischer: Klin. Wschr. 44, 665 (1966).
3. Lindahl-Kiessling, K., and J. A. Böök: Lancet 1964 I, 591.
4. Nowell, P. C.: Cancer Res. 20, 462 (1960).
5. Oehme, J.: In: Fortschritte der Pädologie. Berlin-Heidelberg-New York: Springer 1965.
6. — Mschr. Kinderheilk. 115, 148 (1967).
7. Peiper, A.: Med. Welt 19, 307 (1968).
8. Salge, B. Z.: Kinderheilk. 4, 171 (1912) und 5, 11 (1913).

Prof. Dr. J. Oehme
Kinderklinik des Krankenhauses Holwedestraße
33 Braunschweig, Holwedestraße 16

Bayer-Symposium I, 149—151 (1969)

Cell-Bound Antibodies to Streptococcal Cell-Wall Preparations[1]

OTTO HAFERKAMP, CARL-PETER SODOMANN, BERNO HEYMER, THOMAS B. SMITH, and WILLARD C. SCHMIDT

The walls of streptococci may be considered to have three layers: mucopeptide, polysaccharide, and protein. The mucopeptide is apparently a framework upon which the remainder of the wall is built; it is probably not immunospecific for any of the streptococcal groups. Differences in the structure of the polysaccharide form the basis for the valuable Lancefield serologic classification of haemolytic streptococci. Group A streptococci are responsible for the development of many human diseases, including streptococcal pharyngitis, tonsillitis, rheumatic fever and nephritis. The detailed structure of the protein layer of Group A streptococci is not known, but three protein constituents have been identified, i.e., M-, T-, and R-protein, which are lacking in most of the other groups. Among Group A streptococci there are more than 40 recognized immunologically specific types of M-protein. Type-specific, and group-specific serum antibody formation detectable by serologic methods usually develops after human streptococcal infection but no cytophilic antibodies have been demonstrated against the group-specific and type-specific components of the streptococcal cell-wall.

We began our investigations with the group-specific antigens, using two different methods—the macrophage-disappearance test of Nelson and Boyden (1961) and the cytophilic antibody test of Boyden (1964).

To prepare the group-specific carbohydrate antigen, two different extraction methods were employed. The first consisted of a chemical hydrolysis of trypsinized cell-walls with hot formamide. The formamide-extracted carbohydrate of Group A, and in some instances Group A-variant, was further purified with Sephadex G-25 (Schmidt). The second, an enzymatic extraction method utilizing *Streptomyces albus* enzyme and ethanol or acetone precipitation (McCarty's method, modified by Schmidt, 1965), was used for Group A and Group A-variant.

To prepare antibodies, on the first day of sensitization, the hind footpads of rats were injected with an emulsion consisting of 0.1 ml Freund's complete adjuvant and 0.1 ml of a suspension of either staphylococi or living β-haemolytic streptococci of Groups A, B, C, E, or G. On the following 4 days the rats were given intradermal injections of 0.1 ml of the corresponding suspension of heat killed bacteria. On day 14, all the rats received intraperitoneal injections of oyster glycogen. On day 18, after sterile peritoneal exudates with macrophages had appeared, the animals were divided into different groups for further testing.

For the macrophages-disappearance test, the Group-A-sensitized rats were subdivided into groups and each animal given 50 µg of one of the following pre-

---

[1] These investigations were supported by the Deutsche Forschungsgemeinschaft.

parations intraperitoneally: Formamide cell-wall extract containing Group A or Group A-variant carbohydrate without further purification; formamide-extracted Group A or Group A-variant carbohydrate after purification on a Sephadex G-25 column; ethanol-precipitated preparation containing enzymatically released Group A or Group A-variant carbohydrate; acetone-precipitated enzymatically released Group A carbohydrate; or formamide-extracted Group C carbohydrate without further purification. The last two groups received no further injections. As controls, rats were sensitized with Group B, C, E, or G streptococci or alternatively received no sensitizing injection of bacteria. These control animals were tested with either 50 µg formamide-extracted preparation containing Group A carbohydrate without further purification, or the ethanol-precipitated preparation containing enzymatically released Group A carbohydrate, or, alternatively, the animals received no challenge injection.

Four days after injection of the glycogen and 4 h after injection of the various streptococcal preparations, the animals were given injections of Hanks' solution with heparin and inactivated serum of normal rats for exudate collection. They were then sacrificed, the abdomen gently massaged, the linea alba cut, and the fluid of the peritoneal cavities was collected. A differential cell count (by enumerating 1000 cells) and an absolute macrophage cell count were performed, and results were analyzed in terms of the average macrophage cell count of each group.

Unpurified formamide-extracted preparations containing Group A carbohydrate and the ethanol-precipitated preparation with enzymatically released Group A carbohydrate produced a significant loss of macrophages from the sterile peritoneal exudates following sensitization with streptococci of Group A.

The cytophilic antibody test gave parallel results. This test demonstrates the adherence of tanned, sensitized erythrocytes to macrophages after different streptococcal carbohydrate labeling of the erythrocytes. The macrophages were obtained from animals after the same immunization procedures as those used for the macrophage-disappearance test.

Eighteen days after the beginning of immunization and 4 days after injection of glycogen, the macrophages were isolated from the peritoneal exudates in small Perspex chambers. Thereafter they were brought into contact with tanned erythrocytes coated with the ethanol-precipitated preparation of *Streptomyces-albus*-enzyme-released Group A carbohydrates. According to Schmidt (1965), only ethanol precipitated, *Streptomyces-albus* enzyme preparations of A carbohydrate were effective in the Boyden haemagglutination test; formamide-extracted or acetone precipitated enzyme carbohydrate did not appear to adhere to the tanned cells. After standing for 1 h at room temperature, the chambers were inverted for 5 min in Hanks' solution, during which time the erythrocytes not bound to macrophages were separated by sedimentation. Following this separation period, the number of erythrocytes surrounding individual macrophages in a distribution of 100 macrophages, and in addition, the total number of macrophages with any erythrocyte binding, were enumerated.

The presence of macrophage cytophilic antibodies to an antigen contained in the ethanol precipitated *Streptomyces-albus* enzyme preparation of Group A carbohydrate was demonstrated in rats sensitized with Group A streptococci. Macrophages from rats, sensitized with staphylococci and streptococci of groups other than A, as well as macrophages of nonsensitized rats, revealed significantly lower rates of erythrocyte binding. As another control to demonstrate specific blocking of the fixation of antigen-treated erythrocytes to macrophages, various antigens including the ethanol-precipitated enzymatically released carbohydrate of Group A or Group A-variant were injected into the peritoneal cavities of rats 4 h prior to collection of macrophages. Rats sensitized to Group A streptococci and injected with glycogen were divided into three groups. Four hours before collecting peritoneal exudates, one group was injected with 50 µg per animal of the crude formamide-extracted cell-wall preparation containing Group A polysaccharide without further purification. A second group was given 50 µg per animal of formamide-extracted Group A carbohydrate purified by Sephadex column chromatography, and the last group received 50 µg per animal of the ethanol-precipitated preparation containing enzyme Group A carbohydrate.

The capacity to bind Group A-carbohydrate labeled tanned erythrocytes was significantly decreased by apparent prior combination of the streptococcal cell-wall antibodies on the surfaces of the macrophages with the intraperitoneally injected solutions of unpurified formamide preparation containing Group A carbohydrate and ethanol-precipitated enzyme Group A carbohydrate. Blocking of the cytophilic reaction was not obtained with the purified formamide-extracted Group A carbohydrate.

In summary, these experiments demonstrate that an antigen can be extracted from Group A (and A-variant) streptococcal cell walls, which reacts in the macrophage-disappearance tests with antibody associated with macrophages of rats immunized as described with Group A (or A-variant) streptococci. Similar results were obtained with the cytophilic antibody test in demonstrating an antigen extracted from Group A streptococcal cell-walls. Evidence indicates that this antigen may be a particular form of a carbohydrate or another component also present in these carbohydrate preparations.

References

Boyden, S. V.: Cytophilic antibody in guinea-pigs with delayed-type hypersensitivity. Immunology 7, 474—483 (1964).

Nelson, D. S., and S. V. Boyden: The effect of tuberculin on peritoneal macrophages of normal and BCG-vaccinated guinea-pigs and mice. Med. Res. 1, 20—31 (1961).

Schmidt, W. C.: The lysis of cell walls of group A streptococci by streptomyces albus enzyme treated with diisopropyl fluorophosphate. Characteristics of the lytic reaction and the soluble cell wall fragments. J. exp. Med. 121, 771—792 (1965).

Prof. Dr. O. Haferkamp
Abteilung für Pathologie der Universität
Ulm/Donau

Discussion

WESTPHAL (Freiburg): You said, some of your preparations become fixed to tannin treated erythrocytes only. We have attempted to bind as much material as possible to erythrocytes without tanning them because tanning changes the conditions. We have found that carbohydrate stearoyl esters as a cement can also very firmly bind proteins to erythrocytes. We always wonder why this is possible. If anti-serum against the protein and complement is applied, distinct lysis follows.

FISCHER (Freiburg): But this result is only obtainable with sheep erythrocytes, not with human erythrocytes.

SODOMANN (Bonn): I may add that we used blood group 0 human erythrocytes in our tests. An alteration of the erythrocytes due to the treatment with tannic acid was less important for us, since we in fact used them as an indicator for the used antigen preparations. — Concerning the preparation of antigen I should mention that we used a fairly concentrated form of carbohydrate. The rhamnose content is 51%. From the investigations of Schmidt [J. exp. Med. **121**, 771 (1965)] it is known that these preparations still contain a proportion of mucopeptide, the basic structure of the cell wall. We have attempted to eliminate this mistake by using the purified form of the carbohydrate extract to block the cytophilic antibodies at the surfaces of the macrophages so that antigen coated erythrocytes would no longer become bound to them. Using the purified carbohydrate, however, a reduction of the erythrocyte binding capacity was not observed.

Bayer-Symposium I, 153—155 (1969)

Delayed Hypersensitivity and Tumor Specific Immunity[1]

HERBERT F. OETTGEN, LLOYD J. OLD, ELISABETH P. McLEAN, BARRY R. BLOOM,
and BOYCE BENNETT

Fifteen years ago advances in immunogenetics and in transplantation biology
provided the means by which the antigenicity of tumors was first demonstrated.
Now that several well-defined systems of tumor antigens are available for study,
research has entered the phase of investigation into the origin and nature of these
antigens, and the techniques of classical immunology and of immunochemistry
assume increasing importance. Serological methods, for instance, have played an
important part in the analysis of antigens of virus-induced tumors. By contrast,
they have been of little value in the study of tumors induced by chemical carcinogens,
where it has been shown clearly that tumors induced in mice and rats at the site of
subcutaneous injection of polycyclic hydrocarbons carry antigens capable of
eliciting transplantation resistance in isogenic and even primary hosts (Old and
Boyse, 1964; Prehn, 1965; Klein, Prehn, 1967). These transplantation antigens
are unique for each individual tumor; immunization with any one tumor induces
resistance to that tumor and generally no other. Transplantation immunity can
be transferred to non-immune recipients by means of cells from the spleen, lymph
nodes or peritoneal cavity of immunized donors; serum from such donors does not
confer resistance. Although antibody to surface components of the tumor cell has
been demonstrated (Moeller, Old *et al.*, 1963; Lejneva *et al.*, 1965; Stueck, 1967;
Harder and McKhann, 1968), it is not clear whether the antigens detected by
these techniques are related to the tumor-specific transplantation antigens.

Until recently, the technique of delayed hypersensitivity, as applied to detecting immune reactions to the antigens of chemically induced tumors, has not been
of value as most of the past work with this class of tumors was done in the mouse,
a species where delayed skin reactions are difficult to elicit. The animal of choice
for these reactions is, of course, the guinea pig. Although guinea pigs are generally
less susceptible than mice and rats to chemical carcinogenesis, tumors can be
induced after an extended latent period by subcutaneous injection of polycyclic
hydrocarbons, such as 3-methylcholanthrene (MC), 1,2,5,6-dibenzanthracene
(DBA) and 9,10-dimethyl—1,2-benzanthracene (DMBA) (Mosinger, Blumenthal
and Rogers). Tumors induced by MC, DBA, or DMBA in inbred strain 2 and
strain 13 guinea pigs have been found to be strongly immunogenic. They carry
distinct transplantation antigens, no tumor yet tested being capable of eliciting
transplantation resistance to a tumor other than itself (Morton *et al.*, 1965; Oettgen
et al., 1967). We have studied delayed hypersensitivity to this type of tumor in
guinea pigs of the strain 13.

---

[1] Supported by Grants CA 08748, AIO 7118 and CA 08145 of the National Cancer Institute,
Grant DRG 956A of the Damon Runyon Memorial Fund, and a grant from the Fleischmann
Foundation.

In guinea pigs immunized with isogenic tumor grafts or with a crude tumor homogenate in complete Freund's adjuvant, skin reactions of the delayed type could be elicited by the intradermal injection of a saline extract of tumor of the same antigenic type (Oettgen *et al.*, 1967; Old *et al.*, 1968). No cross reactions between 16 different tumors or with normal adult or foetal tissues were observed. In other words, delayed hypersensitivity reactions, just as induced resistance to tumor grafts, indicated an antigenic individuality for each tumor.

The same pattern of skin reactions was obtained when a soluble antigen preparation—the supernatant after centrifugation at $100,000 \times$ g for 60 min—rather than the crude saline extract was used for immunization and skin tests. Guinea pigs immunized with this soluble material also developed resistance to grafts of the tumor of the same antigenic type but remained susceptible to grafts of other isogenic tumors. Thus, soluble products of chemically induced tumors elicit both delayed hypersensitivity and transplantation immunity in isogenic guinea pigs (Oettgen *et al.*, 1968). Whether the antigens responsible for the skin reactions and for the resistance to transplants are the same cannot for the moment be answered.

In studies with fractions prepared by ammonium sulfate precipitation and column chromatography of the soluble antigen, non-specific irritation made the interpretation of the skin reactions difficult. It seemed desirable, therefore, to determine whether a suitable *in vitro* technique could be developed. The macrophage migration inhibition system, (George and Vaughan, 1962) which has been shown to correlate closely with the delayed-type hypersensitivity *in vivo* (David, 1964), is proving of value in the study of these soluble antigens of guinea pig tumors. Briefly, the method and our initial findings are as follows. Peritoneal cells contained within capillary tubes are incubated in culture medium at 37 °C. If the soluble antigen to which the donor of the peritoneal cells was immunized is present in the medium, the migration of the peritoneal macrophages is inhibited. This inhibition is not due to non-specific toxicity, as the migration of peritoneal cells from non-immunized guinea pigs is not influenced under these conditions. It has been shown (Bloom and Bennett, 1966; David, 1966), that the inhibition of macrophage migration is not caused by a direct interaction of antigen and macrophage, but is mediated by a substance termed "migration inhibitory factor" (MIF) which is produced, in response to the specific antigen, by lymphocytes from animalsthat show delayed hypersensitivity.

In extending these findings to the guinea pig tumor system, lymph node cells from guinea pigs immunized with soluble antigen from a given tumor were incubated with 1) soluble antigen from the same tumor or 2) an antigenically unrelated isogenic tumor. Exposure only to specific antigen resulted in the liberation of MIF, as indicated by inhibition of migration of peritoneal macrophages from normal guinea pigs. Thus, the macrophage migration inhibition system appears to be a method well suited to monitor further fractionation of the guinea pig tumor antigens. On the whole, the detection of tumor antigens by reactions that represent delayed hypersensitivity offers new approaches which facilitate the analysis of the antigens of chemically induced tumors and add another dimension to the study of tumor-specific immune mechanisms.

References

Bloom, B. R., and B. Bennett: Mechanism of a reaction in vitro associated with delayed-type hypersensitivity. Science **153**, 80—82 (1966).

Blumenthal, H. T., and J. B. Rogers: Studies of guinea pig tumors. II. The induction of malignant tumors in guinea pigs by methylcholanthrene. Cancer Res. **22**, 1155—1162 (1962).

David, J. R.: Delayed hypersensitivity in vitro: Its mediation by cell-free substances formed by lymphoid cell-antigen interaction. Proc. nat. Acad. Sci. (Wash.) **56**, 72—77 (1966).

—, S. Al-Askari, H. S. Lawrence, and L. Thomas: Delayed hypersensitivity in vitro. I. The specificity of inhibition of cell migration by antigens. J. Immunol. **93**, 264—273 (1964).

George, M., and J. H. Vaughan: In vitro cell migration as a model for delayed hypersensitivity. Proc. Soc. exp. Biol. (N. Y.) **111**, 514—521 (1962).

Harder, F. H., and C. F. McKhann: Demonstration of cellular antigens on sarcoma cells by an indirect ^{125}I-labeled antibody technique. J. nat. Cancer Inst. **40**, 231—241 (1968).

Klein, G.: Tumor antigens. Ann. Rev. Microbiol. **20**, 223—252 (1966).

Lejneva, O. M., L. A. Zilber, and E. S. Ievleva: Humoral antibodies to methylcholanthrene sarcoma detected by a fluorescent technique. Nature (Lond.) **206** 1163—1164 (1965).

Moeller, G.: Effect on tumour growth in syngeneic recipients of antibodies against tumour-specific antigens in methylcholanthrene induced mouse sarcomas. Nature (Lond.) **204**, 846—847 (1964).

Morton, D. L. L. Goldman, and D. Wood: Tumor specific antigenicity of methylcholanthrene (MCA) and dibenzanthracene (DBA) induced sarcomas of inbred guinea pigs. Fed. Proc. **24**, 684 (1965).

Mosinger, M.: Sur la carcinorésistance du cobaye. Les tumeurs expérimentales du cobaye (seconde partie). Bull. Cancer **48** 546—571 (1961).

Oettgen, H. F., E. A. Boyse u. L. J. Old: Krebs und Immunologie. In: Krebsforschung und Krebsbekämpfung VI, pp. 49—65, H. E. Book, Ed. München: Urban und Schwarzenberg 1967.

—, L. J., Old, E. P. McLean, and E. A. Carswell: Delayed hypersensitivity and transplantation immunity elicited by soluble antigens of chemically induced tumors in inbred guinea pigs. Nature (Lond.) **220**, 295—297 (1968).

Old, L. J., and E. A. Boyse: Immunology of experimental tumors. Ann. Rev. Med. **15**, 167 to 186 (1964).

— —, B. Bennett, and F. Lilly: Peritoneal cells as an immune population in transplantation studies. In: Cell-bound antibodies, p. 89. Amos, B., and H. Koprowski, Eds. Philadelphia: Wistar Inst. Press 1963.

— —, G. Geering, and H. F. Oettgen: Serologic approaches to the study of cancer in animals and in man. Cancer Res. **28**, 1288—1299 (1968).

Prehn, R. T.: Cancer antigens in tumors induced by chemicals. Fed. Proc. **24**, 1018—1022 (1965).

— In: Crossreacting antigens and neoantigens, p. 105. J. J. Trenton, Ed. Baltimore: Williams and Wilkins 1967.

Stueck, B.: Nachweis humoraler Antikörper nach isologer Immunisierung mit einem chemisch induzierten Fibrosarkom der Maus. Z. Krebsforsch. **69**, 236—252 (1967).

Prof. Dr. H. F. Oettgen
Sloan-Kettering Institute for Cancer Research,
410 East 68th Street,
New York, N.Y. 10021, U.S.A.

Discussion

MACHER (Freiburg): I would like to know why inhibition also occurred in your controls in which tuberculin was added to the immunized cells?

OETTGEN (New York): The animals were immunized with the soluble antigen in complete Freund's adjuvant.

HAMMER (Freiburg): I would particularly like to refer to the point of complete Freund's adjuvant. You have very impressively shown that cells which have been sensitized against methylcholanthrene-induced tumors inhibit macrophage migration both with the homologous antigen and with PPD. Is it conceivable that some cross reactions exists between your tumor antigen and PPD?

OETTGEN (New York): The experimental evidence does not support this assumption. In each experiment only one tumor "cross reacts" with PPD — the tumor which was used for the immunization.

HAMMER (Freiburg): Does the possibility exist to substitute for complete Freund's adjuvant any adjuvant which leads to sufficient sensitisation, for eqample aluminium hydroxide or any other material?

OETTGEN (New York): It may be possible but we have not done it.

FISCHER (Freiburg): Is the migration-inhibition factor (MIF) also formed by PHA stimulated lymphocytes?

OETTGEN (New York): No, PHA stimulated lymphocytes do not form MIF; the presence of the specific antigen is necessary.

FISCHER (Freiburg): Should animals which are tumor carriers not be considered as tolerant against their tumors? Further, it would certainly be important to break up this tolerance and thereby achieve tumor defence.

OETTGEN (New York): The question of specific immunological tolerance to tumor-specific antigens is very important. Such tolerance exists in the case of the Gross-virus induced leukemias for example. It has not yet been shown to play a role with respect to chemically induced tumors. In our guinea pigs, we have investigated delayed hypersensitivity in the primary tumor bearing host. The primary tumor was excised, and skin tests using antigen extracted from the primary tumor were performed immediately after the excision and 2 weeks after the excision. Then we immunized the primary host with Freund's adjuvant and the antigen and repeated the test. In none of these three instances was a skin reaction seen. This has been done only with few animals, and it has to be taken into account that many animals in this situation are not in a very good general condition.

DE WECK (Berne): I would like to ask whether you tested the histocompatibility of your guinea pigs. As we know unexpected reactions can be encountered even when transferring normal lymphocytes.

OETTGEN (New York): This is an important point especially since these animals are difficult to breed. We perform skin grafts between these animals; they are tolerated. In some cases we have been able to remove the tumor as well as normal tissues from the same primary host, prepare the antigens and test the normal tissues and the tumor tissue of one and the same animal on animals immunized with tumor tissue. Only the tumor tissues gave a positive test, the normal tissues did not.

Müller-Eberhard (La Jolla): You said that no circulating antibodies appear in the immunized animals. Others however found humoral antibodies in cases of virus induced tumors. This is especially interesting since the cells of such virus induced tumors can be destroyed in vitro by antibody and complement. May I ask you whether in your experiments circulating antibodies occurred after the rejection of the tumor?

Oettgen (New York): We have made every possible effort to detect antibodies. The sera of tumor-bearing animals and of tumor-free animals that were immunized with tumor antigens in different ways were tested for antibody by means of the cytotoxic test, complement fixation, immuno-diffusion, the mixed antiglobulin reaction as well as passive cutaneous anaphylaxis. In no case did we detect circulating antibodies.

Warnatz (Erlangen): We have also carried out investigations concerning cell mediated immunity in tumor cases. We sensitized mice with heat-killed Ehrlich ascites tumor and then incubated lymphocytes of these mice with soluble tumor antigen. No increased lymphocytic transformation was found. If we grew the Ehrlich ascites tumor cells in tissue culture and added lymphocytes of the sensitized animals, these showed a lower mitotic rate than cultures in which lymphocytes of normal animals were incubated with Ehrlich ascites tumor cells.

Oettgen (New York): In a certain sense the production of MIF is also the expression of a stimulation of lymphocytes. Concerning the system itself I would like to say that no histo-compatible host exists for the Ehrlich ascites tumor. The reactions observed are an expression of allo-immunity, not tumor-specific immunity.

Hammer (Freiburg): Is it not conceivable that there are some antibodies against histo-compatibility antigens which bind to some structures within the system but cannot be dissociated. Is it not possible to obtain antibodies against histo-compatibility antigens by the use of dissociation methods and examine them in your in-vitro test? What might happen if, for example, you treat your macrophages with antibodies directed against histo-compatibility antigens and then allow your antigens to act?

Oettgen (New York): In our system, the lymphocyte is responsible for specifity by recognizing the antigen. The macrophage receives a nonspecific message (MIF) from the lymphocyte. It would be interesting to see how a heterologous anti-macrophage serum would affect the reaction.

Macher (Freiburg): Does the migration inhibition test also succeed if you sensitize without adjuvant or do you need the high sensitization rate with Freund adjuvant? Do you have data concerning the physico-chemical properties of your tumor extract?

Oettgen (New York): We have never immunized without using Freund's adjuvant. We are now in the process of preparing fractions in order to purify the antigen.

WESTPHAL (Freiburg): Can it be assumed that every tumor as opposed to the normal cell from which it has stemmed possesses a positively changed immunological spectrum, i.e. actually new determinants.

OETTGEN (New York): The fact that tumor-specific immunological reactions can be demonstrated indicates that there are new determinants.

WESTPHAL (Freiburg): What then really happens in the moment of malignant degeneration, i.e. when the first malignant cell occurs ? Many are of the opinion that this continuously happens in the human body, but that we are able to eliminate these cells, perhaps by specific immune mechanisms.

OETTGEN (New York): We do not know what happens in the early stage of carcinogenesis. A hint may be given by the experience that in mice the stronger antigenic tumors usually have a short latent period, while the less antigenic tumors have a long latent period. From this it may be derived that cells with a very high proliferation potential can win the race against the immune response in spite of a high degree of antigenicity, while the slower growing cells can only form tumors if they are not strongly antigenic. Further clarification of this point must come from in-vitro systems.

GRUNDMANN (Wuppertal): A focal question is, whether so-called "sleeping tumor cells" do exist. In experimental models involving chemical cancerogenesis, e.g. nitrosamine in the rat liver, the first malignant cells can be seen morphologically [Grundmann and Sieburg: Beitr. path. Anat. **126**, 57 (1962)]. Once these cells are present they grow. The question is whether the preliminary stages of the tumor cells can already be demonstrated by immunological methods. Many investigations point in this direction. But they also do not give the answer whether such "sleeping tumor cells" at all occur; for the time being we must call this a hypothesis, in particular in the chemical carcinogenesis.

FISCHER (Freiburg): In-vitro tests should also be applied to chemically induced tumors as soon as possible. In vivo, as we know, the production of malignant tumors always requires a long period of time.

MÜLLER-EBERHARD (La Jolla): With regard to the possible elimination of tumor cells I would like to return to the virus transformed cells.

It has been shown that an antibody directed to the virus is capable, in the presence of complement, of lysing these tumor cells. Maybe, this is a possible mechanism of tumor cell elimination.

OETTGEN (New York): The "sleeping cells" which have not yet formed recognizable tumors are much to the point. There are examples of these in the field of DNA-virus induced tumors: When newborn animals are inoculated with the oncogenic virus, the tumors develop later at a certain rate. Further inoculation, during the latent period, of the same virus into immunologically mature animals results in a decreased frequency of tumors. It has to be assumed that at the time of the immunization with virus transformed cells are already present and that they are eliminated by the immune response.

RIETHMÜLLER (Tübingen): The question is whether the virus originates from the cells against which the antibodies are produced. Maybe the virus is carrying some cell antigens.

WESTPHAL (Freiburg): Is it not possible to produce tolerance artificially ?

OETTGEN (New York): Tolerance is an important factor in the case of certain virus-induced tumors and leukemias due to the natural transmission of the oncogenic virus before or immediately after birth. For animals that have not been exposed to the virus during this critical period, the virus and the tumors which it induces are immunogenic.

ROTHER (Freiburg): Concerning the elimination mechanism: are there differences between the 'taking' of tumors in complement active and complement defective mice ?

OETTGEN (New York): I do not know of any studies of tumor-specific immune reactions in complement defective animals.

HAMMER (Freiburg): One has to be very careful with virus induced tolerance. At any rate, Dixon has recently shown that with LCN virus transferred from mother to offsprings it is possible to obtain some kind of antibody formation.

DRZENIEK (Gießen): I would like to give a comment concerning the problem whether antibodies against virus specific components as well as those against cell specific components can destroy tumors: As mentioned in my lecture experiments, performed by Lindenmann, have shown that in mice the use of influenza viruses which carry ascites tumor antigens on their surface enables antibodies to be produced which prevent the growth of ascites tumor cells.

OETTGEN (New York): At least three types of antigens exist in relation to virus-induced tumors. These are the transplantation antigens of the cell surface, the antigens of the virion and the so called neo- or T-antigens which are located within the cell, not on its surface. They are not part of the virion, although their synthesis appears to be controlled by the viral genome.

Bayer-Symposium I, 160—163 (1969)

Histological Changes in NZB/NZW Mice

H. P. Hobik

With 2 Figures

Evidence of the spontaneous development of an autoimmune disease in laboratory animals was first reported in 1959 by Bielschowsky, Helyer and Howie. Mice of the strain NZB/Bl develop an autoimmune haemolytic anaemia. An incomplete antibody against red blood cells, reticulocytosis, splenomegaly and a depression of haematocrit were found.

In various F_1-Hybrids between NZB/Bl and other inbred strains and alslo in cross-bred strains, kidney lesions, antinuclear antibodies and LE-cells resembing those seen in human systemic lupus erythematosus were also found (Helyer and Howie, 1961; Burnet and Holmes, 1965a; Dubois et al., 1966). We are concerned here with genetically dependent animal models of human autoimmune diseases [Holmes and Burnet, 1963; Burnet and Holmes, 1965b].

The breeding stock of the NZB/NZW cross bred strain were kindly supplied by Mr. W. Hall, Animal Department, University of Otago Medical School, Dunedint They were maintained by brother-sister mating.

45% of the animals gave a positive Coombs-test and in 40% antinuclear antibodies and LE-cells were demonstrable. These findings are age dependent and do not appear until the third month of life and occur more frequently after the first year of life.

As the disease develops, in some animals alopecia is observed in the interscapular region, in the neck and on the head. Ulceration occurs there later. Helyer and Howie 1963 observed similiar changes on NZB/Bl mice. A typical dermatitis is not observed histologically in our animals. The most impressive histopathological changes are seen in the kidneys. They begin between the third and fifth month of life, with a focal glomerulitis. Thickening of the basal membrane results in "wireloops" (Fig. 1) and one can see deposits of PAS-positive material and a proliferation of the cells of the Bowmann's capsule (Hicks and Burnet, 1966).

Later the glomerula becomes sclerosed (Mellors, 1965). First the tubuli are slightly changed and later the dilated tubuli contain hyaline casts of PAS-positive material, and atrophy of the tubular apithelial cells can be seen. During the later stages massive inflammatory infiltrations can be seen.

In all animals with severe nephritic changes, antinuclear antibodies and LE-cells were demonstrable. These changes were more marked in the female animals, also a higher percentage of antinuclear antibodies and LE-cells were demonstrable than in the males (Dubois et al., 1966; Lambert and Dixon, 1968).

Autoimmune diseases are regarded as a disturbance of antibody formation, with proliferation of the cell system which forms autoimmune antibodies.

In our strain of mice, from the eights months at the earliest, we observed with
the progression of the disease, lymphatic follicles and accumulations of reti-
culoepithelial cells in the medulla of the thymus (Burnet and Holmes, 1964;
Vries and Hijmans, 1966) as in humans with, for example, myasthenia gravis and
struma Hashimoto.

Later atrophy of the cortex of the thymus occurs. The spleens of the animals
showed a more marked increase of their relative spleen weight than in other strains
of mice e.g. C57/Bl and CPB/N and NMRI. This is particularly impressive in the
first 8 weeks after birth. The large, indistinct, loosely arranged follicles which are
not sharply defined against the red pulp are notable here, we have not observed

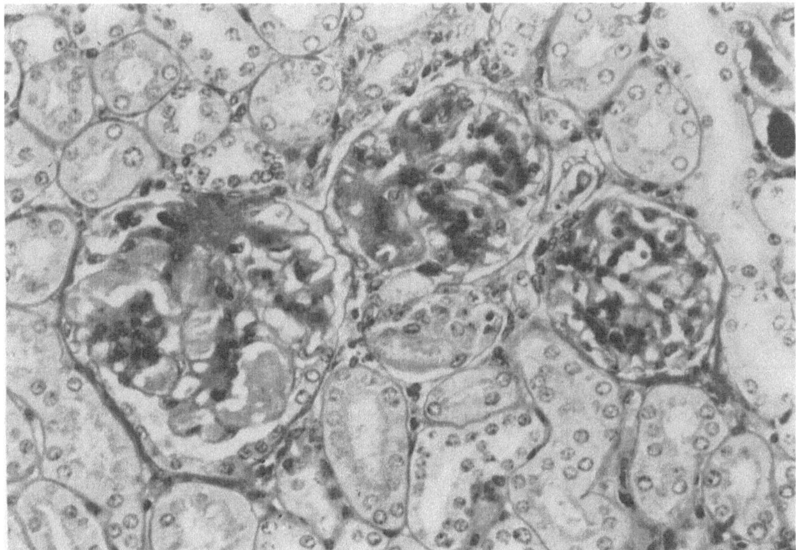

Fig. 1. Kidney section from a 78 week-old male NZB/NZW mouse. Enlargement of the glomeruli, thickening of the basal membranes, wire-loop formations, deposits of PAS-positive
material. (Periodic acid-Schiff, Celestine-blue, 300×)

this in other strains of mice. The germinal centres cannot be clearly recognized.
The cell population is not very uniform, lymphocytes of various size, reticular
hyperplasia and increase in erythropoiesis in the red pulp was seen.

In animals over 1 year old the reticular hyperplasia predominates. This can
also be seen in the lymph nodes. In animals over 2 years old an accumulation of
malignant lymphomas (Fig. 2) is observed (Vries and Hijmans, 1967; East et al.,
1967) starting from the neck or mesenteric lymph nodes, sometimes metastasing
in the liver, lungs and kidneys. These are mostly lymphoreticular sarcomas. We
observed similar tumors in other strains of mice after neonatal thymectomy or
with the GVH-reaction.

These histological changes in NZB/NZW mice look like those in autoimmune
diseases in man: the kidney changes are similiar to those of lupus erythematosus,
the follicle formations in the thymus are similiar to those in myasthenia gravis

and Hashimotos disease. The lymphoreticular hyperplasia in the spleen and lymph nodes and especially the appearance of lympho-reticular tumors as well as reticuloses are found not unlike those in man, e.g. in haemolytic anaemia. We assume that such animal models as demonstrated can contribute to the clarification of immunoproliferative diseases in man.

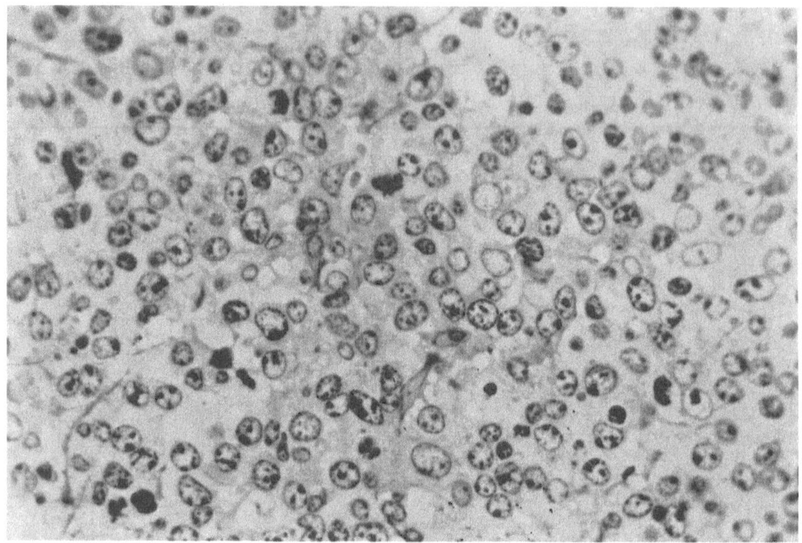

Fig. 2. A 1 μ section through a malignant lymphoma of a mesenteric lymphnode from a 76 week-old femal NZB/NZW mouse. (Epon, methylene blue, 480 ×)

References

Bielschowsky, M., B. J. Helyer, and J. B. Howie: Spontaneous haemolytic anaemia in mice of the NZB/BL strain. Proc. Univ. Otago med. Sch. **37**, 9—11 (1959).

Burnet, F. M., and M. C. Holmes: Thymic changes in the mouse strain NZB in relation to the auto-immune state. J. Path. Bact. **88**, 229—241 (1964).

— — The natural history of the NZB/NZW F₁ hybrid mouse: A laboratory model of systemic lupus erythematosus. Aust. Ann. Med. **14**, 185—191 (1965 a).

— — Genetic investigations of autoimmune disease in mice. Nature (Lond.) **207**, 368—371 (1965 b).

Dubois, E. L., R. E. Horowitz, H. B. Demopoulos, and R. Teplitz: NZB/NZW mice as model of systemic lupus erythematosus. J. Amer. med. Ass. **195**, 285—289 (1966).

East, J., M. A. B. de Sousa, P. R. Prosser, and H. Jaquet: Malignant changes in New Zealand black mice. Clin. exp. Immunol. **2**, 427—443 (1967).

Helyer, B. J., and J. B. Howie: Positive lupus erythematosis tests in a cross-bred strain of mice NZB/BL-NZY/BL. Proc. Univ. Otago med. Sch. **39**, 17—18 (1961).

— — Spontaneous auto-immune disease in NZB/BL mice. Brit. J. Haemat. **9**, 119—131 (1963).

Hicks, J. D., and F. M. Burnet: Renal lesions in the "autoimmune" mouse strains NZB and F1 NZB × NZW. J. Path. Bact. **91**, 467—477 (1966).

Holmes, M. C., and F. M. Burnet: The natural history of autoimmune disease in NZB mice. Ann. intern. Med. **59**, 265—276 (1963).

Lambert, P. H., and F. J. Dixon: Pathogenesis of the glomerulonephritis of NZB/W mice. J. exp. Med. **127**, 507—521 (1968).

Mellors, R. C.: Autoimmune disease in NZB/BL mice. I. Pathology and pathogenesis of a model system of spontaneous glomerulonephritis. J. exp. Med. **122**, 25—40 (1965).

de Vries, M. J., and W. Hijmans: A deficient development of the thymic epithelium and auto-immune disease in NZB mice. J. Path. Bact. **91**, 487—494 (1966).
— — Pathological changes of thymic epithelial cells and autoimmune disease in NZB, NZW and (NZB × NZW) F1 mice. Immunology **12**, 179—196 (1967).

Dr. H. B. Hobik
Institut für experimentelle Pathologie
der Farbenfabriken Bayer AG,
56 Wuppertal-Elberfeld

Discussion

Schubothe (Freiburg): The genetic determination of these changes has not remained undisputed. Thus, a viral cause has been discussed. Virus like particles were found mainly in the immunocompetent cells of these animals. The morphological demonstration of a virus or a virus like particle is no proof that the virus is the cause of the abnormal reaction of the immunocompotent cells. Schwartz in Boston, for example, did not find virus like particles. Have you already undertaken such investigations ?

Hobik (Wuppertal): We have not yet carried out electron microscopic examinations. A genetic cause of this disease is indicated in my opinion by back-crossing experiments with other mouse strains which do not show such diseases.

Springer (Evanston): Incidentally: We have bred NZB mice germ-free and found the same changes. This does not of course exclude the involvement of viruses.

Fischer (Hamburg): Different kinds exist, anti-nucleic factors e.g. an anti-DNA, an anti-nucleoprotein, an anti-histone, an antibody against a saline extract of nucleoprotein, etc. It interests me for example whether a differentiation of the various antibodies has been carried out, that means whether they are 7S- or 19S immune globulins.

Hobik (Wuppertal): In our experiments we have not yet reached that point. We have used the clinically common latex test and therefore cannot say anything about the nature of the antibodies.

Vorlander (Aachen): At the hospital we have observed three cases of visceral lupus erythematosus which developed a lupus nephropathy and at the same time had an acquired auto-immune haemolytic anaemia. In all three cases a reticulo-sarcomatosis occurred later. With the development of the reticulo-sarcomatosis the lupus receded to such a degree that histologically only scars could still be

11*

found in the renal glomeruli. The patients died as a result of the reticulo-sarcomatosis, which is a very similar disease to that of the mice shown here. Can anything
be said to the point whether the same cells which before were responsible for the
auto-immunization pass into malignant degeneration ?

Hobik (Wuppertal): According to the examinations so far, this is quite
possible. In the early stages of the disease, i.e. about the 8th month, atypical cells
are found in the spleen and lymph nodes. One cannot however speak of malignant
degeneration at this stage.

B. Clinical Part

Moderator H.-E. Bock, Tübingen

Bayer-Symposium I, 167—179 (1969)

Clinical and Serological Aspects of the Aetiologic Differentiation of Auto-Immune Haemolytic Anaemias

H. Schubothe

With 7 Figures

The auto-immune haemolytic anaemias are prototypes of auto-agressive diseases due to humoral antibodies. The nature and mechanism of action of these antibodies have been thoroughly investigated and the pathogenesis of the excessive destruction of blood cells has been well elucidated. However, the aetiology of the anti-erythrocytic auto-antibodies has remained a subject of discussion to date.

There are two main hypotheses: according to one opinion the key point of auto-immunisation is the antigen; and the other opinion stresses the decisive role of the immunocompetent cell system. Several variants of both hypotheses have been proposed. Following is a summary of the most important aspects in the genesis of auto-haemantibodies.

1. The hypothesis of the altered erythrocyte antigen is based on the assumption that the antigenic structure of the patient's own blood cells can be changed by various influences such as pathogenic micro-organisms, their metabolic products, or other substances, exogenous or endogenous in origin. This alteration stimulates, in rare cases, the otherwise regularly functioning immune cell system to form antibodies which then react not only with the modified antigens, but also with the unchanged ones. According to Witebsky (1968) and Milgrom (1968), the subject of the postulated change is not the auto-antibody specific antigenic receptor itself, but neighbouring structures, which thereby become effective antigens. Following the principle of Freund's adjuvant, this may through a trigger mechanism potentiate a so far latent or subliminal auto-antigen, which then provokes antibodies reactive with the unchanged autologous receptor.

2. The hypothesis of partial break down of the immune tolerance by various agents presupposes that bacteria, viruses or other substances may exert a nonspecific insult on the regular immunocompetent cells, which leads to a partial loss of their tolerance. In view of the great frequency of bacterial and viral infections, and the rareness of auto-immune haemolytic diseases in human pathology, one must additionally consider the possibility of an endogenous predisposition for such a mechanism. If the active agent and the patient's erythrocytes have an antigen in common, then the specifically provoked antibody can react with host cells. Basically, however, formation of auto-antibodies would be even conceivable without such a common antigen, if the immunocompetent cell system loses its ability to tolerate as "self" one or more autologous erythrocyte antigens.

3. The hypothesis of the occurrence of primary immune intolerant antibody forming cells arises from the idea that, in rare cases, either new immunocompetent cells can result from *somatic mutation* and react against autologous antigens as "not self", or that a similar constellation is brought about by the partial *release* of normally depressed immune intolerant cells ("forbidden clones": Burnet, 1959 a — c).

Causes of such a "release" could be an exogenous insult or the spontaneous waning of an endogenous depressor mechanism. In the first case both, a reversible and an irreversible effect may be possible, however, in the latter case only an irreversible effect is likely. The occurrence of immuneintolerant cells would provide the condition for the formation of antibodies against normal autologous erythrocyte antigens. Auto-immunization would then be the consequence of a primary pathological event in the immunoglobulin forming cell system.

If the synthesis of antibody combining site is not based on information, but is genetically determined (cf. Jerne, 1968), it is then conceivable that hyperplasia, induced by unspecific reaction and autonomous neoplastic proliferation of immune intolerant cell strains, can be associated with a spontaneous auto-antibody formation in which there is no active participation of the auto-antigen.

Which one or which ones of these hypotheses are the most likely is at present not defined. It is possible that the formation of anti-erythrocyte auto-antibodies, in connection with natural diseases, has no uniform aetiology, but is the result of different mechanisms.

In this paper we will present clinical data, as well as serological and haematological findings, which enable conclusions to be drawn with regard to the aetiology of auto-haemantibodies.

In Table 1 the various auto-immune haemolytic diseases and the categories of auto-antibodies responsible for them are summarised for the purpose of a general and specific review.

Recently, other classifications with only serological aspects, have been proposed. They suggest differentiation by the immunoglobulin class of the auto-antibodies without sharp division between the clinical patterns (Weiner, 1967; Gerbal *et al.*, 1967; Engelfriet *et al.*, 1968). These classifications are excellent in their way, but do not fully meet the requirements at the bedside. The treatment of the patient is our most important concern, therefore it is decisive to distinguish between the very different clinical variants of the disease. This differentiation, furthermore, renders important contributions concerning the aetiology of these diseases.

1. When observing auto-immune haemolytic anaemias in general and comparing their incidence with the iso-immune haemolytic anaemias (i.e. haemolytic disease of the new born) or with the hetero-immunizations against bacteria and viruses, one is struck by their relative and absolute rareness. This fact was insufficiently pointed out in aetiological discussions in the past, but cannot be overlooked. It suggests an abnormal predisposition to immune intolerance as the cause of the formation of auto-haemantibodies (however only a few people have this predisposition). The question arises whether such a predisposition is genetically determined or can be acquired by cellular mutation during the individual's life.

2. In fact, several authors reported on the occurrence of auto-immune haemolytic anaemias in several blood relatives (Clough and Richter, 1918; Kissmeyer-Nielsen, 1952; Vajda *et al.*, 1960; Fialkow *et al.*, 1964; Dobbs, 1965; Pirofsky, 1968). Even if in a few of these cases a viral disease may have played a trigger role, the assumption of a genetic disposition for auto-haemantibody formation cannot be dismissed, since certainly many people acquire the same virus diseases without auto-immune haemolytic anaemia. Also concerning alpha-methyldopa therapy, only a number of patients react with the production of incomplete antierythrocyte

Table 1. *Auto-Immune Haemolytic Diseases and the Antierythrocyte Auto-Antibodies Responsible for them*

Clinical patterns	Auto-antibody categories
I. 1. *Idiopathic* chronic and subacute warm auto-antibody anaemia. 2. *Symptomatic* chronic warm auto-antibody anaemia. 3. *Symptomatic acute transient* (postinfectious) warm auto-antibody anaemia.	A. *Antierythrocyte incomplete auto-antibodies of the warm type.* B. *Warm haemolysins.*
II. 1. *Idiopathic* chronic cold agglutinin disease. 2. *Symptomatic chronic* cold agglutinin disease. 3. *Symptomatic acute transient* (postinfectious) cold agglutinin disease.	C. *Antierythrocyte auto-antibodies of the cold agglutinin type.*
III. 1. *Chronic* non-syphilitic cold haemoglobinuria due to DL-haemolysins. 2. *Symptomatic chronic* syphilitic cold haemoglobinuria due to DL-haemolysins. 3. *Symptomatic acute transient* (postinfectious ?) non-syphilitic auto-immune haemolytic anaemia due to DL-haemolysins.	D. *Antierythrocyte cold auto-antibodies of the Donath-Landsteiner type.*

warm auto-antibodies (Carstairs *et al.*, 1966; Worlledge *et al.*, 1966; Dacie, 1967, p. 1088 and others). A genetic disposition is also indicated by the observation that blood relatives of patients with auto-immune haemolytic anaemias are more than coincidentally often affected with other auto-immune diseases or mesenchymal proliferative diseases (Pirofsky, 1968). Furthermore, a patient may present a picture of pluri-auto-immune disease and form, in addition to antierythrocyte antibodies, other auto-antibodies (e.g. against thrombocytes), antinuclear factors, or abnormal immunoglobulins of the "false positive" syphilitic reaction type. Findings of this kind lead to the question of a fundamental disturbance in the immunoglobulin forming cell system as the cause of autohaemantibody formation.

3. The significantly increased incidence of "symptomatic" auto-immune haemolytic anaemias in chronic lymphatic leukaemia, lymphosarcoma, Hodgkin's disease, etc. is another important clinical argument to endorse the previous

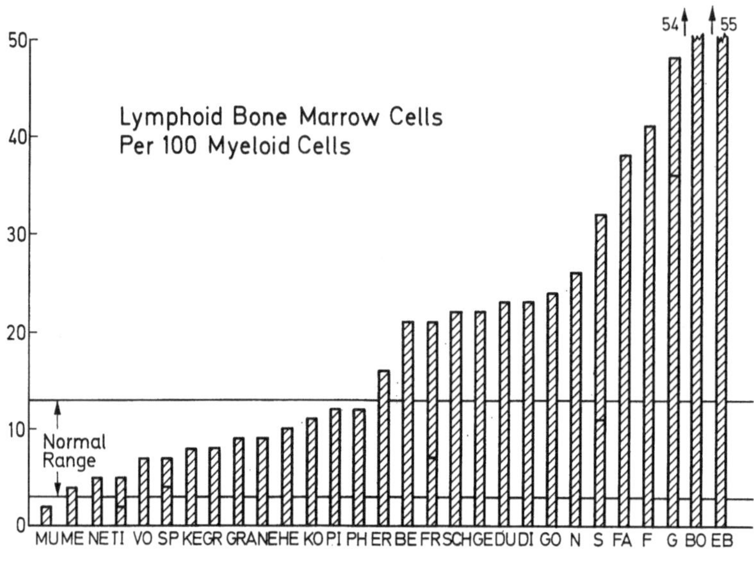

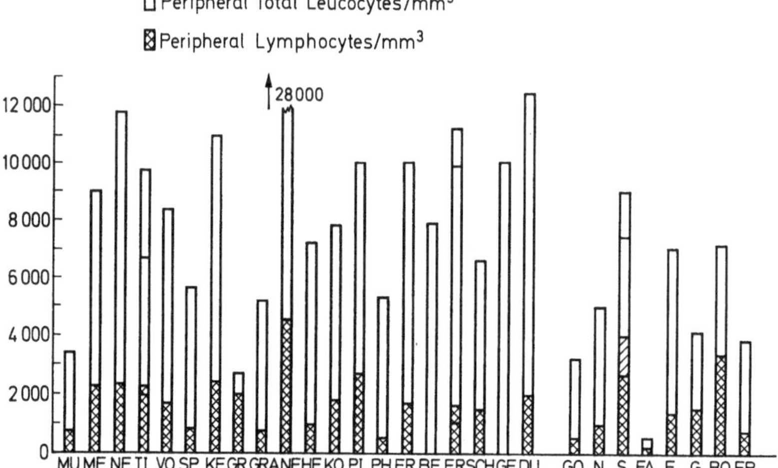

Fig. 1. Number of lymphoid cells per 100 granulopoietic cells in the bone marrow and total peripheral leucocyte and lymphocyte counts in 29 patients with idiopathic warm autoantibody anaemia. ("Normal range" based on controls of six patients with hereditary spherocytosis before splenectomy)

assumption (Ref. Dacie, 1962). Moreover, in the majority of cases of idiopathic chronic warm auto-antibody anaemia, the lymphoid cells in thebone marrow may be increased (Schubothe et al., 1966). This increase can be seen in the upper part of Fig. 1, while the lower part shows a decrease in the absolute lymphocyte count of the peripheral blood in 12 out of 28 cases, a finding mentioned already by Schwartz and Costea (1966).

In idiopathic chronic cold agglutinin disease the increase in lymphoid cells in the bone marrow can be even greater (Fig. 2, Schubothe, 1967). The cytological picture can look like a lymphatic leukaemia or Waldenström's macroglobulin anaemia, a condition closely related to idiopathic chronic cold agglutinin disease.

Thus, limited proliferations of lymphoid cells are characteristic of the discussed variants of auto-immune haemolytic anaemias. Unfortunately the bone marrow

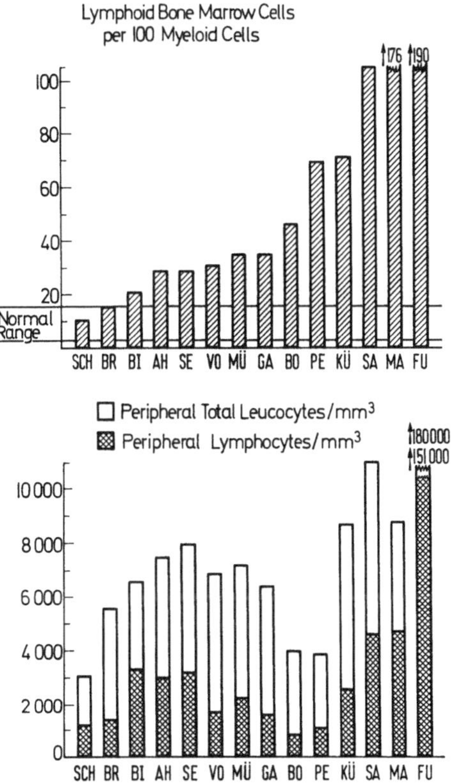

Fig. 2. Number of lymphoid cells per 100 granulopoietic cells in the bone marrow and total peripheral leucocyte and lymphocyte counts in 14 patients with idiopathic chronic cold agglutinin disease

cytology of the reversible forms of warm, cold and Donath-Landsteiner groups of diseases have not sufficiently enough been investigated to afford valid comparison with chronic variants.

4. Clinically, there exist two basically different forms of auto-immunehaemolytic anaemias: a *chronic* one which can last for years, and in some instances is amenable to therapy, however is often treatment-refractory; and an *acute transient* form, usually associated with a febrile infection, which, with the exception of a few fatal cases, within a few weeks clears spontaneously (the auto-antibodies subsiding and disappearing). This shows clearly the possibility of primary autonomous

172   H. Schubothe

production of auto-antibodies which in the case of treatment-resistance is a irreversible processe. This resistant form differs principally from the spontaneously reversible type cases by the individually abnormal reactions to a sometimes definable, but sometimes aetiologically obscure infection. Typical examples are demonstrated in Fig. 3. The stated patient age is that at which the disease began.

The first patient (RA) had a therapy resistant *idiopathic chronic warm auto-antibody anaemia* and after 8 years of illness, died in hepatic coma following transfusion hepatitis. Similar courses can be observed in chronic symptomatic variants, e.g. those in connection with lymphatic leukaemias, Hodgkin's disease, etc.

The second patient (SO) was a boy of three. In association with a Coxsackie virus infection he developed an *acute transient warm auto-antibody anaemia* which cleared without specific treatment, and within 8 weeks was Coombs negative (cf. Betke, Richarz, Schubothe and

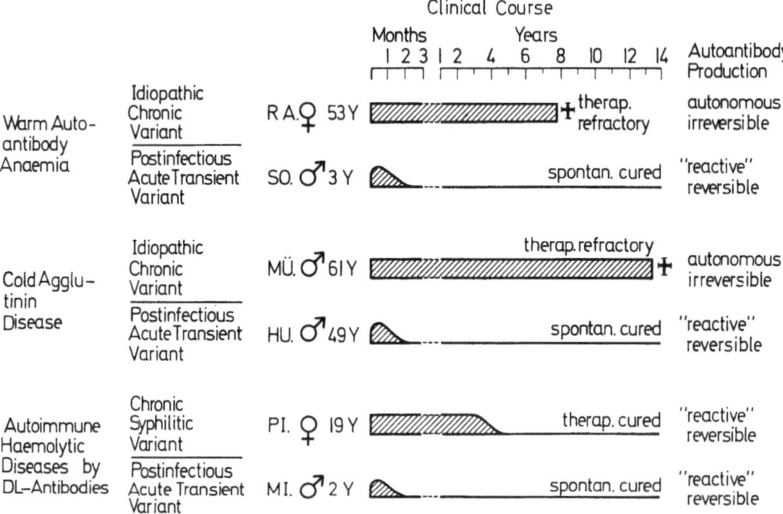

Fig. 3. Typical examples of the clinical course and the duration of various auto-immune haemolytic anaemias. Variants of autonomous, irreversible and spontaneously or therapeutically reversible auto-antibody production

Vivell, 1953). Similar to this variant is the formation of warm auto-antibodies induced by alpha-methyldopa therapy although its spontaneous remission (after the termination of medication) lasts often over several months (Carstairs et al., 1966; Worlledge et al., 1966; Dacie, 1967, p. 1088 and others). It develops gradually and leads only rarely to a haemolytic anaemia which ceases soon after discontinuation of the therapy. Apparently it is also reversible.

The third case (MÜ) is a representative example of therapy resistance in an *idiopathic chronic cold agglutinin disease*. After suffering from the disease for almost 14 years, the patient died of a chronic urinary tract infection with pyelonephritis. A similar course is taken by symptomatic chronic cold agglutinin diseases in malignant lympho-reticular disorders, the difference being, that the *basic* disease usually leads to a more rapid death.

On the other hand, the fourth patient (HU) had a pneumonia of the Mycoplasma type with *acute transient haemolytic anaemia due to high titre cold agglutinins*, which without any specific therapy, returned to normal levels within a few weeks with no sign of continued anaemia.

It is possible that the rare *auto-immunehaemolytic disease due to Donath-Landsteiner antibodies* in the *chronic non-syphilitic form* is an idiopathic autonomous variant of the disease, but this has not been proven. Therefore, we have not included it in the graph. Both of the demonstrated courses represent reversible types of disease. The female patient (PI) had a *chronic syphilitic variant*, which in untreated syphilis can remain active for decades while the chronic infection maintains abnormal auto-antibody formation. The patient was cured of the paroxymal cold haemoglobinuria by consequent therapy of the basic disease.

The last patient (MI) was ill with an aetiologically undefined febrile infection and severe *transient autoimmune haemolytic anaemia due to DL haemolysins*, the latter disappearing and the blood picture returning to normal without specific treatment within a few weeks (Schubothe and Gädeke, 1960).

Fig. 3 demonstrates important clinical conditions for development of auto-immune haemolytic anaemias. Immunehaematological tests carried out during the course of the disease proved with absolute certainty the possibility of two different mechanisms of auto-haemantibody production: a primary autonomous irreversible one and a reversible one. Since antibodies are produced in cells, the basic factor in the group of transient variants of disease must be a time limited increase of antibody synthesis, either with or without increase in number of the antibody producing cells. To say which mechanism applies, is not yet possible. Classification requires a large number of cases in which during the course of the disease, several bonemarrow examinations have to be carried out, the immunoglobulin forming cells have to be demonstrated by specific fluorescence technique or culture, and analyses of the antibodies these cells produce are necessary in vitro.

Since autohaemantibody formation induced by viruses or alpha-methyldopa is not an obligatory reaction, but requires an individual predisposition, the stimulation of auto-immune competent cells is probably non-specific rather than antigen-specific. Reinforcing this interpretation is the already demonstrated non-identity of cold agglutinins and specific Mycoplasma antibodies (Feizi, 1967). In an rare few individual cases of Mycoplasma infection patients produce, in addition to the regular infection-specific antibodies, temporarily excessive amounts of antierythrocyte cold agglutinins. This possibly non-specific provocation ceases with the subsidence of the infection-specific stimulus. The model example of alpha-methyldopainduced warm auto-antibody production can be interpreted similarly; noting that after cessation of the drug use the antibody production slowly subsides.

Basically different are the conditions in the group of idiopathic chronic auto-immune haemolytic anaemias. In these, a limited (but in terminals stages sometimes progressive) poliferation of auto-immune competent cells must be assumed, resulting from either mutation of an individual cell or the (genetically determined ?) failure of a supracellular feedback regulator (Altmann, 1966). A great deal more research and classification is needed to define the pathological significance of the lymphoid cell increase in the bone marrow of the above mentioned group of diseases. The same is true of the question of whether the specific synthesis of the antibody combining sites of abnormal immunoglobulins *depends* on or is *independ* of the antigen. The latter process could be considered possible because the auto-antibodies of this disease group are either paraproteins or resemble paraproteins in some properties (Schubothe, 1967). Furthermore, it has been sometimes observed that specific haemantibodies may be formed in some patients disregarding blood transfusions or pregnancies, the corresponding antigens of which lack in the patients erythrocytes. Nevertheless, sometimes these antibodies attach themselves to the patients erythrocytes which is a remarkable phenomenon ("Pseudo-auto-antibodies": Spielmann, 1968). The higher incidence of iso-haemantibodies, long known in patients suffering from warm auto-antibody anaemia, which has been until now interpreted by an increased tendency to iso-specific immune response to blood transfusions should therefore be revised. Perhaps these iso-antibodies could be immunoglobulins which were not provoced by a specific stimulus but arose spontaneously independent of an antigen.

5. Remarkable is the great difference in reaction mechanism of the auto-haemantibodies of different categories with erythrocyte receptors (Dacie, 1962; Schubothe, 1968). Out of these many differences we want to stress here the very impressive temperature dependence of antibody fixation and blood cell alteration. Fig. 4 schematically shows the four categories of auto-antibodies. The dots indicate the temperature range, and the dense dotted area demonstrates the optimum antibody fixation zones. Hatchmarks indicate lysis by complement or blood cell alteration without the participation of complement. The width of the

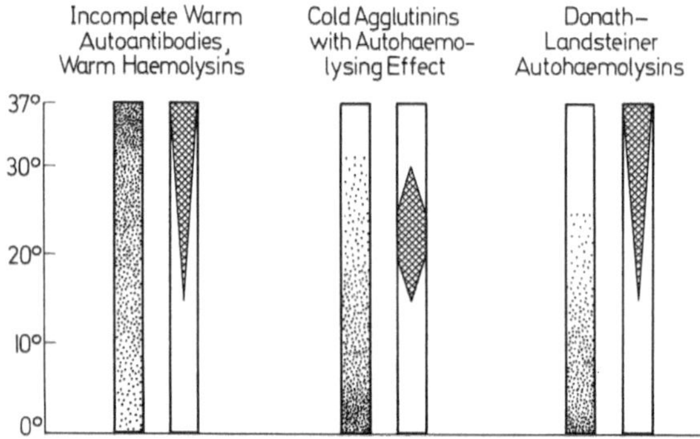

Fig. 4. Diagram showing temperature dependence of fixation of and blood cell damage by autohaemantibodies. ⊡ Adsorption of the auto-antibody to the blood cell surface. ▩ Blood cell damaging effect

hatched area on a temperature level shows the degree and extent of cell damage. In the case of the incomplete warm auto-antibodies and the warm haemolysins the temperature ranges of both phases (antibody fixation to the erythrocyte surface and damage of the red cell) are approximately concordant. While in the case of Donath-Landsteiner antibodies they are extremely discordant. The cold agglutinins have a peculiar complement lysis optimum temperature range between 20 and 25 °C, which is due to the rapid dissociation of antibody binding at higher temperatures (Schubothe, 1958). Such differences in the biological activity of immunoglobulins require corresponding fundamental differences in the synthesis at the cellular basis. Thus, there could be different cell races, which under corresponding conditions, are enabled to form antierythrocyte auto-antibodies. This is also indicated by the observation that incomplete warm auto-antibodies are produced as immunoglobulin classes G, A or M (Engelfriet et al., 1968), and that pathological cold agglutinins are of classes M or A (Angevine et al., 1966; Roelcke and Dorow, 1968). The few Donath-Landsteiner antibodies that have been examined so far belong to the IgG class (van der Hart et al., 1964), some warm haemolysins (which in vitro were only active against enzyme treated test erythrocytes) to the IgM class (Engelfriet et al., 1968).

6. But even within one category an auto-antibody can show greater serological differences from patient to patient than had been detected, as far as we know, among regular iso- or hetero-antibodies. This variability phenomenon has been reported already (Schubothe, 1968). Here are mentioned only examples of the very different pathogenicity of various auto-antibodies. Fig. 5 demonstrates a case of incomplete warm auto-antibodies disease of very mild pathogenicity — despite a highly positive direct Coomb's test, no significant anaemia or reticulocytosis. Secondly, a case of highly pathogenic auto-antibodies is shown with a slightly positive direct Coomb's test, severe anaemia and vigorous reticulocytosis. Lo Buglio *et al.* (1964) using an radioactive chromium technique obtained comparable results by correlating the T/2 value of the survival span of erythrocytes with incomplete warm auto-antibodies to the antibody nitrogen content/ml of red blood cells. There is wide scattering of the values from case to case, far exceeding that noted in testing incomplete anti-D-isoantibodies. Constantoulakis *et al.* (1963) and Schwartz and Costea (1966) ascribed this scattering to individual differences in

	Hb g%	Reti‰	Direct Antiglobulin Test																Ind. AGT
			Reciprocal Dilution of Antiglobulin Serum																
			2	4	8	16	32	64	128	256	512	1000	2000	4000	8000	16000	32000	NaCl	
BO ♀	13.7	24	(+)	+	++	+++	+++	+++	+++	+++	+++	++!	+!	+	(+)	Sp	Ø	Ø	Ø
KÄ ♀	6.2	489	(+)	(+)	+	+	+!	+!	(+)	Sp	Ø	Ø	Ø	Ø	Ø	—	—	Ø	Ø

Fig. 5. Typical examples of a mildly pathogenic warm auto-antibody with strong positive antiglobulin test and a highly pathogenic warm auto-antibody with relatively weak positive antiglobulin test

the avidity of the auto-antibodies, which ultimately reflects the sharpness of the chemical structure of the antibody combining site. Although these findings appear convincing the question remains whether avidity and pathegeneity have to be *always* proportional (cf. Fig. 5). Furthermore, in this connection those cases have to be mentioned in which healthy people, free of anaemia (mostly blood donors), were found by random to give a strong positive direct Coombs test of the Ig G type (Stratton and Tovey, 1959; Weiner, 1965; Hennemann, 1967; Spielmann, 1968 and others). In these instances the blood cell coating auto-antibodies have clinically no pathologic significance. Generally, the incomplete warm auto-antibodies exhibit a wide scatter from fully "benign" to very "malignant" variants.

Great individual differences are also found between chronically increased cold agglutinins. Fig. 6 shows three different types of relationships between agglutinating and haemolytic activity. The middle example does not haemolyse untreated test erythrocytes or patient erythrocytes in vitro, but only fermented blood cells, and clinically does not lead to anaemia. This situation is, however, rare. Among 36 sera of patients with chronic cold agglutinin disease that we have tested up to now, there were only three cases in which haemolytic activity against untreated red blood cells was absent. In this instance, presumably the molecule of the cold agglutinin is present in a variant form which is only capable of binding incomplete amounts of complement (cf. Schubothe, 1967, p. 565). The enormous differences in the molar agglutinating activity between pathological cold agglutinins (Schubothe *et al.*, 1965; Schubothe, 1967) can be seen in Fig. 7. In addition it has been possible to demonstrate by the agar-gel double diffusion technique individual differences in the antigenic structure of the heavy chains of pathological cold agglutinins (Mehrotra, 1960 and others) and by means of starch-gel electrophoresis different band patterns of the light chains have been found (Cooper, 1968), although the anti-I-specific modifications, as far as it is known, are always kappa-chains.

Also the Donath-Landsteiner auto-antibodies do not behave similarly in different patients. Besides the long known differences in their temperature ranges

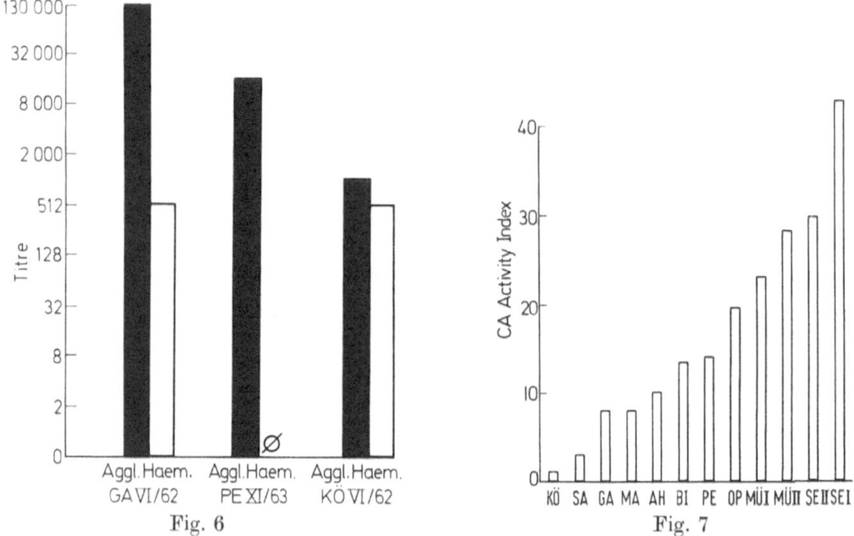

Fig. 6. Different correlation of cold agglutinating and haemolysing activity of the sera of three patients with idiopathic chronic cold agglutinin disease

Fig. 7. Individually varying degrees of effect of cold agglutinin-active macroglobulins.

$$\text{Index} = \frac{\text{CA Titre} \times 10^{-3}}{\text{Amount of CA-active macroglobulins}}$$

variability in the temperature stability of its fixation and its optimum pH binding are encountered (Schubothe, unpublished findings).

All the above discussed variabilities and anomalies are further arguments in substantiation of a primary pathological immunological condition as the basic factor for the production of auto-haemantibodies.

7. Finally, some findings are mentioned which point to a "monoclonal" origin of chronic, irreversible auto-antibody formation, and a "polyclonal" origin of transient reversible auto-antibody formation. Data in these respects are, however, still incomplete, because the necessary examinations have not yet been systematically carried out in all variants of disease. Incomplete warm auto-antibodies are noted for their high frequency of light chain monotypic representatives (Leddy and Bakemeier, 1965; Bakemeier *et al.*, 1965). Table 2 shows two examples of light chain monotypic patterns found by the direct Coombs' test with antisera of different specificity.

In the first case the pattern of the erythrocyte fixed incomplete warm auto-antibody corresponds to an IgG of the K type, in the second case to an IgG of the L type. From other patients with chronic warm auto-antibody anaemia we obtained light chain bitypic reaction patterns. This does not, however, prove by itself that antibodies are of polyclonal origin, because it is known, that occasionally in such patients, several auto-antibodies of different specificity occur at the same time. Several monoclonal auto-antibodies, belonging to different light chain types, could certainly produce a bitypic reaction pattern. Analogous investigations have not yet been carried out in acute transient disease, as far as we know. The pathological cold agglutinins of idiopathic chronic cold agglutinin disease have always been proven to be light chain monotypic. It is remarkable that all representatives with anti-I-specificity that have been examined so far, belonged to the K type. In acute transient variants of the disease, monotypic and bitypic mixtures of cold agglutinins have been described, and in this manner they rather resemble the

Table 2. *Results of the direct Coombs' test with antisera possessing different specificity in two patients with warm auto-antibody anaemia*

Antiserum	Direct Coombs' test	
	Case 1	Case 2
Anti-Ig	+	+
Anti-IgG	+	+
Anti-IgA	∅	∅
Anti-IgM	∅	∅
Anti-kappa	+	∅
Anti-lambda	∅	+
Anti-C' (β_1 C β_1 A)	∅	∅

always reactive iso- or hetero-antibodies and are, therefore, suggestive of a polyclonal origin. As yet however, no definite statements can be made on this account. The Donath-Landsteiner auto-antibodies, being very rare and technically difficult to isolate, have not yet been examined as to whether they are of light chain type.

References

Altmann, H.-W.: Der Zellersatz, insbesondere an den parenchymatösen Organen. Verh. dtsch. Ges. Path. 50, 15 (1966).

Angevine, C. D., B. R. Andersen, and E. V. Barnett: A cold agglutinin of the IgA class. J. Immunol. 98, 578 (1966).

Bakemeier, R. F., J. P. Leddy, and J. H. Crookston: Structural aspects of human antierythrocyte antibodies: an unusual anti-Rh_0 iso-antibody. Blood 26, 881—882 (1965).

Betke, K., H. Richarz, H. Schubothe und O. Vivell: Beobachtungen zu Krankheitsbild, Pathogenese und Ätiologie der akuten erworbenen hämolytischen Anämie (Lederer-Anämie). Klin. Wschr. 31, 373 (1953).

Burnet, F. M.: The clonal selection theory of acquired immunity. Cambridge: University Press 1959 a.

— Autoimmune disease I. Modern immunological concepts. Brit. med. J. 1959 b II, 645.

— Autoimmune disease II. Pathology of the immune response. Brit. med. J. 1959 c II, 720.

Carstairs, K., S. M. Worlledge, C. T. Dollery, and A. Breckenridge: Methyldopa and haemolytic anaemia. Lancet 1966 I, 201.

Clough, M. C., and J. M. Richter: A study of an autoagglutinin occurring in a human serum. Bull. Johns Hopk. Hosp. **29**, 86 (1918).

Cooper, A. G.: Purification of cold agglutinins from patients with chronic cold haemagglutinin disease. Evidence of their homogeneity from starch gel electrophoresis of isolated light chains. Clin. exp. Immunol. **3**, 691 (1968).

Constantoulakis, M., N. Costea, R. S. Schwartz, and E. Dameshek: Quantitative studies of the effect of red blood cell sensitization on in vitro hemolysis. J. clin. Invest. **42**, 1790 (1963).

Dacie, J. V.: The haemolytic anaemias. Congenital and acquired. Part. II. The autoimmune haemolytic anaemias. 2nd. Ed. London: Churchill 1962.

— The haemolytic anaemias congenital and acquired. Part IV. Drug-induced haemolytic anaemias. 2nd Ed. London: Churchill 1967.

Dobbs, C. E.: Familial auto-immune hemolytic anemia. Arch. intern. Med. **116**, 273 (1965).

Engelfriet, C. P., A. E. G. Kr. van der Borne, M. van der Giessen, D. Beckers, and J. J. van Loghem: Autoimmune haemolytic anaemias I. Serological studies with pure anti-immuno-globulin reagents. Clin. exp. Immunol. **3**, 605 (1968).

Feizi, T., and D. Taylor-Robinson: Cold agglutinin anti-I and mycoplasma pneumonia. Immunology **13**, 405 (1967).

Fialkow, P. J., H. Fudenberg, and W. V. Epstein: "Acquired" antibody hemolytic anemia and familial aberrations in gamma globulins. Amer. J. Med. **36**, 188 (1964).

Gerbal, A., J. C. Homberg, H. Rochand, G. Liberge, F. Delarue et Ch. Salmon: Nouvelle classification immunologique des anémies hémolytiques avec autoanticorps. Nouv. Rev. franç. Hémat. **7**, 401 (1967).

Hart, M. van der, M. van der Giessen, M. van der Veer, F. Peetom, and J. H. van Loghem: Immunochemical and serologic properties of biphasic haemolysins. Vox Sang. (Basel) **9**, 36 (1964).

Hennemann, H. H.: Positiver Coombstest bei klinisch Gesunden. Dtsch. med. Wschr. **92**, 1179 (1967).

Jerne, N. K.: The antibody dilemma. Conference in commemoration of the 25th anniversary of the Central Laboratory of the Netherlands. Red Cross Blood Transfusion Service. Amsterdam 1968.

Kissmeyer-Nielsen, F., K. Bent-Hansen, and J. Kieler: Immuno-hemolytic anemia with familial occurrence. Acta med. scand. **144**, 35 (1952).

Landois, L., u. R. Rosemann: Lehrbuch der Physiologie des Menschen, p. 430. Berlin/Wien: Urban und Schwarzenberg 1932.

Leddy, J. P., and R. F. Bakemeier: Structural aspects of human erythrocyte autoantibodies. J. exp. Med. **121**, 1 (1965).

Mehrotra, T. N.: Individual specific nature of the cold auto-antibodies of acquired haemolytic anaemia. Nature (Lond.) **185**, 323 (1960).

Milgrom, F.: Autoimmunity. Conference in commemoration of the 25th anniversary of the Central Laboratory of the Netherlands Red Cross Blood Transfusion Service. Amsterdam 1968.

Pirofsky, B.: Hereditary aspects of autoimmune hemolytic anemia; a retrospective analysis. Vox Sang. (Basel) **14**, 334 (1968).

Roelcke, D., u. W. Dorow: Besonderheiten der Reaktionsweise eines mit Plasmozytom -γA-Paraprotein identischen Kälteagglutinins. Klin. Wschr. **46**, 126 (1968).

Schubothe, H.: Antikörperbedingte haemolytische Anämien. Verh. dtsch. Ges. inn. Med. **58**, 679 (1952).

— Serologie und klinische Bedeutung der Autohämantikörper. Basel: Karger 1958.

— The paraproteinaemia — like features of cold and warm autoantibody anaemias. In: Gamma-Globulins. Killander, J., Ed. Structure and control of biosynthesis, p. 555. Nobel Symposium 3. Stockholm: Almquist and Wiksell 1967.

— Das Phänomen der Variabilität erythrozytärer Autoantikörper. Verh. dtsch. Ges. inn. Med. **74**, 506 (1968).

—, W. Baumgartner und H. Yoshimura: Makroglobulinvermehrung und lymphoide Zell-proliferation bei der chronischen Kälteagglutininkrankheit. Schweiz. med. Wschr. **91**, 1154 (1961).

—, u. R. Gädeke: Die akute passagere hämolytische Anämie durch nichtsyphilitische Donath-Landsteinersche Hämolysine. Verh. dtsch. Ges. inn. Med. **66**, 1026 (1960).

—, K. Kitahama, D. Klemm und G. Erpenbeck: Quantitative und qualitative Untersuchungen der Makroglobuline in Seren von Patienten mit chronischer Kälteagglutininkrankheit. Proc. 10th Congr. europ. Soc. Haemat., Strasbourg 1965, part II, p. 1469. Basel/New York: Karger 1967.

—, S. Raju und F. Wendt: Hyperplasie lymphoider Retikulumzellen im Knochenmark bei idiopathischer autoimmunhämolytischen Anämien vom Wärmetyp. Klin. Wschr. **44**, 1319 (1966).

Schwartz, R. S., and N. Costea: Autoimmune hemolytic anemia: clinical correlations and biological implications. Sem. Hémat. **3**, 2 (1966).

Spielmann, W.: Personal communication 1968, published in: Ursachen und Bedeutung des positiven direkten Coombstestes unter besonderer Berücksichtigung von Alpha-Methyl-Dopa. Klin. Wschr. 1969 **47**, 325 (1969).

Stratton, F., and J. H. Tovey: Positive Coombs tests in normal donors. Brit. med. J. **1959** I, 115.

Vajda, I., L. Aszodi, B. Hajdu, E. Stenszky, P. Barzo, and E. Howath: Familial relationships in acquired hemolytic anemia. Magy. belorv. Arch. **13**, 121 (1960). Zit. nach Pirofsky (1968).

Weiner, W.: Coombs positive normal people. Proc. 10th Congr. int. Soc. Blood Transf. Stockholm 1964, p. 35, 1965.

— Classification of immune haemolytic anaemias. Proc. 10th, Congr. europ. Soc. Haemat. Strasbourg 1965, Part II, p. 327. Basel/New York: Karger 1967.

Witebsky, E.: Introductory remarks to the panel discussion: Autoimmunity in mice and man. Conference in commemoration of the 25th anniversary of the Central Laboratory of the Netherlands Red Cross Blood Transfusion Service. Amsterdam 1968.

Worlledge, S. M., K. C. Carstairs, and J. V. Dacie: Autoimmune haemolytic anaemia associated with alpha-methyldopa therapy. Lancet **1966** II, 135.

Prof. Dr. H. Schubothe
Abteilung für klinische Immunpathologie
der Medizinischen Universitätsklinik,
78 Freiburg i. Br., Hugstetter-Straße 55

Discussion

HILSCHMANN (Göttingen): These monoclonal cells which chiefly occur in the chronic forms of haemolytic anaemia are they monoclonal from the beginning ? For an understanding of auto-immune diseases it would be important whether these diseases originate from antibody forming cells or lastly from the antigens. If they originate from the cells a mutation might be envisaged in the direction of a forbidden clone. In this case they would have to be monoclonal from the beginning.

SCHUBOTHE (Freiburg): A direct answer to this question is not possible since we receive only chronic forms for clinical treatment and then the first stages are already past. But indirectly an answer is possible in respect to the idiopathic chronic cold agglutinin disease: The Waldenström macroglobulinaemia with biologically inert IgM is surely based on a primary monoclonal cell proliferation. And the chronic cold agglutinin disease is surely a variant of the Waldeström macroglobulinaemia, however, with an anti-I specific modifid IgM. So the cells producing it must also be monoclonal from the beginning.

Müller-Eberhard (La Jolla): I should like to return again the question concerning complement fixation by antibodies generally. In order to induce cell damage the antibody must have the ability to react at least with the first component of complement. The other steps of the complement reaction can then take place directly on the cell membrane. Of 7S-gammaglobulin we know that the four heavy chain subgroups, G_1, G_2, G_3 and G_4 differ greatly in their ability to react with C1. Gamma G_1 and G_3 react readily with the first component, Gamma G_2 less so and Gamma G_4 probably not at all. We can also expect such differences to occur in the case of Gamma M-globulins. One molecule of the Gamma-M type antibody suffices to induce a complement reaction. However at least two molecules of Gamma-G-globulin in close proximity are necessary for binding the first component.

Fischer (Hamburg): On the question of influencing the formation of auto-antibody: For quantitative studies of the erythrocytic binding we have mentioned a test which allows changes of the erythrocytic antibody load to be followed up. For this, the patient's erythrocytes are initially washed five times. Of one portion we prepare a 5% suspension, the other portion we use for the absorption of anti-globulin serum. Then we test, using the patient's erythrocytes which have the positive Coombs' test, the titre difference before and after absorption. In this way we gain a measure of the erythrocytic charge, always using half sediment and half anti-globulin serum, so that any existing anaemia cannot have an influence [Fischer, K.: Transact. 6th Cong. Europ. Soc. Haemat., p. 671—674. Copenhagen 1957. Basel/New York: Karger]. I can show you the results of a child whose antibody load we have followed up for 12 years. At the age of 4 the child became ill with a warm auto-antibody anaemia which comprised an auto-anti-D-antibody and a non-specific auto-antibody of the IgG type. Initially, under the influence of corticosteroids, the erythrocytic survival span decreased but after the administration of unwashed blood a haemolytic reaction occurred. The haptoglobins disappeared and some time later we saw a marked increase in the antibody load. It may be that the haemolysis led to an enhanced auto-antibody formation — possibly induced by complement factors. After renewing treatment with corticosteroids the antibody load again gradually decreased. When the corticosteroids were interrupted for 24 h autoantibody formation was again enhanced, probably due to an accelerated phagocytosis of the reticulo-histiocytic system. Employing the labelled chromium test it was found that the breakdown took place chiefly in the spleen. Following splenectomy 3 more years were required for the Coomb's test to become negative.

Westphal (Freiburg): Against which chemical groups are the antibodies in fact directed ? Is anything known about the erythrocytic fraction ?

Schubothe (Freiburg): Many warm auto-antibodies are directed against receptors of the rhesus system. Most cold auto-antibodies are directed against the so-called I-receptor. They are now being more differentiated [Roelcke: Klin. Wschr. 46, 1174 (1968); Roelcke, u. Uhlenbruck: Z. Immun.-Forsch. (in press)]. The Donath-Landsteiner antibodies are anti- Tj^a (P + P$_1$) specific. These symbols designate serologically defined blood group antigens.

Westphal (Freiburg): What do these letters mean chemically, are they protein receptors ?

Springer (Evanston): The chemistry of the cell-bound blood-group substances has not as yet advanced far enough to answer this question. Yesterday we spoke about the M and N-substances. The A-B-O-substances have been obtained mainly from secretions. Morgan and Watkins determined that the P-antigen is a substance containing hexosamine.

Oehme (Braunschweig): Where is the post-infectious anaemia of the type Lederer/ Brill to be classified ?

Schubothe (Freiburg): Most of the cases described by Lederer and Brill in 1926 probably belong to the acute transient warm auto-antibody anaemias.

Oettgen (New York): Is anything known about the reason why antibody bound in the cold dissociates in the warmth ? Has it been considered, for example, if something like antigenic modulation occurs in the presence of antibody ?

Schubothe (Freiburg): This question cannot yet be clearly answered. Firstly, further clarification of the antigenic nature of the I-receptor is required. Maybe we are concerned with a prevailing physical adsorption. Maybe the cold agglutinin exists in the cold in a form which is somewhat different from that which exists in the warmth, perhaps a polymerized state, since there are cases in which genuine cryoprecipitates occur.

Hilschmann (Göttingen): I would like to refer to the work of S. Cohn (Heterogenicity of immunoglobulin light chains. In: Killander, Nobel Symp. 3, Gamma globulins, Stockholm 1967) who isolated and analyzed the L-chains of different cold haemagglutinins. The differences he found correspondended to those found in different Bence-Jones proteins. Obviously, the same specificity can be achieved by different structures.

Bock (Tübingen): Not only cryoglobulins but also cryofibrinogen is a reality. Dr. Schubothe can you say something about the cryofibrinogenaemia and about its active mechanisms ?

Schubothe (Freiburg): I myself have not yet examined cases of cryofibrinogenaemia.

Walford (Los Angeles): Is the cold dependent haemolytic anaemia age-dependent and does a preferential sex distribution exist ?

Schubothe (Freiburg): Chronic idiopathic cold agglutinin disease is a disease of the 3rd to the 7th decade of life but elderly subjects are more frequently affected. The warm auto-antibody anaemia on the other hand covers the entire scale of life, even cases in very young children have been reported. In cold agglutinin disease a sex difference is not known for certain, while warm auto-antibody anaemia, similar to lupus erythematosus, shows some preference for the female sex.

RICKEN (Bonn): How for example may one envisage the production of cold agglutinins in adenovirus infections ? Does the surface of the erythrocytes undergo an alteration mediated by the virus ?

SCHUBOTHE (Freiburg): Such an alteration of the erythrocytic surface is in fact often supposed. In my opinion however, at least a possibility exists that the infectious impetus stimulates nonspecifically an abnormal immunopotent cell population which afterwards returns to its balanced state. A similar mechanism may be supposed when α-methyldopa induces a positive Coombs' test. Also the fact that not all patient with a mycoplasma infection show a pathologically increased production of cold agglutinins may suggest that a particular disposition in the immunopotent system is prerequisite.

Bayer-Symposium I, 183—193 (1969)

The Pathogenesis of Hemolytic Diseases of the ABO-System of the Newborn[1]

K. Fischer

With 8 Figures

Levine and Stetson [18] had been aware of the pathogenesis of hemolytic disorders of the newborn, due to antibodies of the Rh-system, already in 1939: The mother produces irregular isoantibodies; these react after passage through the

Table 1. *Clinical and serological differences between hemolytic disorders of the newborn in ABO- and Rh-systems*

	Hemolytic disease of the newborn	
	ABO-system	Rh-system
Affliction of the first child	common	rare
Progressiveness of damage with the number of children	no	frequent
Intrauterine death	does practically	relatively frequent
Hydrops	not occur	
Affliction of premature babies	rare	usually severe
Anemia	usually little	often severe
Spherical cells	often numerous	a few
Direct Coombs test	usually negative	usually positive
Correlation of disease with serological findings	poor	good

placenta with receptors of the infantile erythrocytes, which have been inherited from the father, and cause hemolysis with anemia, icterus gravis, and congenital generalized hydrops. Discovery of rh-antibodies (that normally are not present) in the mother and on infantile cells (direct Coombs test is regularly positive) correlates well with the above clinical picture.

Hemolytic disorders of the newborn of the ABO-system (ABO-erythroblastosis) are different. I observed these in 0.62% (of those 48.5% boys, 51.5% girls) of newborn in 18130 confinements at the University Hospital for Women, Hamburg: antibodies of anti-A- and/or anti-B-specificity—in accordance with Landsteiner's rule—are always demonstrable in the mother, independent of any disorder of the child. The normal direct Coombs test is usually negative and thus has no great diagnostic significance. Table 1 shows the clinical and serological differences between ABO- and Rh-erythroblastosis.

How can these differences be explained? Initially it was known that not all antibodies of the ABO-system enter the fetal circulation. The macromolecular

[1] Supported by grant from the Deutsche Forschungsgemeinschaft.

antibodies of the IgM-type, which present as complete antibodies and hemolysins, do not pass the placenta, and only the IgG-antibodies, which are able to pass the placenta, are the potential pathogenic agents. They may be demonstrated to be incomplete agglutinins, hemolysins, and also complete agglutinins in a NaCl milieu [1, 11, 17, 21, 28—31].

Fig. 1 shows the antibodies that occur in maternal serum. For the selective assay of antibodies of the IgG-type two methods are particularly used: the AB-γ test, described by me in 1959 [8, 9] and the indirect Coombs test with mono-specific anti-IgG after absorption with water-soluble AB-substance, described in

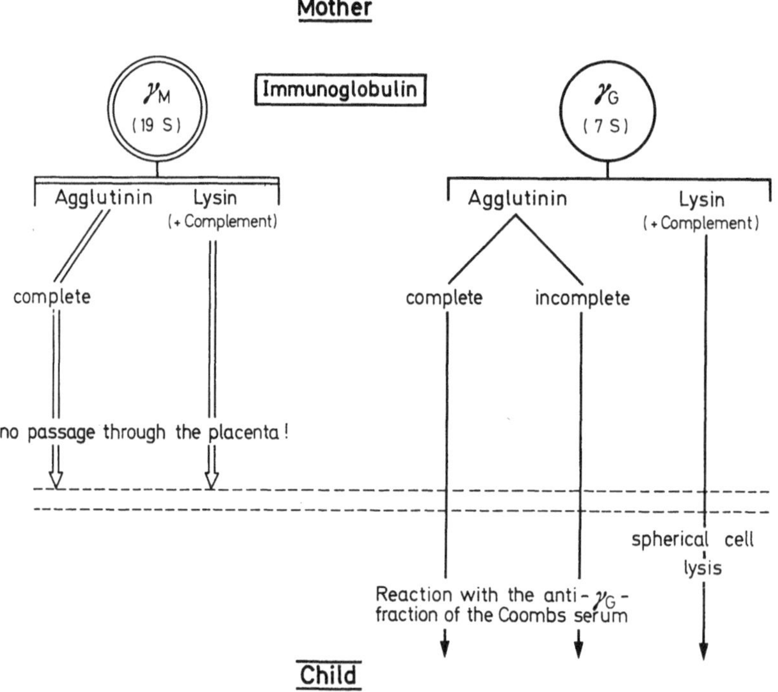

Fig. 1. Antibodies of the ABO-system and their passage through the placenta

1965 by Polley, Mollison, Rose, and Walker [22]. Water-soluble substance binds IgM-antibodies 20 times more strongly than it does IgG-antibodies. In this respect blood group substances of human or animal provenance behave similarly as I have shown [1]. According to Schellong [23] the serum bilirubin levels of mature new-born babies agree well with the results of the AB-γ test (from 1:10), in contrast to findings in premature babies (Fig. 2).

I was able to demonstrate the placental passage of IgG-antibodies in a twin pregnancy (Fig. 3).

The IgG-anti-A titer, as demonstrated by the indirect Coombs test, of the twin with blood group 0 corresponded with that of the mother, whilst the agglutinating (complete) A-antibodies consisted mainly of the immunoglobulin M, which does not pass the placenta. In twin I (blood group A), whose illness was minor, small quantities of A-antibodies were discovered on the erythrocytes. These were demonstrated by the normal Coombs test and by the more sensitive "coagglutination Coombs test," as described by me [6]. The other antibodies were probably attached to the extraerythrocytic blood group receptors, which may also be found dissolved in the blood of non-excretors [14]. These dissolved A- and B-receptors that are not demonstrable in the rh-system, prevent the antibodies from attach-

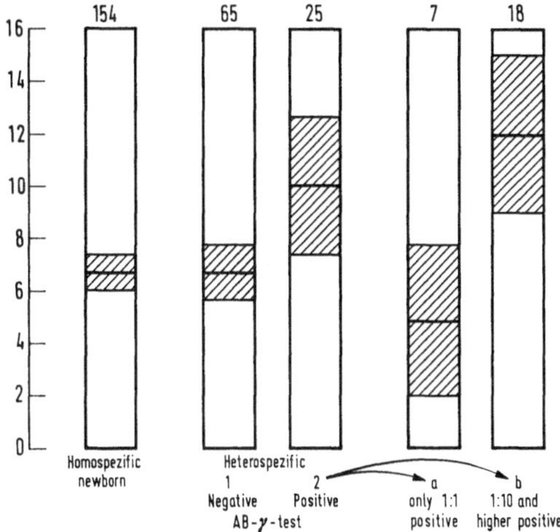

Fig. 2. Means and confidence limits of the maximal bilirubin values of 90 ABO-heterospecific newborns, which were classified according to the results of the AB-gamma test of the mother. The 2nd group (with positive AB-gamma test) was further classified according to the titer of the AB-gamma test [23]

Mother

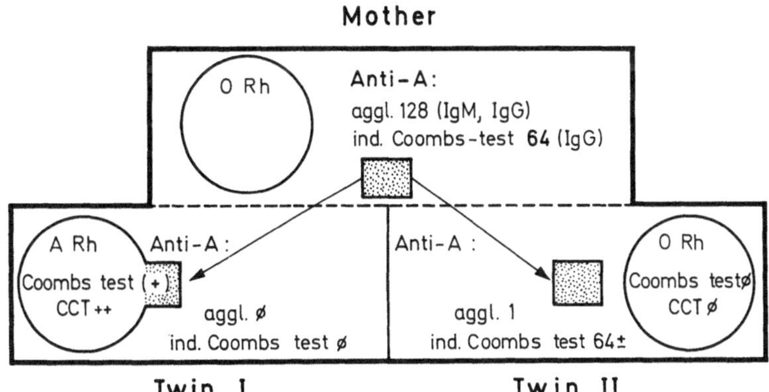

Fig. 3. Passage through the placenta of IgG-anti-A (= "immuno-anti-A")

ment to fetal erythrocytes. Henke and I [13] were able to demonstrate the presence of A-anti-A complexes in retroplacental and umbilical blood serum by heating the sera to 70 °C after dilution 1:1 for 10 min. This leads to dissociation of antigen and antibody, and the thermolabile antibody is denatured. It is now possible to ascertain the binding ability of the liberated thermostable A-substance for anti-A with anti-A test serum and anti-test erythrocytes. The assay of B-blood groups is carried out similarly. Fig. 4 shows the results.

Although proof of the presence of IgG-antibodies is correlated with an increase, albeit only slight, of bilirubin, prediction of severe ABO-erythroblastosis, which might require treatment, merely from the results of tests of maternal blood is very difficult and uncertain. As the A-antibodies of the ABO-system are directed against A-receptors of varying specificity, which may also be found in animals, an effort has been made to demonstrate an antibody that might particularly well correlate with the disorder of the child. Borel [2] systematically determined antibodies against A^{P1}-erythrocytes (pig), R-erythrocytes (sheep), J^C-erythrocytes (cattle), and Forssman antigen in pregnant women, without succeeding to obtain definite predictability.

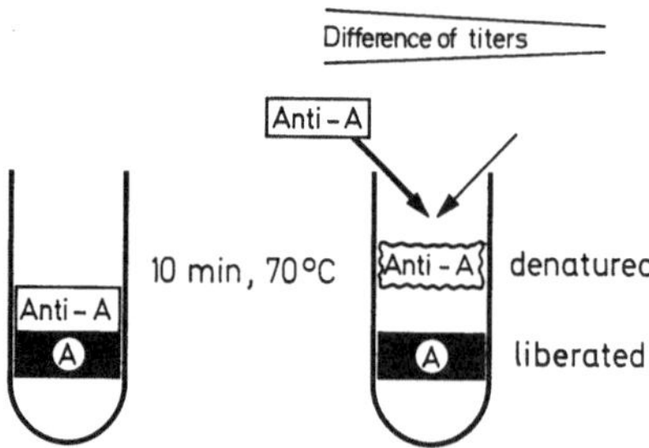

n	Mother	Child	Inhibition of agglutination (steps)
Retroplacental blood			
45	0	A	2.8 (0—5)
16	0	B	2.1 (0—4)
20	0	0	0
Umbilical vein blood			
36	0	A	1.4 (0—4)
32	0	B	1.4 (0—4)
6	0	0	0

No A-/B-blood group substance was demonstrated in the serum of the mothers (0/A = 100, 0/B = 30).

Fig. 4. Demonstration of antigen-antibody complexes in ABO-heterospecific pregnancy

It will not do to explain the poor correlation of the serological findings in the mother with the disease of the child merely by the protecting extraerythrocytic AB-receptors. Both healthy and sick A-children with anti-A in plasma may be observed, who have a negative normal direct Coombs test. I evolved a hypothesis in 1961 [6], which explains all peculiarities of the pathogenesis of ABO-erythroblastosis and which has been supported by further investigations.

As Fig. 5 shows, the IgG-antibodies reach the fetal erythrocytes, the ability of which to bind antibodies may vary greatly, after passage through the placenta and partial neutralization by extraerythrocytic A-/B-receptors.

Erythrocytes with many A- or B-receptors are particularly quickly destroyed, whilst macrocytic erythrocytes, which are usually older, have much less well-developed A-/B-receptors. Obviously, in such an erythrocyte population the direct Coombs test will be usually negative. Extreme anemia with hydrops is hardly ever seen on account of the residual erythrocyte population, which is not open to a great deal of attachment. Premature babies have only few erythrocytes with strong ability to bind antibodies and therefore only very rarely become ill [24]. I found hat the group of premature babies that are afflicted consists chiefly of babies with

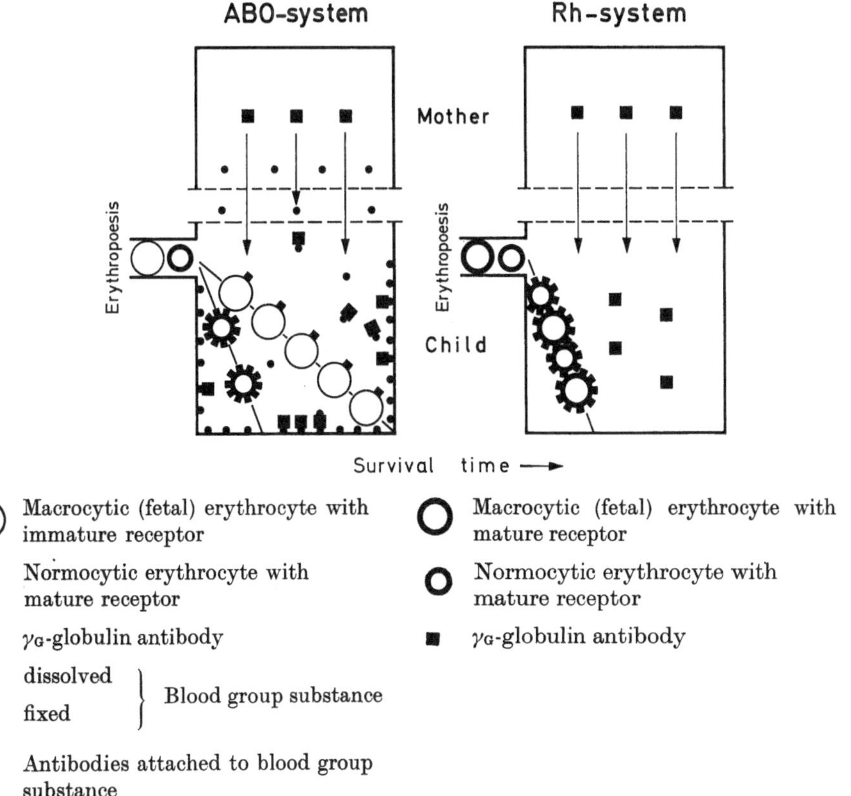

Fig. 5. Reaction of IgG-antibodies of the ABO- and Rh-systems after passage through the placenta [6]

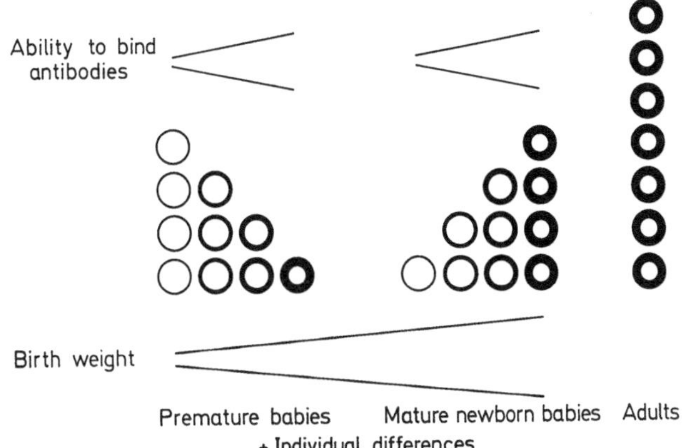

Fig. 6. Development of the ability of erythrocytes to bind anti-A and anti-B during fetal life

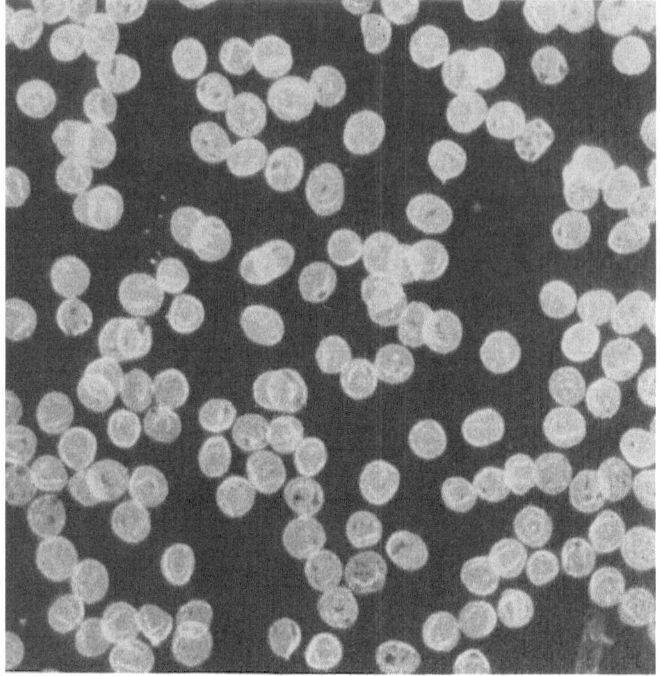

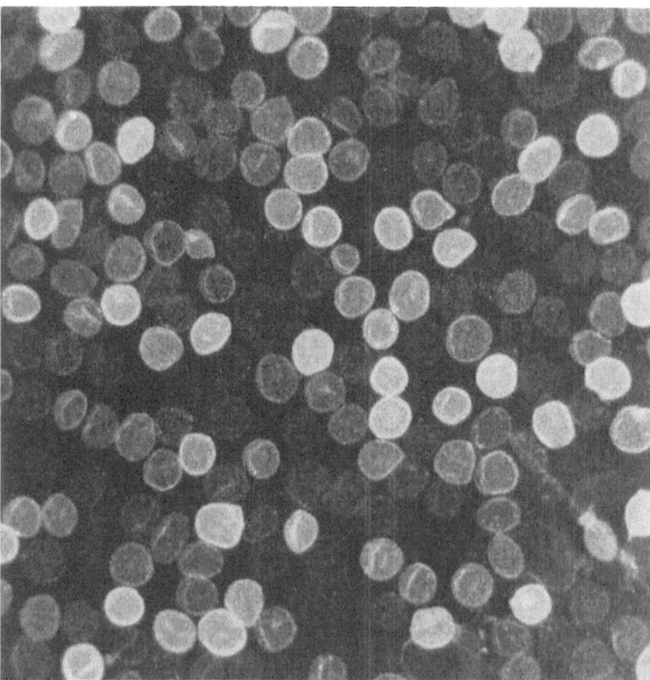

Fig. 7a—d. Demonstration of erythrocytic IgG-anti-A binding by indirect immunofluorescence technique. a A_1-adult blood; b Mature A_1-newborn; c A_1-premature; d Mature A_1-newborn with anti-A erythroblastosis

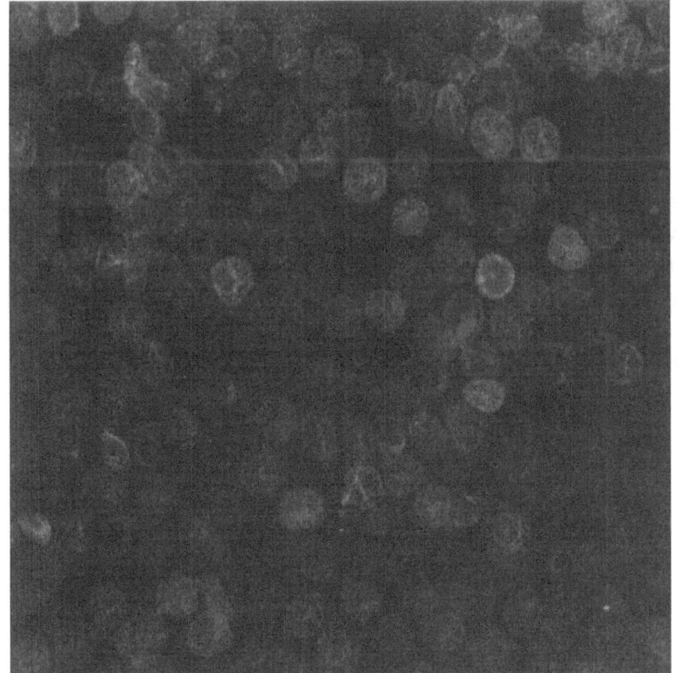

c

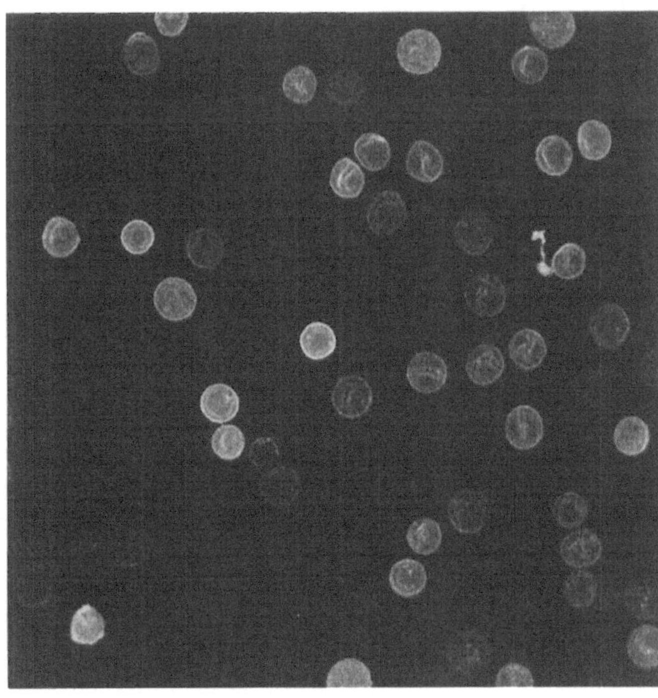

d

intrauterine dystrophy, whose low body weight is only apparently due to immaturity (Fig. 6).

I was also able to demonstrate with a special technique using indirect immunofluorescence the linkage of IgG-anti-A and IgG-anti-B to individual erythrocytes on a blood smear [10].

Fig. 7a shows the even and strong attachment of antibodies to adult erythrocytes. There are, in contrast, various erythrocyte populations in the mature newborn with variegated antibody attachments. Through the influence of maternal A-hemolysins a number of erythrocytes become spherical, as shown in Fig. 7d. Finally, Fig. 7c shows the weak attachment of antibodies in a premature baby.

My fellow-worker Möllnitz-Schier carried out the immunofluorescence technique in 49 blood samples of mature A_1-newborn of 0-mothers before and after

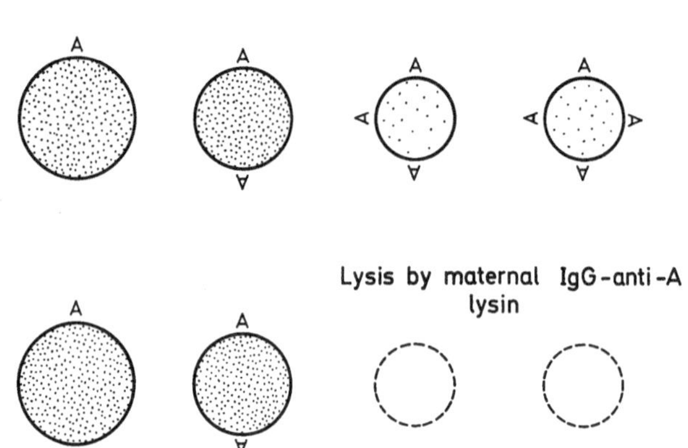

Fig. 8. Indirect action of anti-A hemolysin on the activity of erythrocyte acetylcholinesterase of the newborn. Effect of partial lysis: Preponderance of old macrocytic erythrocytes (Hb_E-rise) with reduced acetylcholinesterase activity

interaction with A-hemolysin in vitro, to discover whether the erythrocytes that shine brighter, are dissolved preferentially by hemolysins [19]. The ratio of particularly bright shining erythrocytes before the action of lysin was $22.3 \pm 8.1\%$, after the action of lysin it was only $2.8 \pm 3.2\%$. This proved the parellelism of strength of fluorescence and sensitivity to lysin. Grundbacher [12] had also found diminished sensitivity of erythrocytes of newborn to anti-A hemolysin with great individual variability. Finally, I should like to mention a further finding, that can be explained by my pathogenetic concepts: Kaplan, Herz, Ku Shin Hsu, Stevenson, and Scheye [15] had found in ABO-erythroblastosis a diminished activity of erythrocyte acetylcholinesterase, whilst this was not the case in Rh-erythroblastosis. It is well known that young erythrocytes possess greater acetylcholinesterase activity than old cells [16].

It may well be that these findings are due to selective dissociation of young erythrocytes with strongly developed A-receptors, whilst the older macrocytic erythrocytes with less acetylcholinesterase activity remain.

In contrast, owing to the very early maturity of Rh-receptors no selective destruction of erythrocytes will occur and acetylcholinesterase activity will not diminish. Brandenburg [3] and I in the Enzyme Laboratory of Dr. W. Schröter (University Lecturer, Children's Hospital, University of Hamburg) determined acetylcholinesterase activity in parallel with serological findings. We used the following serological methods: AB-γ test [6, 9], modified direct Coombs test according to Speiser (Sp.C.C.[2]), coagglutination Coombs test [6], and indirect Coombs test of the infantile serum and A_1 and B-adult erythrocytes, according to the blood group of the child. Table 2 shows a particularly great diminution of erythrocytes in terms of acetylcholinesterase activity, when all serological tests had become positive. This confirmed the results of Kaplan and fellow workers, who had not published their detailed serological findings. Further investigations

Table 2. *Activity of erythrocyte acetylcholinesterase and IgG-antibody findings in the ABO-system* [3]. *(idCT = indirect Coombs test, SpCT = Speiser's modified direct Coombs test)*

		n	$M \pm t_s \cdot \dfrac{s}{\sqrt{n}}$	Normal range — limits P = 0.05	
Healthy adults	1	18	165 $\pm$ 10.4	134.8	195.2
Women during confinement	2	20	184.5 $\pm$ 11.6	147.3	221.7
Normal newborn O/O	3	36	100.0 $\pm$ 4.8	79.6	120.4
Non-immunized newborn (O/A and O/B)	4	24	99.2 $\pm$ 4.8	82.7	115.7
Mature newborn All tests positive	5	16	62.4	39.5	89.6
As 5, but idCT negative	6	10	89.0 $\pm$ 13.5	62.5	115.5
As 5, but idCT and ABγT negative	7	18	93.9 $\pm$ 12.3	59.6	128.2
Mature immunized newborn with positive SpCT	8	34	77.3 $\pm$ 12.6	24.3	130.3
Newborn with Rh-erythroblastosis	9.1	7	96.0	67.8	120.4
Newborn with hyperbilirubinemia	9.2	6	90.0	67.2	113.2
Premature babies	10	21	92.8 $\pm$ 10.1	61.1	124.5

will show how far it is possible to obtain a diminution of erythrocyte acetylcholinesterase activity also by lysin action in vitro.

The aim of all these investigations in ABO-erythroblastosis, when, as indicated, a great variety of immunological methods may be used, was to enable prediction of this disorder. If the present methods of investigation (AB-γ test, modified, direct Coombs test according to Speiser, etc.) give positive results, then treatment by exchange transfusions on account of very high serum bilirubin levels is needed only in every 3rd to 4th child.

References

1. Bärwolf, Ch.: Untersuchungen über das physikochemische Verhalten von 19S- und 7S-Antikörpern gegenüber verschiedenen A- und B-Blutgruppenrezeptoren. Thesis, Hamburg 1966.
2. Borel, J. F.: Serological analysis of anti-A antibodies in relation to the ABO Morbus haemolyticus neonatorum. Z. Immun.-Forsch. **132**, 72 (1967).

---

[2] [5, 25—27, 4, 7].

3. Brandenburg, I.: Der diagnostische Wert der Erythrozyten-Acetylcholinesteraseaktivität beim Morbus haemolyticus neonatorum im ABO-System. Thesis, Hamburg 1968.

4. Dorszewski, E.: Eine Methode zur Identifizierung erythrozytär gebundener inkompletter Antikörper bei haemolytischen Neugeborenenerkrankungen. Z. Immun.-Forsch. **129**, 13 (1965).

5. Dugge, E., u. K. Fischer: Blutgruppenserologische und therapeutische Fragen bei Morbus haemolyticus neonatorum. Ärztl. Lab. **14**, 68 (1968).

6. Fischer, K.: Morbus haemolyticus neonatorum im ABO-System. Stuttgart: Thieme 1961.

7. — Zur Pathogenese und Diagnose der ABO-Incompatibilität. Pädiat. Pädol. **1**, 306 (1965).

8. — III. Die ABO-Inkompatibilität. Bibl. gynaec. (Basel) **38**, 79 (1966).

9. —, u. M. Lurati: Eine Methode zur Unterscheidung natürlich vorkommender Antikörper von Immunantikörpern für die Diagnose der ABO-Erythroblastose („AB-Gamma-Test"). Klin. Wschr. **37**, 493 (1959).

10. —, and N. Stege: On the pathogenesis of ABO erythroblastosis: Demonstration of quantitative variations in the power of neonatal erythrocytes to combine with antibody, using the immuno-fluorescent-technique. Vox Sang. (Basel) **12**, 145 (1967).

11. Fong, S. W., A. Nuckton, and H. H. Fudenberg: Characterization of maternal isoagglutinins in ABO hemolytic disease in the newborn. Blood **27**, 17 (1966).

12. Grundbacher, F. J.: Quantitative variation of the A antigen at birth; its significance in ABO hemolytic disease and in the infant's development. Acta paediat. (Uppsala) **54**, 550 (1965).

13. Henke, I., u. K. Fischer: Über den Nachweis von Antigen-Antikörperkomplexen des ABO-Blutgruppensystems im Retropalzentarserum und im Serum Neugeborener. In Vorbereitung.

14. Höstrup, H.: Influence of foetal A and B blood-group substances on the immunization of pregnant women. Vox Sang. (Basel) **9**, 301 (1964).

15. Kaplan, E., F. Herz, Ku Shin Hsu, J. Stevenson, and E. Scheye: Erythrocyte acetylcholinesterase activity in ABO hemolytic disease of the newborn. Pediatrics **33**, 205 (1964).

16. —, J. T. Tildon, J. Stevenson, and C. Fluharty: Changes in red cell enzyme activity in relation to red cell survival in infancy. Pediatrics **32**, 371 (1963).

17. Konugres, A., and R. R. A. Coombs: Studies on human anti-A sera with special reference to so-called immune anti-A. 2. Identification of the antibody detected by Witebsky's "partial neutralization" test as anti-A^P and the occurrence of the A^P antigen on human and animal red cells. Brit. J. Haemat. **4**, 261 (1957).

18. Levine, P., and R. E. Stetson: An unusual case of intragroup agglutination. J. Amer. med. Ass. **113**, 126 (1939).

19. Möllnitz-Schier, P.: Thesis, Hamburg (in preparation).

20. Oelschläger, M.: Untersuchungen zur Differenzierung von IgM- und IgG-Blutgruppenantikörpern durch Disulfidbrückensprengung mit Penicillamin. Thesis, Hamburg 1967.

21. Polley, M. J., M. Adinolfi, and P. L. Mollison: Serological characteristics of anti-A related to type of antibody protein (7S γ or 19S γ). Vox Sang. (Basel) 8, 385 (1963).

22. Polley, J. M., P. L. Mollison, J. Rose, and W. Walker: A simple serological test for antibodies causing ABO haemolytic disease of the newborn. Lancet **1965**, 291.

23. Schellong, G.: Icterus neonatorum. Stuttgart: Thieme 1962.

24. — Über den Einfluß mütterlicher Antikörper des ABO-Systems auf Retikulozytenzahl und Serumbilirubin Frügeborener. Z. Kinderheilk. **90**, 134 (1964).

25. Speiser, P.: Die Serologie des ABO-bedingten Morbus haemolyticus neonatorum. Bibl. haemat. (Basel) **20**, 249 (1965).

26. — Welche Antigene führen zum Morbus haemolyticus neonatorum? Pädiat. Pädol. **1**, 302 (1965).

27. — Der modifizierte Coombs-Test bei ABO-bedingter Erythroblastose Mkurs. ärztl. Fortbild. **16**, 591 (1966).

28. Tovey, G. H., J. W. Lockyer, A. N. Blades, and H. C. G. Flavell: Ante-natal prediction of ABO haemolytic disease. Brit. J. Haemat. 8, 251 (1962).

29. Vlahovic, V., O. Beleznay, and M. Juretic: Serological findings in ABO hemolytic disease of the newborn. Vox Sang. (Basel) **15**, 59 (1968).

30. Winstanley, D. P., A. Konugres, and R. R. A. Coombs: Studies on human anti-A sera with special reference to so-called immune anti-A. 1. The A^P-antigen and the specificity of the haemolysin in anti-A sera. Brit. J. Haemat. **3**, 341 (1957).
31. Yokoyama, M., and A. Stegmaier: A new method for detection of immune-type of anti-B antibody. Proc. Soc. exp. Biol. (N. Y.) **119**, 854 (1965).

Prof. Dr. K. Fischer
Abteilung für klinische Immunpathologie,
Universitäts-Kinderklinik und -Poliklinik,
Universitäts-Krankenhaus Eppendorf,
2 Hamburg 20, Martinistraße 52

Discussion

DRZENIEK (Gießen): Using erythrocytes from blood of the umbilical cord we have observed that in some cases it is difficult to obtain clear-cut agglutination patterns with commercial anti-A- and anti-B-sera. Treatment of the erythrocytes with neuraminidase, however, improves the agglutination pattern and leads to higher titers. It could be conceivable that in the newborn A, B-receptors on the erythrocytic surface are blocked by N-Acetylneuraminic acid.

SPRINGER (Evanston): This suggestion seems somewhat complicated. — It should be stressed that ABO antigens are universally distributed not only in cells but also in secretions. This is different from the Rh antigen which is confined to red cells. The haemolysins probably play a decisive role in A-B-O damage. For example, the examination of commercial influenza vaccine regularly reveals that these viruses possess A-substance. The vaccine is able to elicit A-antibodies. These agglutinate and produce haemolysis. Cross reacting anti-B-haemolysins then also occur. Many abortions are found in families with heamolysins, essentially more than in families without haemolysins.

Bayer-Symposium I, 194—210 (1969)

From the Medical Clinic, University of Tübingen
(Director Prof. Dr. H.-E. Bock)

Immune Phenomena in Pernicious Anaemia

W. Hartl

With 12 Figures

The clinical observation of patients with pernicious anaemia who ceased to respond to hog-intrinsic factor preparations after prolonged oral treatment (Schwartz, Taylor) suggested almost 10 years ago that immune processes may play a role in the pathogenesis of this disease. In early trials with pernicious anaemia patients Schwartz, Denmark, succeeded in 1958, simultaneously with Taylor in England, in inhibiting the therapeutical effect of intrinsic factor by previous contact with the serum of certain pernicious anaemia patients. With refined immunological in vitro techniques it was possible to confirm and more closely to investigate the antibody nature of this serum factor blocking intrinsic factor activity (Ardeman, Chanarin, Abels *et al.*, Gottlieb *et al.*, Herbert *et al.*, Jeffries, Sleisinger). Besides the immunological principle active against intrinsic factor, English authors (Taylor *et al.*, Irvine) found another antibody system reacting specifically with antigens of the gastric mucosa in pernicious anaemia and also in certain forms of chronic atrophic gastritis which are now considered as subclinical stages of pernicious anaemia (Dagg, Markson, Moore). This duality of antibody systems in pernicious anaemia shows distinct parallels to the immunological background of Hashimoto's thyroiditis. In both diseases chronic inflammatory processes in the "target organ" of the immunological process, i.e. thyroid or gastric mucosa, lead to destruction of the organ parenchyma and thus cause cessation of secretory function. In view of the obvious relationship between the immunological phenomena, expressed also in a mutual overlapping of serological findings in pernicious anaemia and autoimmune thyroiditis, pernicious anaemia was soon regarded as belonging to the group of autoimmunopathies, before it was possible to provide exact serological proof of the autospecificity of the antibodies.

With the development of adequate in vitro methods in recent years it finally became possible more closely to define and classify the antibodies in pernicious anaemia and atrophic gastritis with regard to their immunological properties.

I. Serology

Two antigen-antibody systems are now of special importance for the clinical immunology of pernicious anaemia (Fig. 1).

1. Antibodies against Intrinsic Factor

Among the immunoglobulins reacting specifically with intrinsic factor there are two variants which differ with regard to their action on the intrinsic factor molecule and thus in their serological specificity (Bardhan *et al.*, Roitt *et al.*, Schade *et al.*, Schwartz, Taylor *et al.*) (Fig. 2).

Antigens	Methods of demonstration

Intrinsic factor	Biological tests
	    (Schwartz, 1960)
	Electrophoresis retention test
	    (Jeffries, 1963)
	Dialysis method
	    (Abels, 1963)
	char coal essay
	    (Ardeman, Chanarin, 1963)

Cytoplasmatic antigens of fundus mucosa	Complement fixation Immunofluorescent essay

Fig. 1. Antibodies in pernicious anaemia

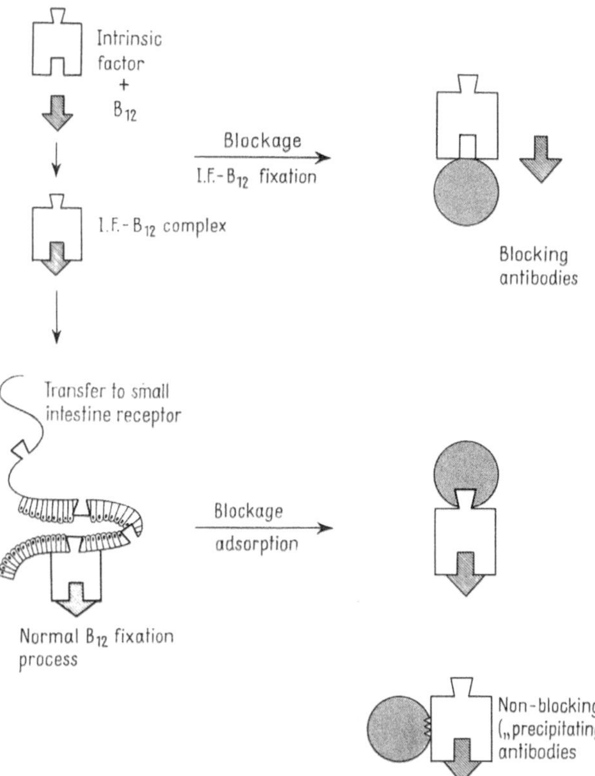

Fig. 2. Different types of intrinsic-factor-specific antibodies, modified from Schwartz, 1960

13*

The most thoroughly examined are the so-called blocking, intrinsic-factor-specific antibodies which by their reaction with intrinsic factor block its "combining site" for vitamin B_{12} ("blocking type antibody").

Two methods, especially, have been developed for the determination of this antibody—the dialysis technique according to Abels *et al.* and the charcoal adsorption method ("charcoal technique") according to Ardeman and Chanarin. The latter method was further improved in recent years (Herbert *et al.*, Gottlieb *et al.*) and owing to its simple technique has become increasingly popular in serological practice[1].

In our own investigations (Hartl, Genth) the gel filtration method (Abels *et al*) was modified for the demonstration of blocking, intrinsic-factor-specific antibodies (Fig. 3).

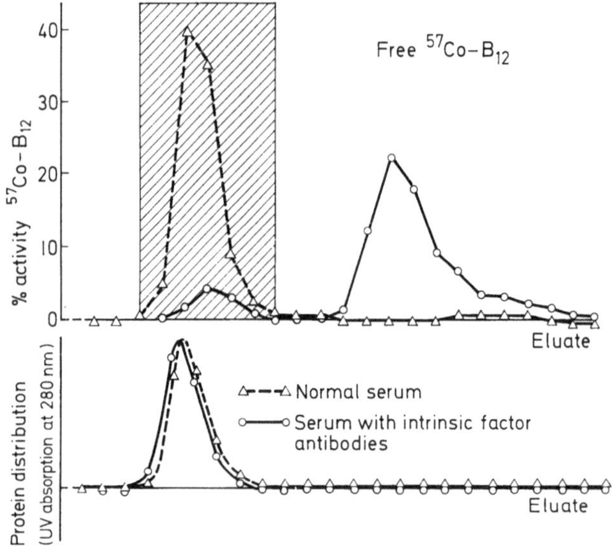

Fig. 3. Demonstration of blocking intrinsic factor antibodies by means of gel filtration on Sephadex G-25 fine

When normal serum and intrinsic factor are mixed and ^{37}cobalt labeled vitamin B_{12} is added, the radioactivity of vitamin B_{12}-intrinsic factor complex is found in the protein fraction of the eluate after passage over a column of the gel Sephadex G-25. If, however, with the addition of intrinsic factor to antibody-containing serum the binding of vitamin B_{12} by intrinsic factor is blocked, the free vitamin B_{12} enters the gel and therefore appears in the eluate later.

Fig. 4 summarises the results in a total of 15 sera of patients with pernicious anaemia and 4 other patients with various other conditions. It shows that the method of gel filtration on Sephadex G-25 is suitable for the demonstration of intrinsic-factor-specific antibodies of the blocking type. The results are comparable with those obtained by means of the charcoal adsorption method according to Ardeman and Chanarin.

---

[1] With the use of a standardised antibody preparation this method is also suitable for the quantitative determination of intrinsic factor (Irvine *et al.*).

Besides the blocking type of intrinsic factor antibody there is in pernicious anaemia another antibody variant which reacts with intrinsic factor even after its saturation with vitamin B_{12}. This specific antibody reaction occurs with the intrinsic factor-vitamin B_{12} complex ("complex binding type", Fig. 2).

Antibodies of this type were demonstrated in recent years by electrophoretic methods (Jeffries, Sleisinger) and radio-immune diffusion techniques (Gullberg et al.). The immunological or physico-chemical co-precipitation of the immuno-

				Charcoal technic %	Gel filtration Sephadex G-25 fine Inhibition[a] %
1	Schr., M.	f [b]	Pernicious anaemia	100.0	100.0
2	Mül., A.	f	Pernicious anaemia	76.9	84.4
3	Orz., E.	f	Pernicious anaemia	87.6	93.9
4	Schr., E.	m	Pernicious anaemia	0.7	0.2
5	Gal., D.	m	Pernicious anaemia	0.7	0
6	Sei., M.	m	Pernicious anaemia	0.5	0
7	Epp., O.	m	Pernicious anaemia	0.2	0
8	Kup., G.	f	Pernicious anaemia	0.9	0
9	Schw., K.	f	Pernicious anaemia	0.8	1.4
10	Str., M.	f	Pernicious anaemia	0.4	0
11	Schä., E.	f	Pernicious anaemia	0.9	0
12	Mär., W.	m	Pernicious anaemia	0.7	0
13	Hal., K.	f	Pernicious anaemia	0.2	2.5
14	Gen., Ch.	f	Pernicious anaemia	0	4.8
15	Sta., K.	m	Pernicious anaemia	0.6	2.5
16	Fra., R.	f	Achlorhydria	99.1	99.0
17	Käch., A.	f	Hyperthyroidism	38.4	39.6
18	Mach., R.	f	Addison's disease	48.3	50.3
19	Ste., L.	f	Megaloblastic anaemia	77.8	65.9
20—29		5 f/5 m	Blood donors (n = 10)	$\bar{x} \triangleq 0$; s = 0.95	$\bar{x} \triangleq 0$; s = 1.82

Correlation (Spearman) $r_s = + 0.964$; $\alpha < 0.01$

[a] maximal ^{57}Co-B_{12}-Inhibition [$\triangleq 0.002097$ IE intrinsic factor]

[b] f = female, m = male

Fig. 4. Results with the charcoal method and gel filtration for blocking type intrinsic factor antibodies

globulins of pernicious anaemia serum is also suitable for the demonstration of non-blocking intrinsic factor antibodies (Schade et al.).

In our own investigations (Hartl, Genth) the method of gel filtration on Sephadex G-200 was used for the demonstration of complex-binding, intrinsic-factor-specific antibodies.

With the passage of a mixture of antibody-containing serum and intrinsic factor-vitamin B_{12} complex over a Sephadex G-200 gel the immune complex appears in the eluate distinctly earlier than the vitamin B_{12}-intrinsic factor complex added to normal serum, which is of smaller molecular size (Fig. 5).

As shown in Fig. 6, in the comparison between the methods of gel filtration and immunological co-precipitation using antihuman-IgG rabbit serum a good correlation between positive and negative results is found.

                               W. Hartl

Intrinsic-factor-specific antibodies from the serum of pernicious anaemia patients as a rule belong to the 7S or IgG type of immunoglobulins (Ardeman, Chanarin) as confirmed by our own investigations (Hartl *et al.*) and are therefore transmissible via the placenta (Bar Shany, Herbert, Fisher *et al.*). With regard to the genetic structure they are heterogenic, as shown by Bernier and Hines in investigations with precipitating anti-BJK- and BJL-sera. Intrinsic-factor-

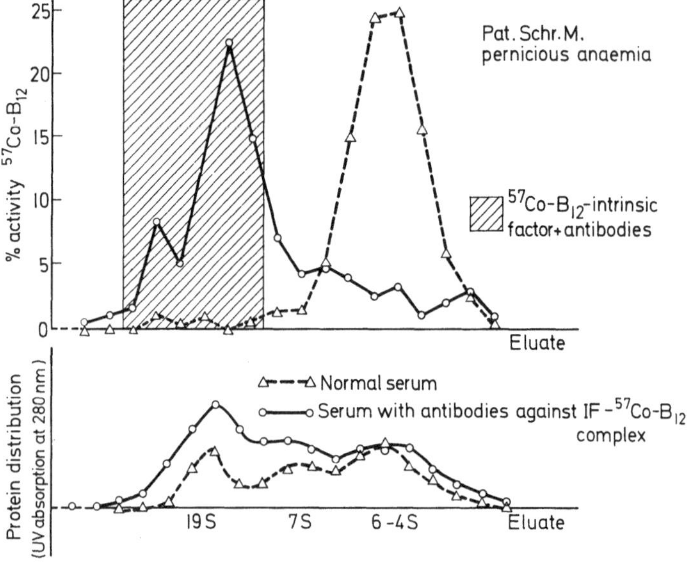

Fig. 5. Demonstration of antibodies against intrinsic factor-B$_{12}$ complex by means of gel filtration on Sephadex G-200-fine

			Co-precipitation (anti-human IgG) %	Gel filtration Sephadex G-200 % activity[a]
1. Schr., M.	f[b]	Pernicious anaemia	45.3	67
2. Mül., A.	f	Pernicious anaemia	24.6	61
3. Orz., E.	f	Pernicious anaemia	22.1	32
4.—14. (n = 12)	f	Pernicious anaemia (cases without IF-B$_{12}$-antibodies)	$\bar{x}=1.58; s=0.619$	$\bar{x} = 3.3; s = 0.4$
15. Mach., R.	f	Adrenal insufficiency	0.7	3.0
16. Käch., A.	f	Hyperthyroidism	1.0	3.5
17. Ste., H.	f	Megaloblastic anaemia	0.4	4.3
18.—27.	5f/5m	Blood donors (n = 10)	$\bar{x} = 1.36; s = 0.65$	$\bar{x} = 3.2; s = 2.36$
Ratio: Serum/^{57}Co-B$_{12}$ standard gastric juice			0.2	1.25

[a] Activity IF-B$_{12}$ antibody complex/total activity $\times$ 100
[b] f = female, m = male

Fig. 6. Results of co-precipitation and gel filtration for antibodies against intrinsic factor-B$_1$[2] complex

specific antibodies demonstrated in the gastric juice of pernicious anaemia patients belong to the immunoglobulin type IgA (South, Cooper).

Intrinsic factor antibodies are strongly species-specific (Ramsey, Herbert), and only the antibody with human specificity is typical of pernicious anaemia (Gullberg *et al.*). Antibodies against hog-intrinsic factor are generally rare in patients. We found no seropositive cases of this kind in 15 pernicious anaemia patients. The more frequent occurrence of hog-intrinsic-factor-specific antibodies in Northern Europe is attributed to the formerly common therapeutic use of preparations from hog stomach in the oral treatment of pernicious anaemia in these regions (Gullberg *et al.*).

2. Antibodies against Antigens of the Gastric Fundus Mucosa

Besides the intrinsic-factor-specific immunoglobulins, antibodies against antigens of the gastric fundus mucosa are of special importance for the clinical immunology of pernicious anaemia and chronic gastritis.

Antibodies against gastric mucosa antigens in the serum of pernicious anaemia patients were at first demonstrated by means of the complement fixation test (Markson, Moore), using homogenates of the gastric fundus mucosa. Far more sensitive than this technique is the immuno-fluorescent essay on frozen sections of gastric fundus mucosa. This procedure was adapted by Irvine to the immuno-pathology of pernicious anaemia and atrophic gastritis from the method suggested earlier by Coons and Kaplan in 1950. With this technique it is possible to localise the antibody reaction with mucosa antigens in the parietal cells of the gastric fundus mucosa (Fig.7). As shown in further investigations with gastric mucosa homogenates, the mucosa antibody reacts with cytoplasmatic antigens of the parietal cells and more particularly with the microsomal fraction of the mucosa extract (Baur *et al.*). Examinations by the electron-microscope of the antigen substrate (Ward, Nairn) further showed that the antigen-antibody reaction takes place only with the smooth membranes and not with the rough ones or the ribosomes.

The mucosa antibodies in pernicious anaemia or immunogastritis are, in the majority of cases, immunoglobulins of the 7S or IgG type (Baur *et al.*, Fisher, Taylor, Irvine, Jeffries *et al.*) and can pass the placenta. In only 2 out of a total of 41 seropositive cases in our own material we were able to demonstrate IgM type antibodies. All the other sera contained IgG-antibodies. In this serological study we did not find IgA-type antibodies against parietal cells. Although mucosa-specific antibodies are organ-specific, they are not as strictly species-specific as e.g. the antimicrosomal thyroid antibodies in Hashimoto's thyroiditis.

Parietal cell antibodies can also be demonstrated by immunofluorescence using rat stomach as substrate. However, this method is not quite as sensitive as with the use of stomach of human origin (Jeffries *et al.*).

Like the intrinsic factor antibodies, parietal cell antibodies are structurally heterogenic and polyclonal, as we could show by immunofluorescence techniques.

After incubation of gastric mucosa sections with patients sera containing parietal cell antibodies the tissue is treated with monospecific anti-BJK- und BJL-sera from rabbit of SEVAC, Prag. The preparation is developed with fluoresceinated anti-rabbit serum from the goat. With all of 14 seropositive pernicious anaemia sera a positive immunofluorescence

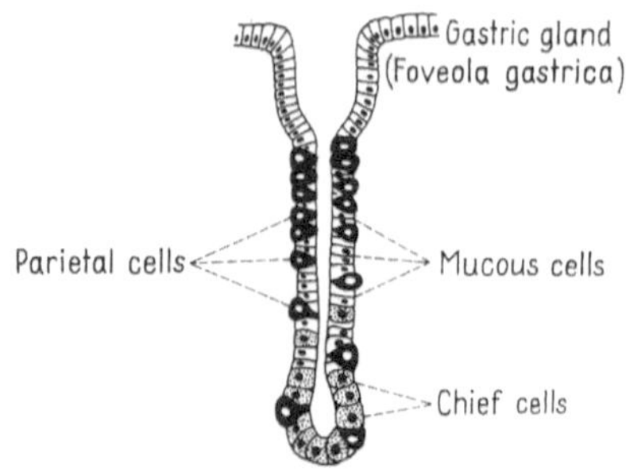

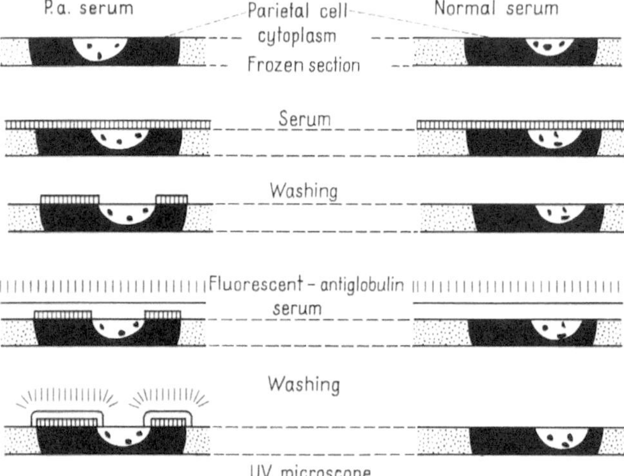

Fig. 7. Demonstration of parietal cell antibody by the indirect immunofluorescent essay according to Coons and Kaplan, 1950

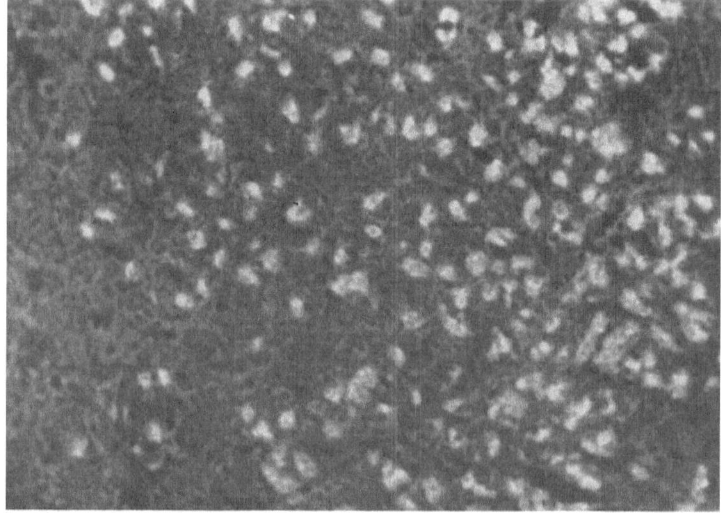

Fig. 8. Positive immunofluorescence of parietal cells with the serum of a patient with pernicious anaemia

of the parietal cells could be produced with anti-BJK and BJL sera. The tests with sera of healthy blood donors remained negative.

In a different immuno-histological set up we were able to show, that the antigen-antibody reaction on the cytoplasma of the parietal cells fixes complement.

A frozen section of gastric fundus mucosa is first treated with the patient's serum containing parietal-cell-specific antibodies. Fresh human serum of the AB blood group is used

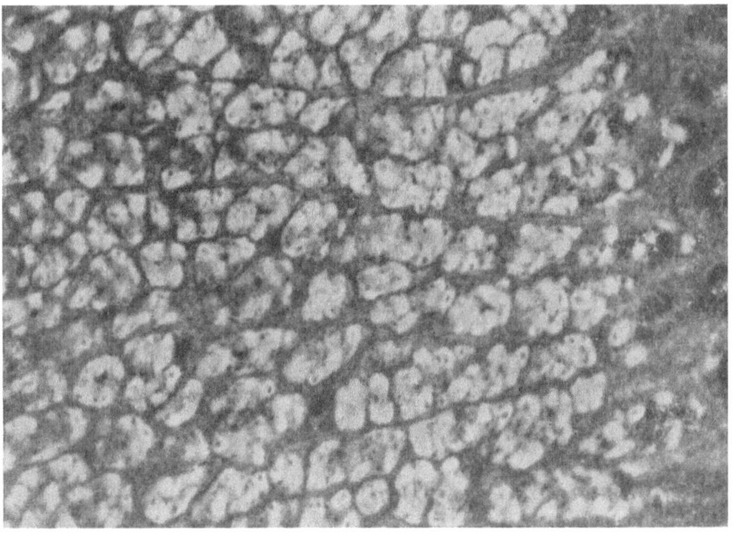

a

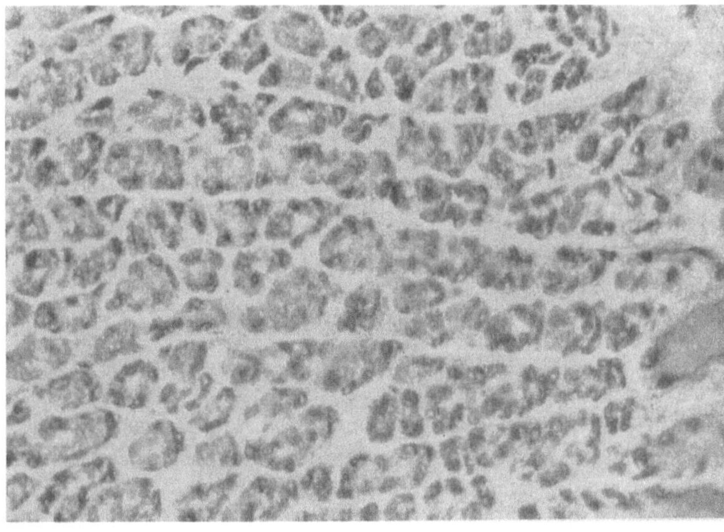

b

Fig. 9. Demonstration that cells giving positive immunofluorescence are parietal cells: The gastric mucosa section was photographed after the fluorescent-antihuman-globulin test (a), stained afterwards with PAS-haematoxylin-aurantia and then rephotographed (b). The stained parietal cells are identical with the immunofluorescence-producing cells

as complement source. The parietal cells show specific immunofluorescence when the preparation is developed with a fluorescein-labelled anti-β_{1A} serum. (Negative results with the addition of EDTA to the test system an with the use of previously inactivated sera.)

II. The Importance of Immunological Findings for the Clinical Diagnosis of Pernicious Anaemia

Biermer's disease, of course, represents an etiologically heterogenic clinical picture in which a vitamin B_{12} deficiency state develops on the basis of insufficient intrinsic factor production. Characteristic disturbances of haemopoiesis with a megaloblastic anaemia, achlorhydria of the gastric juice resistant to stimulation and various defects of neurological functions dominate the clinical picture.

How can the clinician use the serological findings for the diagnosis of pernicious anaemia ?

Decrease of depth of gastric mucosa by atrophy of gastric glands.

Replacement of differentiated mucosa epithelium (chief and parietal cells) by undifferentiated or mucous secreting cells, intestinal metaplasia.

Inflammatory infiltration of mocusa layers with lymphocytes (lymph follicles) and plasma cells (Russel bodies).

Reduction in the secretion of hydrochloric acid, pepsin, and intrinsic factor into the gastric juice.

Fig. 10. Criteria of chronic atrophic gastritis according to Hafter, 1965

Chronic atrophic gastritis, closely connected pathogenetically with the development of pernicious anaemia, can be very well diagnosed clinically by bioptic and functional criteria.

Chronic atrophic gastritis is characterised histologically by a loss of height of the mucosa epithelium on the basis of an atrophy of the gland ducts (Fig. 10). The secretorily active chief and parietal cells of the fundus mucosa are replaced by cells of minimal differentiation or producing mucin (intestinal metaplasia). According to the stage of gastritis, there is a more or less marked infiltration of all mucosa layers with lymphocytes and plasma cells. The functionally prominent symptom is the diminution of hydrochloric acid, pepsin and intrinsic factor secretion which in pernicious anaemia can lead to complete cessation of secretory function (Hafter, Sielaff, James *et al.*).

The evaluation of immunological parameters enables the clinician to differentiate more closely the diagnosis of a chronic gastritis, taking into account etiological points of view (Brus *et al.*).

As shown in a tentative classification of chronic atrophic gastritis (Fig. 11), gastritis in a pernicious anaemia patient is very often associated with the demonstration of intrinsic-factor-specific antibodies. Concerning the blocking type of this antibody, the figures reported in the literature fluctuate between 30% and 60%, depending on the method used (Abels *et al.*, Fisher *et al.*, Irvine *et al.*). In our own investigations (Hartl *et al.*), carried out by means of the charcoal-technique and gel filtration with Sephadex G-25, blocking intrinsic factor antibodies were demonstrated in about $^1/_4$ (5 out of 19) of pernicious anaemia cases. Three of these seropositive sera also contained complex-binding-type intrinsic factor antibodies, as shown with the co-precipitation technique and gel filtration on Sephadex G-200. The corresponding figures for intrinsic factor antibodies of the complex-binding type in pernicious anaemia patients are between 20% and 45% (Bardhan et al., Irvine et al.) in the literature. The fact that a relatively large proportion of pernicious anaemia sera, despite definitely confirmed clinical diagnosis, contained no intrinsic-factor-specific antibodies—the percentage of seronegative cases in our own material was over 75%—provides further evidence that certainly not all cases of pernicious anaemia are of immunological origin. We were able to demonstrate blocking intrinsic factor antibodies in 4 cases where clinically pernicious anaemia did certainly not exist. (Diagnoses: achlorhydria, hyperthyroidism, adrenal in-

	Pernicious anaemia	"Idiopathic gastritis"	Gastric neoplasia, peptic ulcer
Antibodies (serum) to intrinsic factor			
blocking type:	5/19 [30—60%]	2/40 [O]	O
complex binding type:	3/17 [20—45%]	0/25 [O]	O
mucosa antigen			
CFT	12/18 [40—75%]	11/18 [20—40%][b]	O
immunofluorescent test	17/20 [75—96%]	15/24 [20—60%][b]	O
Decrease of serum complement levels[a]	++	O	O
IgA globulin deposits in mucosa infiltrates	+	++	+

[a] acc. to Brus, Glass et al., 1968.

[b] with achlorhydria.

[] Roitt et al., 1966; Irvine, 1965; Fisher et al., 1965; Jeffries et al., 1965; Markson et al., 1962; Brus, Glass et al., 1968.

Fig. 11. Tentative classification of chronic atrophic gastritis on the basis of immunological findings (Hartl, Genth, Waldeck, 1968)

sufficiency, megaloblastic anaemia of uncertain origin.) The serological finding in regard to the presence or absence of intrinsic-factor-specific antibodies therefore neither proves nor excludes pernicious anaemia and can be interpreted only in close consideration of the clinical state.

In forms of atrophic gastritis called "idiopathic" more definite information on their etiology is still lacking. Intrinsic factor-specific antibodies are usually not found in this condition. The same applies to atrophic gastritis in gastric carcinoma or certain gastric ulcers (Finlayson et al., Brus et al.).

Antibodies against parietal cells are demonstrable in a high percentage of cases of pernicious anaemia; 75% to 96% when immunofluorescent techniques are employed (Irvine et al., Jeffries et al., Roitt et al., Taylor et al.). In our own material 17 out of 20 pernicious anaemia patients had parietal-cell-specific antibodies in their sera. With the use of the less sensitive complement fixation test mucosa-specific antibodies were found, according to the literature, in 40% to 75% of pernicious anaemia cases (Irvine, Taylor et al.). The importance of the demonstration of mucosa-specific antibodies for the diagnosis of pernicious anaemia is stressed by some authors (Bernhard *et al.*), who suggest to reconsider the diagnosis of pernicious anaemia if, with sufficiently sensitive techniques, parietal cell antibodies cannot be demonstrated.

In the idiopathic forms of chronic gastritis the proportion of seropositive cases with parietal cell antibodies is distinctly lower than in the pernicious anaemia group, i.e. 20% to 60% with the use of fluorescent techniques and 20% to 40% with the complement fixation test (Fisher, Taylor, Roitt *et al.*). The largest proportion of seropositive cases in this group is represented by gastritis cases with achlorhydria and those with iron deficiency states (Dagg *et al.*, Markson, Moore). Women with "idiopathic" gastritis are more likely to be seropositive than men (Coghill *et al.*, Roitt *et al.*). With higher age of the patients the proportion of positive serological findings increases (Roitt *et al.*). 15 out of 24 of our own patients with histamine-refractory achlorhydria had parietal cell antibodies in their serum. Impressed by these immunological findings, numerous authors to-day believe that seropositive forms of gastritis represent early stages of pernicious anaemia (Dagg, Goldberg *et al.*, Irvine). Patients with "concomitant gastritis" (Begleitgastritis) in gastric neoplasm or ulcer as well as after gastrectomy as a rule have no mucosa-specific antibodies (Brus *et al.*, Finlayson *et al.*, Kravetz *et al.*) in their blood. Positive serological findings may be seen only in carcinoma patients where the gastric tumor has developed in association with pernicious anaemia on the basis of atrophic gastritis (Shearman *et al.*).

Pernicious anaemia patients very often have in their blood antibodies reacting specifically with thyroid antigens. The incidence of positive thyroid antibody findings in pernicious anaemia is reported to be about 40% (Irvine). Conversely, in about 5% of cases with hyperthyroidism intrinsic-factor-specific antibodies may be found (Roitt *et al.*) and parietal cell antibodies in about 30% of the cases (Evans *et al.*, Irvine, Williams *et al.*). In autoimmune thyroiditis the percentage of positive parietal cell antibody findings is about 15 to 30% (Irvine, Irvine *et al.*, Markson, Moore). The overlapping of serological findings in pernicious anaemia and certain thyroid conditions (hyperthyroidism, primary myxoedema, hypothyroidism) is in accordance with the findings of a syntropy of certain symptoms in both clinical pictures, as has been emphasized in the literature repeatedly. According to Tudhope as well as Markson and Moore, about one half of all cases of hypothyroidism have a histamine refractory achlorhydria, with a considerable incidence of pathological Schilling tests. In accordance with the findings of Roitt *et al.*, Faber and Elling, we have not observed any overlapping of serological findings with antibodies typical for lupus erythematosus in our pernicious anaemia patients.[2]

Glass and his group (Brus *et al.*, Jakob *et al.*) discuss as a further immunological criterium of atrophic gastritis in pernicious anaemia the lowering of the blood complement level in this condition. By the determinations of the β_{1A}-globulin concentrations in the serum of 17 pernicious anaemia patients we were unable to

---

[2] Cytoplasmatic antibodies in lupus erythematosus or biliary liver cirrhosis (Roitt, Doniach) can lead to false positive results in immunofluorescent tests on gastric mucosa sections despite a slightly different fluorescent pattern. The anticytoplasmatic antibodies in lupus erythematosus are not, however, organ-specific and can easily be identified by control tests, e.g. on thyroid sections or leucocyte preparations.

confirm a decrease of serum complement levels as postulated by these authors. As shown in Fig. 12, the majority of β_{1A}-levels of pernicious anaemia sera was low but within the normal range. The individual values did not correspond to the antibody titres.

A final judgement on the usefulness of serum complement determinations in patients with atrophic gastritis will probably be possible only after more extensive studies on a wider scale. The same applies to the observation of an increase in IgA-globulin-producing plasma cells and of an increased deposition of this globulin in the cellular infiltrates of the gastric mucosa in pernicious anaemia (Crabbé). These findings may be of special interest in regard to the pathogenesis of chronic atrophic gastritis.

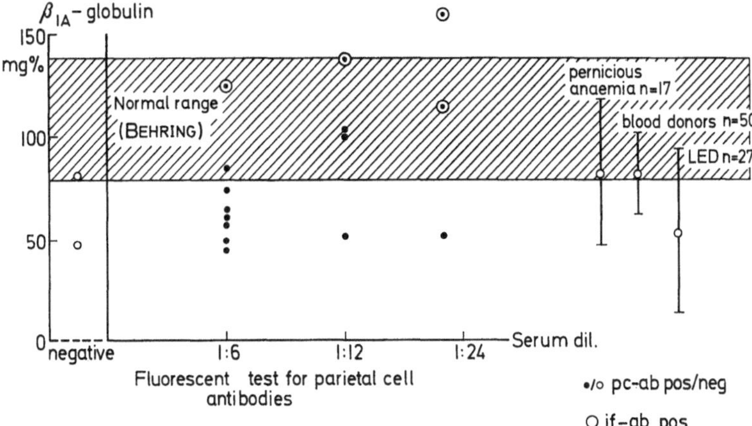

Fig. 12. β_{1A}-globulin serum levels and intrinsic factor antibodies or parietal cell antibodies in 17 patients with P. A.

The validity of serological findings for the diagnosis of pernicious anaemia can briefly be summarised as follows:

The finding of intrinsic-factor-specific antibodies and the demonstration of antibodies against parietal cells of the gastric fundus mucosa are, as a rule, associated with

1. histological changes of chronic atrophic gastritis and

2. a diminution of secretory function of the gastric mucosa with regard to hydrochloric acid and intrinsic factor.

There is no proportionality between the serological findings and the histological degree of gastritis and certain clinical parameters, such as the duration of pernicious anaemia, the manifestation of the neurological complications, the result of the Schilling test and the degree of the diminution of secretory function of the gastric mucosa (Adams et al., Coghill et al.). Serological findings which reflect chronic inflammatory processes of atrophic gastritis, may precede the manifestation of pernicious anaemia by years and may be recognised even before the gastric secretion of hydrochloric acid and intrinsic factor ceases. Clinical serology of pernicious anaemia should therefore be important also for prophylactic medicine, e.g. for the recognition of prepernicious stages of Biermer's disease or for studies in relatives of pernicious anaemia patients (Irvine *et al.*, te Velde *et al.*, Wangel, Schiller).

Scandinavian authors (Schwartz, Bastrup Madsen) recently observed that after the injection of certain vitamin B_{12}-preparations a high blood level of this vitamin was maintained for a prolonged time in some patients. This phenomenon was explained as an antibody like principle, directed against the serum protein transcobalamine II which is important for the transport of vitamin B_{12} in the blood. (Hom *et al.*, Olesen *et al.*). Thus another very interesting immune phenomenon in pernicious anaemia has become known whose importance for pathophysiological relationships of the disease is still not clear.

III. Concepts of the Immunopathogenesis of Pernicious Anaemia

As in most autoimmunopathies, almost nothing is known so far about the immunological pathomechanisms underlying the manifestations of atrophic gastritis and pernicious anaemia. The lack of any strict correlation of antibody titres with the clinical condition is a rather strong argument against the concept, that circulating antibodies against intrinsic factor or mucosa antigens in the patient's serum may play a major role in the pathogenesis of these diseases. A further argument against the pathogenic role of humoral antibodies are observations in babies of mothers with pernicious anaemia in whose blood the antibodies transmitted via placenta were demonstrated in the absence of any clinical symptoms of the disease.[3]

While intrinsic factor antibodies circulating in the serum of patients apparently do not interfere with vitamin B_{12} transport from the food via the intestinal wall into the blood, the demonstration of these antibodies in the gastric juice has again focused interest on humoral immune reactions in regard to the pathogenesis of pernicious anaemia (Schade *et al.*). These intrinsic factor antibodies in the gastric juice of pernicious anaemia patients are IgA-immunoglobulins. Proteins of this type may be produced locally in the gastric mucosa, as was recently shown by Crabbé *et al.* employing immunofluorescent techniques. It may be tempting to speculate that in pernicious anaemia intrinsic-factor-specific antibodies, produced locally in the same place as intrinsic factor itself, can immunologically block the biological functions of the latter, thus causing the vitamin B_{12} deficiency state so characteristic of the disease.

A cytotoxic effect of parietal cell antibodies has not been proved convincingly so far. We do not share therefore the opinion of some gastro-enterologists (Glass *et al.*) who postulate a relation between the lowering of blood-complement levels in pernicious anaemia patients as observed by them and an antigen-antibody reaction taking place in the parietal cells of the fundus mucosa. We are confirmed in our opinion by the so far unsuccessful attempts to demonstrate locally complement or complement factors in stomach biopsy specimens from patients with seropositive atrophic gastritis.

Since the pathogenic role of immune reactions of the humoral type cannot be proved yet convincingly in pernicious anaemia the pathogenesis of autoimmune

---

[3] Only Bar Shany and Herbert report on a child who went through a temporary vitamin B_{12} deficiency state with positive serological findings caused by transplacentally transmitted intrinsic factor antibodies of the mother.

gastritis and Biermer's disease was explained on the basis of immune reactions of the delayed type. But also this theory has to be proved.

Certain cases of pernicious anaemia respond to the administration of gluco-steroid preparations not only with an increase of reticulocytes (Bock *et al.*) but also with a regeneration of the fundus mucosa demonstrable by biopsy and with re-establishment of intrinsic factor secretion. This clinical observation may not yet contribute anything concrete to the pathogenesis of immunogastritis, but nevertheles appears to be of interest in this connection.

The present state of knowledge in regard to the immunopathogenesis of atrophic gastritis and pernicious anaemia, is restricted to some antibody systems which react specifically with autologous antigen substrates in vitro. Since it is not yet possible to produce by immunological methods either a progressive gastritis or a condition resembling pernicious anaemia in animals, the premisses for a study of the pathogenesis of the diseases are even worse than e.g. in autoimmune thyroditis. The latter can be induced very well in animal experiments and transmitted to other animals by immune-competent cells in transfer experiments. The criteria formu-lated by Milgrom and Witebsky as prerogatives for recognising a disease as an autoimmunopathy are even less fulfilled in the case of pernicious anaemia than in most other autoimmune diseases.

In the scope of a working hypothesis the pictures of immunogastritis and pernicious anaemia have been classified among the so-called organ-specific auto-immunopathies. In support of this view are the character and specifity of the antibodies demonstrable in these conditions and the numerous immunological parallels with Hashimoto's disease. Other subjects of hypotheses are disturb-ances of immune tolerance postulated in these concepts, disturbances which cause a normally functioning immune system not to recognise autologous sub-strate as "self" any more and to initiate auto-aggressive immune processes, with the final result of extensive organ destruction. It has been discussed whether this failure of the immune system is a basically genetic error (te Velde *et al.*, Sharpstone, Chanarin, Ardeman).

Summary

Of special importance for the clinical immunopathology of chronic atrophic gastritis and pernicious anaemia are intrinsic-factor-specific antibodies and anti-bodies against parietal cells of the gastric mucosa. The serological findings allow a further etiological differentiation in cases of chronic atrophic gastritis. Gastritis in pernicious anaemia is often associated with intrinsic factor antibodies whereas parietal cell antibodies are found in nearly all cases. In the heterogenic group of so-called "idiopathic" gastritis intrinsic factor antibodies are usually not demon-strable while parietal cell antibodies may be found especially in cases where the gastritis is associated with achlorhydria. In concomitant gastritis ("Begleit-gastritis") of gastric ulcer or neoplasia antibodies usually are not demonstrable.

The role of intrinsic factor antibodies in the gastric juice with regard to the pathogenesis of pernicious anaemia is not yet clear. Since these antibodies are possibly produced in the gastric mucosa they could react with intrinsic factor at its site of formation and interfere with its biological function on vitamin B_{12} transport.

References

Abels, J., W. Bouma, A. Jansz, M. G. Woldring, A. Bakker, and H. O. Nieweg: Experiments on the intrinsic factor antibody in serum from patients with pernicious anemia. J. Lab. clin. med. **61**, 893—906 (1963).

Adams, J. F., A. I. M. Glen, E. H. Kennedy, I. L. Mackenzie, J. M. Morrow, J. R. Anderson, K. G. Grey, and D. G. Middleton: The histological and secretory changes in the stomach in patients with autoimmunity to gastric parietal cells. Lancet **1964 I**, 401—403.

Ardeman, S., and I. Chanarin: A method for the assay of human gastric intrinsic factor and for the detection and titration of antibodies against intrinsic factor. Lancet **1963 II**, 1350—1354.

— — Steroids and Addisonian pernicious anemia. New Engl. J. Med. **273**, 1352—1355 (1965).

— — Intrinsic factor antibodies and intrinsic factor mediated vitamin B_{12} absorption in pernicious anaemia. Gut **6**, 436—443 (1965).

Bar Shany, and V. Herbert: Transplacentally acquired antibody to intrinsic factor with vitamin B_{12} deficiency. Blood **30**, 777—784 (1964).

Bardhan, K. D., J. R. Hall, G. H. Spray, and S. T. E. Callender: Blocking and binding type autoantibody to intrinsic factor. Lancet **1968 I**, 62—64.

Baur, S., I. M. Roitt, and D. Doniach: Characterization of the human gastric parietal cell autoantigen. Immunology 8, 62—68 (1965).

Bernhardt, H., L. L. Burkett, M. L. Field, and J. Kilian: The diagnostic significance of parietal cell immunofluorescent test. Ann. intern. Med. **63**, 635—641 (1965).

Bernier, G. M., and J. D. Hines: Immunological heterogeneity of autoantibodies in patients with pernicious anemia. New Engl. J. Med. **277**, 1386—1391 (1967).

Bock, H. E.: Fortschritte in der Erkennung und Behandlung megalozytärer Anämien. Regensburg. Jb. ärztl. Fortbild. 8, 1—4 (1959/60).

Brus, I., G. B. J. Glass, J. E. Siegel, H. I. Tanaka, H. Weisberg, and N. Yamaguchi: Immunological differentiation of etiologic types of atrophic gastritis. 8th International Congress of Gastroenterology, Prag 1968.

Chanarin, I., A. Jakobs, L. Griffiths, and S. Ardeman: Family study in Addisonian pernicious anemia. Blood **27**, 599—610 (1966).

Clark, R., K. Tornyos, V. Herbert, and J. J. Twomey: Studies on 2 patients with concomitant pernicious and immunoglobulin deficiency. Ann. intern. Med. **67**, 403—410 (1967).

Coghill, N. F., D. Doniach, I. M. Roitt, D. L. Mollin, and A. W. Williams: Autoantibodies in simple atrophic gastritis. Gut **6**, 48—56 (1965).

Coons, A. H., and M. H. Kaplan: Localisation of antigen in tissue cells. J. exp. Med. **91**, 1—13 (1950).

Crabbé, E. A., A. O. Carbonera, and J. F. Heremans: The normal human intestinal mucosa as major source of plasma cells containing IgA immunoglobulin. Lab. invest. **14**, 235—248 (1965).

Dagg, I. M., A. Goldberg, W. N. Gibbs, and J. R. Anderson: Detection of latent pernicious anemia in patients with iron deficiency anemia. Brit. med. J. **1966 II**, 619—621.

Dagg, J. H., A. Goldberg, J. R. Anderson, J. S. Beck, and K. G. Gray: Autoimmunity in iron deficiency anaemia. Brit. med. J. **1964 II**, 1349—1350.

— — — — — Auto-immunity in iron deficient anaemia. Ann. N. Y. Acad. Sci. **124**, 692—695 (1965).

Doniach, D., I. M. Roitt, and K. B. Taylor: Autoimmune phenomena in pernicious anemia. Brit. med. J. **1963 I**, 1374—1379.

Evans, A. W. H., J. C. Woodrow, C. C. M. McDougall, A. R. Chew, and R. W. Evans: Antibodies in the families of thyrotoxic patients. Lancet **1967 I**, 636—641.

Faber, V., and P. Elling: Anti-nuclear-factors (ANF) as determined by the immunofluorescent-antibody technique. Acta med. scand. **177**, 309—319 (1965).

Finlayson, N. D., D. J. C. Shearman, and R. H. Girdwood: Intrinsic factor production and immunological status in patients with gastric carcinoma. 8th International Congress of Gastroenterology, Prag 1968.

Fisher, J. M., and K. B. Taylor: A comparison of autoimmune phenomena in pernicious anemia and chronic atrophic gastritis. New Engl. J. Med. **272**, 449—503 (1965).

— — Placental transfer of gastric antibodies. Lancet **1967 I**, 695—698.

Fisher, J. M., I. R. Mackay, K. B. Taylor, and B. Ungar: An immunological study of categories of gastritis. Lancet **1967 I**, 176—180.

Goodman, D. H., and R. S. Smith: Hypogamma-globulinemia, allergy and absence of intrinsic factor. J. Allergy **40**, 131—134 (1967).

Gottlieb, C., K. S. Lau, L. R. Wasserman, and V. Herbert: Rapid charcaol assay for intrinsic factor, gastric juice unsaturated B_{12}-binding capacity, antibody to IF and serum unsaturated B_{12}-binding capacity. Blood **25**, 884 (1965).

Gullberg, R., S. Kistner, L. E. Böttiger, and U. Evaldsson: Precipitating serum antibodies to intrinsic factor in pernicious anemia. Acta med. scand. **180**, 87—94 (1966).

Hafter, E.: Praktische Gastroenterologie, pp 165—166. Stuttgart: Thieme 1965.

Hartl, W., u. E. Genth: Zum Nachweis intrinsic factor-spezifischer Antikörper mit Hilfe der Gel Filtration. Klin. Wschr. **47**, 89—93, 1969.

— — und H.H. Waldeck: Autoimmunphaenomene bei perniziöser Anämie und atrophischer Gastritis. Dtsch. med. Wschr. **93**, 641—652 (1968).

Herbert, V., C. Gottlieb, Kam-Seng-Lau, and R. L. Wasserman: Intrinsic factor assay. Lancet **1964 II**, 1017—1018.

Hom, B. L., H. Olesen, and M. Schwartz: Turnover of ^{57}Co labelled vitamin B_{12}-transcobalamin II and autologeous ^{131}J labelled IgG in a patient with antibodies to transcobalamin II. Scand. J. haemat. **5**, 107—115 (1968).

Irvine, W. J.: Gastric antibodies studied by fluorescence microscopy. Quart. J. exp. Physiol. **48**, 427—444 (1963).

— Immunologic aspects of pernicious anemia. New Engl. J. Med. **273**, 432—438 (1965).

—, S. H. Davies, I. W. Delamore, and A. W. Williams: Immunological relationsship between pernicious anemia and thyroid disease. Brit. med. J. **1962 II**, 454—456.

— —, R. C. Haynes, and L. Scarth: Secretion of intrinsic factor in response to histamine and to gastrin in the diagnosis of Addisonian pernicious anemia. Lancet **1965 II**, 397—401.

— —, S. Teitelbaum, I. W. Delamore, and W. W. Williams: The clinical and pathological significance of gastric parietal cell antibody. Ann. N. Y. Acad. Sci. **124**, 691 (1965).

Jakob, E., and G. B. J. Glass: Complement participation in parietal cell antibody antigen reaction in the gastric mucosa. XIIth Congress International Society of Hematology, New York 1968.

James, W. B., A. G. Melrose, J. W. Davidson, and R. I. Russel: Radiological diagnosis of gastritis. Gut **6**, 372—375 (1965).

Jeffries, G. H.: Parietal antibodies. Ann. intern. Med. **63**, 717—719 (1965).

—, and M. H. Sleisinger: The immunologic identification and quantitation of human intrinsic factor in gastric secretions. J. clin. Invest. **42**, 442—449 (1963).

— —, and S. Margolis: Studies of parietal cell antibodies in pernicious anemia. J. clin. Invest. **44**, 2021—2028 (1965).

Kaplan, M. A., R. Zalusky, J. Remington, and V. Herbert: Immunologic studies with intrinsic factor in man. J. clin. Invest. **42**, 368—382 (1963).

Kiossoglou, K. A., W. J. Mitus, and W. Dameshek: Chromosomal aberrations in pernicious anemia. Blood **25**, 662—682 (1965).

Kravetz, R. E., S. van Norden, and H. M. Spiro: Parietal cell antibodies in patients with duodenal ulcer and gastric cancer. Lancet **1967 I**, 235—237.

Markson, J. L., and J. M. Moore: Thyroid antibodies in pernicious anemia. Brit. med. J. **1962**, 1352—1355.

— — Autoimmunity in pernicious anemia and iron deficient anemia. Lancet **1962 II**, 1240 to 1243.

Milgrom, F., and J. Witebsky: J. Amer. med. Ass. **191**, 706—716 (1962).

Olesen, J., B. L. Hom, and M. Schwartz: Antibody to transcobalamin II in patients treated with long acting vitamin B_{12} preparations. Scand. J. haemat. **5**, 5—16 (1968).

Ramsey, C., and V. Herbert: Dialysis essay for intrinsic factor and its antibody: Demonstration of species specificity of antibodies to human and hog intrinsic factor. J. Lab. clin. Med. **65**, 143—152 (1965).

Roitt, I. M., and D. Doniach: Diskussionsbemerkung. Immunopathology, 4. Int. Symp., p. 420. Monte Carlo 1965. Basel, Stuttgart: Schwabe u. Co. Publ. 1966.

— —, and C. Shapland: Intrinsic factor antoantibodies. Brit. med. J. **1964 II**, 469—470.

Roitt, I. M., D. Doniach, and C. Shapland: Autoimmunity in pernicious anemia and atrophic gastritis. Ann. N. Y. Acad. Sci. **124**, 644—656 (1965).

— — — Antoimmune phenomena in relation to gastric mucosa in human disease. Immuno-pathology, 4. Int. Sympos., pp 314—324. Monte Carlo 1965. Basel/Stuttgart: Schwabe u. Co, Publ. 1966.

Schade, S. G., P. Frick, M. H. Irvine, and R. F. Schilling: In vitro studies on antibodies to intrinsic factor. Clin. exp. Immunol. **2**, 399—413 (1967).

— —, M. Muckerheide, and R. F. Schilling: Occurence in gastric juice of antibody to a complex on intrinsic factor and vitamin B_{12}. New Engl. J. Med. **275**, 528 to 531 (1966).

Schwartz, M.: Intrinsic factor inhibiting substance in serum of orally treated patients with pernicious anemia. Lancet **1958 II**, 61—62.

— Intrinsic factor antibody in serum from patients with pernicious anemia. Lancet **1960 II**, 1263—1267.

—, and P. Bastrup Madsen: A new vitamin B_{12}-binding protein in serum causing excessively high serum vitamin B_{12} levels. Scand. J. Haemat. **5**, 35—40 (1968).

Sharpstone, P., and D. G. James: Pernicious anemia and thyrotoxicosis in a family. Lancet **1965 I**, 246—248.

Sherman, D. J. C., N. D. C. Finlayson, R. Wilson, and R. R. Samson: Carcinoma of the stomach and early pernicious anemia. Lancet **1966 II**, 403—404.

Sielaff, H. J.: Die Bedeutung der bioptischen Untersuchung des Intestinaltraktes für die Diagnose und Therapie intestinaler Störungen. Internist **2**, 479—489 (1961).

South, M. A., M. D. Cooper, F. A. Wolheim, R. Hong, and R. A. Good: The IgA-System. J. exp. Med. **123**, 615—627 (1966).

Taylor, K. B.: Inhibition of intrinsic factor by pernicious anemia sera. Lancet **1959 II**, 106 to 107.

—, I. M. Roitt, D. Doniach, K. G. Couchman, and C. Shapland: Autoimmune phenomena in pernicious anemia: Gastric antibodies. Brit. med. J. **1962 II**, 1347—1352.

Tudhope, G. R., and G. M. Wilson: Deficiency of vitamin B_{12} in hypothyroidism. Lancet **1962 I**, 703—706.

te Velde, K., J. Abels, G. J. P. A. Anders, A. Arends, P. J. Hoedemaeker, and H. O. Nieweg: A family study of pernicious anemia by an immunologic method. J. Lab. clin. Med. **64**, 177—187 (1964).

Wall, A. J., S. Whittingham, T. R. Mackay, and B. Ungar: Prednisolone and gastric atrophy. Clin. exp. Immunol. **3**, 359—366 (1968).

Wangel, A. G., and K. F. Schiller: Diagnostic significance of antibody to intrinsic factor. Brit. med. J. **1966 I**, 1274—1276.

Ward, H. A., and R. C. Nairn: Extraction of gastric parietal cell autoantigen. Clin. exp. Immunol. **2**, 565—571 (1967).

Williams, M. J., and G. B. Scott: Antigastric antibodies in hyperthyroidism: Their relation-ship to impaired acid secretion. Brit. med. J. **1966 I**, 388—391.

Priv.-Doz. Dr. W. Hartl
Medizinische Universitätsklinik
74 Tübingen, Olfried-Müller-Straße

Discussion

Müller-Eberhard (La Jolla): Is the antigen localised in the mucosa, is it a membrane associated antigen or a cytoplasmic antigen ? And further: is complement bound in the mucosa ?

Hartl (Tübingen): The antigen has been found in the microsomal fraction of homogenates of gastric mucosa. It is difficult to demonstrate complement bound in the mucosa in patients with pernicious anaemia and advanced gastritis because the mucosa in these cases contains no longer parietal cells. Glass (8th Int. Congress of Gastroenterology, Prague, 1968) interpretes a reduced level of serum complement in sera of patients with pernicious anaemia as an indication of immunologic activity.

ROTHER (Freiburg): It is an open question whether such a reduction of the complement titre indicates a consumption of complement by an antigen-antibody reaction. Even in nephritis in which huge surfaces react, one finds a lowering of the peripheral complement titre only during massive acute reactions.

SPRINGER (Evanston): Are such antibodies also found in people who do not have pernicious anemia ? As we know, the gastric mucosa contains plenty of blood group substances ?

HARTL (Tübingen): We have found intrinsic factor specific antibodies besides in pernicious anaemia only in rare instances e.g. in Addison's disease, in hypo-thyroidism and in one case of megaloblastic anaemia of unknown etiology. On the other hand, one cannot draw any diagnostic conclusion from the absence of intrinsic factor antibodies with regard to pernicious anaemia. Parietal antibodies however are widespread and not specific for pernicious anaemia. I would like to point out, that the absence of mucosa antibodies renders the diagnosis of perni-cious anaemia highly improbable from the serologic point of view.

BOCK (Tübingen): From the cessation of resorption of intrinsic factor until the break-out of a pernicious anaemia, a period of 8 to 16 years may elapse. How-ever, it is by no means permissible to classify pernicious anaemia always as an immunological disease.

FISCHER (Hamburg): In similar studies using immunofluorencence techniques we have great difficulties in eliminating the non-specific reactions. Which techni-que have you used ?

HARTL (Tübingen): I used the procedure of Roitt, Doniach, and Shapland [Ann. N. Y. Acad. Sci. 124, 644—656 (1965)]. Unfixed cryostat sections were developped in the indirect essay of Coons with fluoresceinated antisera of Hyland Inc., Div. Travenol Laboratories, Los Angeles, Calif., USA. With techniques of conjugating sera with fluorescein makers I have no personal experiences.

MÜLLER-EBERHARD (La Jolla): Are the auto-antibodies that have been found in fact pathogenic ?

HARTL (Tübingen): It is known that the IgG antibodies in pernicious anaemia do not probably possess pathogenicity. The intrinsic-factor antibody of the IgA type which may be secreted into the gastric juice can supposedly have a neu-tralising action in vivo. If it could be proved that in chronic gastritis the plasma cells secrete an intrinsinc-factor specific IgA-antibody, some knowledge would be gained with regard to the pathogenesis of pernicious anaemia. For the time being everything remains open.

ROITT (London): If I may make one or two comments to back up what Dr. Hartl has said. Ramsey and Herbert injected a patient with pernicious anemia with Freund's adjuvant mixed with hog intrinsic factor. They produced a very good

14*

circulating antibody to intrinsic factor and a very good delayed hypersensitivity reaction. When they fed hog intrinsic factor by mouth, this was able to mediate the absorption of vitamin B_{12} as well as if the patient had not been immunised. The significance is that intrinsic-factor antibodies, if they are going to neutralise intrinsic factor, have to be in the lumen of the gut. To the question whether these were pathogenic: this is of course a basic question particularly in all organ-specific autoimmune diseases. The earliest experiments showed that feeding intrinsic factor antibodies with gastric juice to a pernicious anaemia patient prevented the intrinsic factor from mediated B_{12} absorption. Later studies have shown the presence of intrinsic factor antibodies in the gastric juice where they would be able to effectively neutralize intrinsic factor.

Ardeman and Chanarin have treated a patient with pernicious anaemia with high doses of prednisone, about 40 mg a day for a few weeks. They found that after this time the production of gastric acid and intrinsic factor in response to histamine had recovered somewhere near normal whereas before the prednisone there had been virtually no production of either. Furthermore, a biopsy showed regeneration of mucosal elements. One reasonable interpretation is that the prednisone was inhibiting the attack by the inflammatory cells and was allowing an underlying regeneration of the mucosal elements to become apparent. I would say that this is reasonable evidence in favour of an aggressive role of the autoimmune reaction.

Bayer-Symposium I, 213—231 (1969)

From the Department of Pathology, Mount Sinai School of Medicine of The City University
of New York, New York 10029

Immune Reactions in Chronic Liver Diseases[1]

F. PARONETTO, and H. POPPER

With 9 Figures

The question of whether or not human liver diseases may be initiated or per-
petuated by immune processes has been raised by a number of observations, not
necessarily related. Among these may be included:

1. Lack of knowledge of the etiology of many acute liver diseases and particularly of such chronic disorders as cirrhosis. The absence of a specific etiologic test
for viral hepatitis hampers progress here.

2. The tendency of chronic liver disease to progress even if a known etiologic
factor has disappeared (self-perpetuation).

3. Appearance of abnormal serologic reactions as well as immunofluorescence
observations in liver diseases.

4. Similarities between histologic manifestations in liver diseases and reactions
known to be on an immunologic basis.

5. The fact that immunosuppressive agents are presumably effective in the
therapy of liver diseases.

While it has been established that abnormal immunologic reactions occur in
liver diseases, their pathogenetic role is still unproven. A review of the available
evidence should therefore consider:

1. The question of liver specific or nonspecific antigens.

2. Existence of antibodies or cell-bound immunity related to liver.

3. Attempts to reproduce chronic perpetuating liver disease by immunologic
reactions in animals and thus establish the pathogenetic role of immunologic
factors.

4. The diseases in which immunologic processes may play a role, particularly
chronic active or aggressive hepatitis, primary biliary cirrhosis and drug-induced
liver injury.

A liver specific antigen, preexisting or resulting from liver damage, is the first
line of investigation for hepatic autoimmune reactions. Its demonstration depends
upon the technique applied and purification. Agar gel diffusion, hemagglutination,
complement fixation, precipitation, γ globulin consumption test, and other
techniques have been applied to study the reactions of serum and normal and
damaged human and animal liver tissue. Most positive reactions have also been
obtained with tissue from other organs, or with serum from patients without

---

[1] This investigation was supported by Grant No. AM 03846, U.S.P.H.S., National Institutes of Health.

hepatic diseases. Fractionation of hepatocytes has shown presumptive evidence of liver-specific antigens in the alcohol-insoluble extracts, in microsomes, and in the supernatant fraction; in the last named these antigens possibly represent hepatocellular carrier proteins, for instance those active in the binding of bilirubin. Bile specific proteins have also been described (Table 1). Immunofluorescent techniques have shown binding of the serum of patients with liver diseases and animals with experimentally induced liver injury to: a) nonspecies nonorgan-specific antigen in inner membranes of mitochondria (Berg *et al.*), (Pinckard and Weir) (Fig. 1), b) nonidentified, nonspecies specific smooth muscle antigens (Johnson *et al.*, 1965) (Fig. 2), c) nuclei which appears to be also nonorgan and species specific, except for one report (Elling and Faber) (Fig. 3), d) to proliferated bile ductules (Paronetto

Table 1. *Liver specific antigens*

Localization	Investigators
Liver extracts	Asherson and Dumonde
	Engelhardt *et al.*
	Nairn *et al.*
	Sargent *et al.*
	Weiler
Cytoplasm hepatocytes Kupffer cells	Lundkvist *et al.*
Microsomes	Emetarom *et al.*
	Vogt
	Whitbeck and Rosenberg
Thermostabile alcohol insoluble extract	Milgrom *et al.*
105,000 G supernatant	Dorner *et al.*
	Meyer zum Büschenfelde
Biliprealbumin, Alpha-1 Biliprotein-Biliproalbumin	Yoon *et al.*

et al., 1964a) (Fig. 4). The latter binding seems to be organ-specific but poorly related to the clinical picture, and corresponds to an antigen of carbohydrate nature in the bile, so far not isolated but which has been demonstrated by serologic reactions. Antigens characteristic of or missing in hepatic cancer, are omitted from this discussion. A pathogenetic role of nonliver specific antigens in liver diseases similar to that in lupus erythematosus has not yet been proven, since antigen/ antibody complexes have not been demonstrated in human liver diseases, with the exception of primary biliary cirrhosis.

A discussion of circulating antibodies should first refer to the elevation of the various γ globulin fractions in chronic human and experimental liver injury. This reflects both chronicity and activity of liver cell injury. Formation of γ globulin in the liver itself by plasma cells has been demonstrated. These may not be recognizable by light microscopy (Paronetto *et al.*, 1962a). All γ globulin fractions are elevated to varying degrees, most consistently IgG; IgA is high in alcoholic liver injury. IgM values are very high in primary biliary cirrhosis, less so in chronic active hepatitis or acute viral hepatitis. Nevertheless, γ globulin fractionation has little diagnostic value in view of the heavy overlap (Feizi), (Walker and Doniach).

Presumably, almost all γ globulin fractions are antibodies and the multiclonal elevation of γ globulin raises the question of the antigen against which these antibodies are directed. In experimental liver injury, nonliver specific antibodies are increased upon immunization when compared with those in animals without liver cell injury (Paronetto and Popper, 1964). Liver damage has been considered to have an adjuvant effect similar to that found after the destruction of macrophages by silica (Pernis and Paronetto). A similar increased response to immunization in patients with liver diseases has been claimed by some investigators, and denied by others (Havens *et al.*, 1951 and 1957; Cherrick). Erratically abnormal serologic reactions have been reported in a group of chronic liver diseases; here, the antigen is quite variable and not liver-specific. Such reactions tend to cluster in patients with the specific diseases mentioned above, and occur frequently together though not necessarily so. The positive reactions in question include various types of antinuclear antibodies (Doniach *et al.*), a positive LE test (Mackay *et al.*), positive serologic reactions for syphilis (Bartholomew *et al.*), high levels of rheumatoid factors (Atwater and Jacox; Badin *et al.*; Bonomo *et al.*), (Dresner and Trombly), complement-fixing and antimitochondrial antibodies which are found in all immunoglobulin fractions (Doniach *et al.*; Paronetto *et al.*, 1967). Also by immunofluorescence antibodies to smooth muscle only found in the γ globulin fraction and not complement-binding, are detected (Johnson *et al.*, 1967), (Whittingham *et al.*). Antibodies to renal glomeruli and bile canaliculi have likewise been found (Johnson *et al.*, 1966). The significance of antibodies to liver tissue has so far been clouded by common cross-reactions with other organs which does, in effect, indicate an excess of an antitissue antibody not necessarily specific for liver. Antibodies to ductules were previously mentioned.

The possibility of a cell-bound immunity or delayed hypersensitivity reaction specific to liver tissue has been raised. In chronic liver diseases inflammation, particularly in and around the portal tract, reveals under the light microscope an appearance similar to established histologic pictures in delayed hypersensitivity reactions in other organs, and to early changes in homotransplantation reactions. In the latter conditions, as in chronic hepatitis, electron microscopy demonstrates the presence of large lymphoid cells rich in polysomes, indicating cytoplasmic protein formation, but devoid of the endoplasmic reticulum seen in plasma cells suggesting protein secretion (Klion and Schaffner). In chronic active hepatitis, primary biliary cirrhosis and some types of drug-induced liver injury, autologous liver tissue induces transformation of cultured lymphocytes to lymphoblasts (Tobias *et al.*; Warnatz, 1969; Paronetto, unpublished observations), suggesting a liver-specific, cell-bound immunity reaction.

Summarizing the evidence, some liver diseases, with particular frequency those listed above, are characterized by hypergammglobulinemia and erratic immunoserologic reactions, some of which suggest specificity for the liver. They could reflect simple mesenchymal hyperactivity, since liver cell injury, particularly a chronic one, induces such activation of hepatic, splenic and lymphoid mesenchyma. Chronic liver injury results in hypergammaglobulinemia also in germfree animals, so bacterial antigens seem not to play a dominant role (Bauer *et al.*). However, the clustering of the reaction in specific diseases suggests a pathogenetic role beyond simple mesenchymal stimulation.

With the question of hepatic specific antigen and the pathogenetic significance of the serologic and lymphocyte reactions unsettled, attempts to reproduce chronic liver disease in experimental animals by immunologic means become import. Such

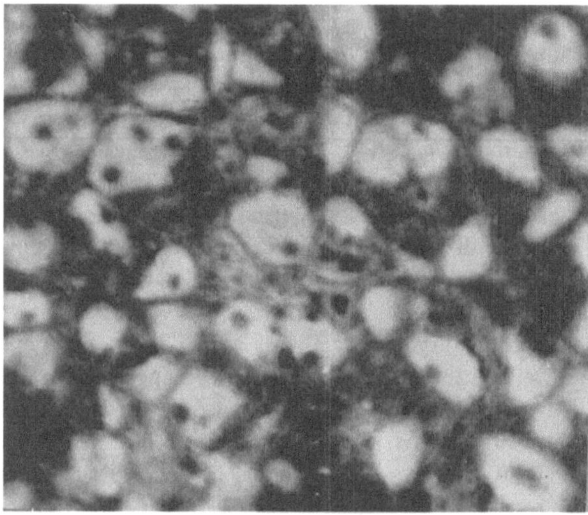

Figs. 1—4. Antibodies in sera of patients with chronic active hepatitis or primary biliary cirrhosis detected by applying 1:10 dilution of patient's sera on cryostat sections of liver and stomach followed by fluoresceinated antihuman γ globulin

Fig. 1. Antimitochondrial antibodies. The parietal cells of stomach are stained (substrate: unfixed rat stomach, × 250)

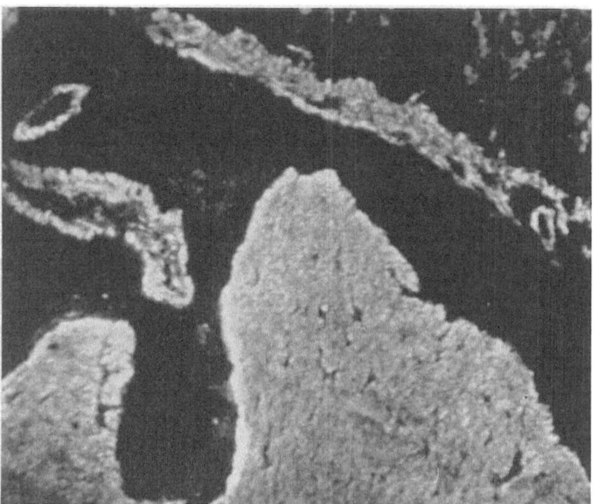

Fig. 2. Antismooth muscle antibodies. The muscularis mucosae, muscle coat and vessel wall are stained (substrate: unfixed rat stomach, × 100)

experiments might decide whether demonstrated autoimmune or heteroimmune hyperactivity represent a feature accompanying liver disease, an epiphenomenon induced, for instance, by liver cell breakdown, or a pathogenetic factor in initiating or perpetuating it. The latter might be accomplished if a specific etiologic factor should permit the abnormal access of hepatic antigens to lymphoid tissue or alter

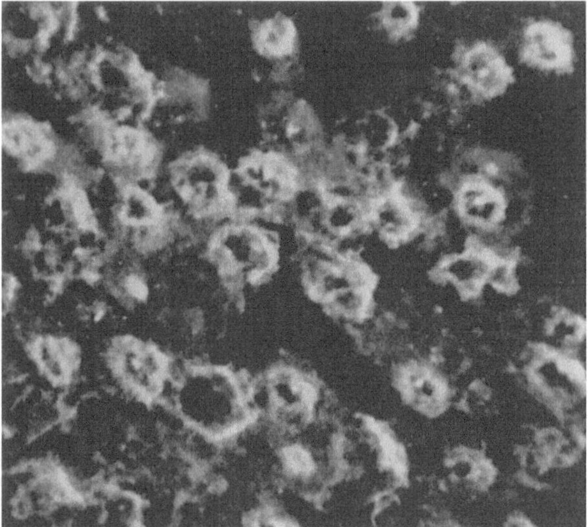

Fig. 3. Antinuclear antibodies. The binding is mainly on the nuclear membrane and nucleoli (substrate: aceton-fixed rat stomach, × 560)

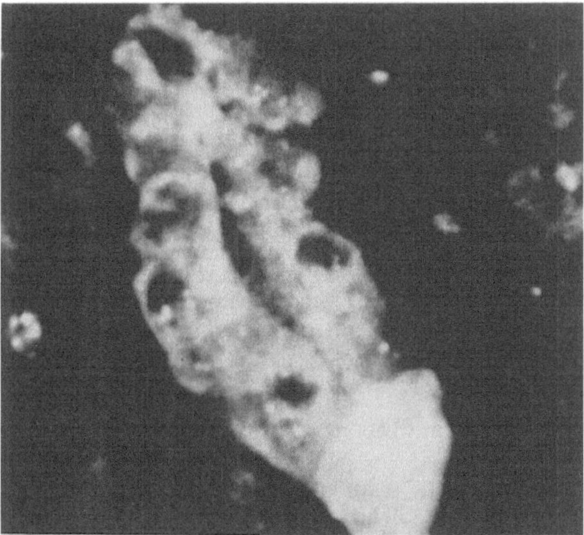

Fig. 4. Antiductular cell antibodies (substrate: liver from a patient with chronic active hepatitis, × 560)

hepatic protein so that it becomes antigenic, or unmasks new antigenic determinants. The literature abounds with observations, speculations and working hypotheses—the usable evidence is slight. There is no doubt that acute liver injury can be created by various hetero- and autoimmunologic techniques. Liver cell injury does not, as a rule, persist in experimental animals after removal of an offending agent, immunologic or not. Various chronic experimental injuries may bring an elevation of γ globulin, some erratic serologic reactions and reticuloendothelial hyperplasia in spleen and regional lymph nodes, but all these parameters return to normal after discontinuation of the offending regime; while scarring and epithelial hyperplasia persist, the inflammation so characteristic of human chronic hepatitis subsides. It is interesting that plasma cells are seldom found in experimental liver injuries of nonimmunologic character although they are commonly present in most types of human liver disease.

The injection of antigens in the liver of presensitized animals results in hepatic necrosis. This Arthus phenomenon implies a locally cytotoxic effect of antigen/antibody complexes combining with complement. The Kupffer cells, however, exert a protective effect in phagocytizing antigen/antibody complexes. Effective production of this necrosis is obtained by administering the material in high concentration directly to the liver, e.g., via portal vein or common bile duct (Paronetto et al., 1962 a). Preceding liver injury favors the accumulation of antigen/antibody complexes in hepatocytes; this deposition is associated with an aggravation of the hepatic necrosis (Auer reaction), particularly when the Kupffer cells do not phagocytize these complexes (Paronetto and Popper, 1965). These observations raise the possibility that, in analogy to renal diseases, the ratio between antigens not necessarily liver specific, and antibodies may decide the solubility of the complexes. These may thus, under some circumstances, be deposited in damaged liver tissue and perpetuate liver injury. However, γ globulin, complexes or complement have so far been found by immunofluorescence only in the damaged liver tissue in primary biliary cirrhosis (Paronetto and Popper, 1968). By contrast known antigens, such as schistosomal protein complexed with antibody, account for characteristic lesions of the liver in schistosomiasis (Andrade et al.).

Injection of the sera of animals sensitized with normal and abnormal liver has not resulted in prolonged hepatic lesion as in Masugi nephritis, and attempts to produce chronic liver injury by sensitization with normal or abnormal liver with or without the Freund's adjuvant have also failed (Table 2). Freund's adjuvant alone induces activation of hepatic macrophages, granulomas and focal necrosis, all of transient character; the lesion is only accentuated if liver tissue is added (Paronetto; Scheiffarth et al., 1967). Since it can be transferred to normal animals by lymphocytes, a cell-bound immunity is probable. Injections of chemically modified supernatant with Freund's adjuvant into the guinea pig leads to larger but still transient necroses (Paronetto), rabbits exhibit the features of active chronic hepatitis (Kössling and Meyer zum Büschenfelde). Injection of foreign protein in the rat produces a fibrosis with superficial resemblance to cirrhosis, but without progression (Paronetto and Popper, 1966). That the injection of rat mitochondria causes a peribiliary fibrosis is interesting in view of primary biliary cirrhosis (Dóbiás and Balázs). Administration of canine hepatitis virus to partially immune dogs induces chronic active hepatitis without rendering the liver infec-

Table 2. *Attempts to reproduce in animals chronic perpetuating liver disease*

Administration of:	Animal	Results	Investigators
Liver extracts with Freund's adjuvant	Guinea pig	Focal area necrosis	Reviewed by Paronetto and Popper (1968)
	Mouse	Lesion transferred by leucocytes to normal recipients	Scheiffarth *et al.* (1967)
Chemically modified 100,000 G supernatant of Guinea pig liver and Freund's adjuvant	Guinea pig	Focal area necrosis	Paronetto
Chemically modified human liver specific proteins and Freund's adjuvant	Rabbit	Chronic active hepatitis	Kössling and Meyer zum Büschenfelde
Foreign proteins	Rat	Diffuse fibrosis — no progression	Paronetto and Popper (1966)
Rat mitochondria	Rabbit	Fibrosis around bile ducts	Dóbiás and Balázs
Canine viral hepatitis	Dog, partially immune	Chronic active hepatitis. Liver not infective	Gocke *et al.*

tious. This is an interesting model of an immunologic reaction, possibly implying virus-liver interaction (Goecke *et al.*).

Thus, experimental attempts to produce immunologic liver injury have thrown less light on the pathogenesis of chronic liver disease than such attempts did in allergic encephalomyelitis, or thyroiditis. Although in some human liver diseases the complement titer drops (Zlotnick and Rodnan), an attack by circulating antibodies is improbable—as a matter of fact they may protect. An injury from the localization of specific and nonspecific antigen/antibody complexes is possible but also improbable; one from chemically altered protein via haptenes is not excluded. Cell-bound immunity may play a role; this might be substantiated through tissue culture studies. Alteration of the lymphoid tissue in the sense of forbidden clones is an intriguing hypothesis as far as the liver is concerned.

Turning to clinical liver diseases, in acute viral hepatitis it remains to be established whether or not antigens common to virus and liver account for the hypersensitivity, clinical and histologic manifestations as well as for certain serologic reactions.

As already mentioned, the main interest concerns a group of diseases termed chronic active, aggressive or periportal hepatitis (De Groote *et al.*). These show a tendency to progress to cirrhosis in contrast to other types of chronic hepatitis which are basically restricted to the portal tracts and are designated "persisting hepatitis." Chronic aggressive hepatitis may follow icteric viral hepatitis or develop insidiously; cholestatic jaundice may or may not appear later. Histologically, it is characterized by piecemeal necrosis, indicating portal infiltration by macrophages, lymphocytes and plasma cells producing γ globulin, as well as erosion of the limiting plate of the parenchyma (Fig. 5). The lesion in this context can be considered to consist of four groups of phenomena, each of which represents a circle with various clusters of findings (Table 3). The participation of each circle varies in the individual patient. The first circle encompasses hypergammaglobulinemia which may simply represent a response to sustained liver injury. The second circle reflects a number of abnormal serologic reactions. These include antinuclear antibodies, with or without the LE reaction, antimitochondrial antibodies, usually present in low titer, high titers of rheumatoid factors, antismooth muscle antibodies in high titer, positive serologic reactions for syphilis, and a high incidence of complement-fixing antibody to liver. The positive reaction for LE in some patients has led to applying the term "lupoid hepatitis" (Mackay *et al.*) to this group, but a relation to lupus erythematosus is now denied by most investigators. A third circle concerns those systemic reactions—fever, skin rashes, arthralgia, renal and thyroid involvement—all of which resemble symptoms present in lupus erythematosus. These may be related to antigen/antibody complexes deposited in tissue because of immunologic hyperactivity stimulated by liver cell damage. Altered serologic reactions need not be present. The fourth circle represents fibrosis leading to cirrhosis with fibroplasia another, clinically more important, manifestation of mesenchymal hyperactivity. Present evidence suggests that the transition into cirrhosis depends more on the fibroplastic than the immunologic component since even patients with fullblown immunologic reactions ("lupoid hepatitis") have fully recovered. A designation of chronic aggressive hepatitis as "lupoid" is confusing, but separation of the group by the systemic manifestations is useful from both the symptomatic and prognostic viewpoints.

The initial stage of primary biliary cirrhosis is a chronic destructive nonsuppurative cholangitis (Rubin *et al.*), characterized clinically by itching, hyperlipemia, bromsulphalein retention and high alkaline phosphatase activity, but not

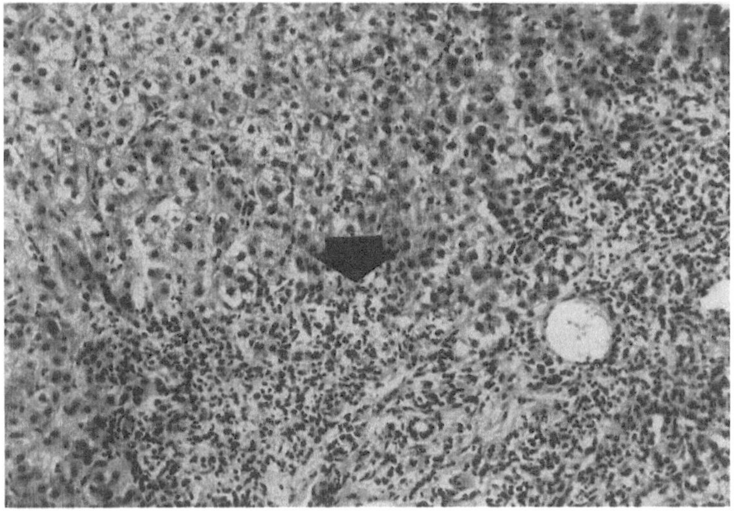

a

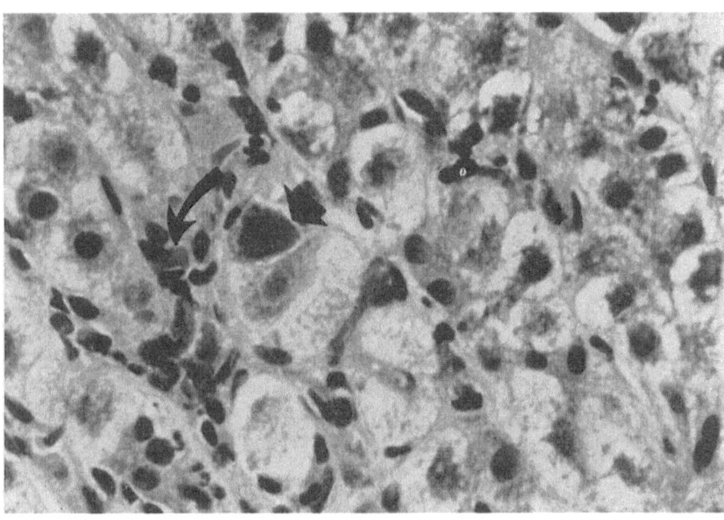

b

Fig. 5. a Peripheral piecemeal necrosis in a liver biopsy of a patient with chronic aggressive hepatitis. Border between parenchyma and portal tract not sharp because of erosion of limiting plates of parenchyma (arrow). Proliferation of bile ductules and accumulation of inflammatory cells is noted (hematoxylin and eosin, × 100). b Close approximation between normal and abnormal hepatocytes and inflammatory cells, including lymphocytes, plasma cells (curved arrow), and macrophages (straight arrow) (hematoxylin and eosin, × 400)

necessarily by jaundice which usually begins later. In many instances viral hepatitis or a nonicteric bile passage disease such as cholecystitis precedes the onset by a few years. In the acute stage the histologic picture shows destruction of the epithelium of the bile ducts associated with accumulation of macrophages (Fig. 6), occasionally progressing to granuloma, with lymphocytes and plasma cells forming characteristically (Fig. 7). PAS-positive glycolipoproteins may also escape from the bile duct lumen (Rubin *et al.*), and extracellular γ globulin and complement have been noted (Table 4), (Fig. 8). The serum contains antiductular

Table 3

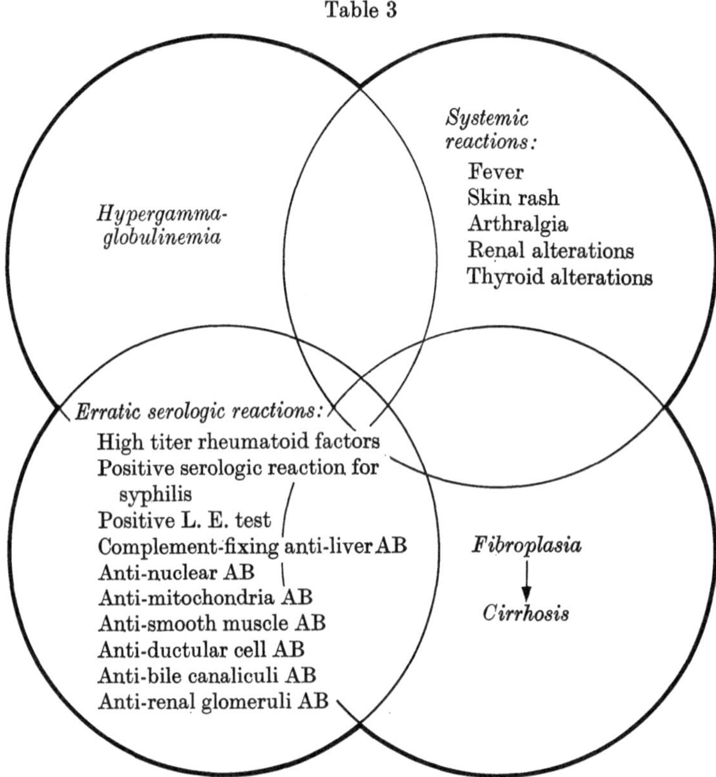

and antimitochondrial antibodies, with the latter serving to differentiate the condition diagnostically from extrahepatic biliary obstruction (Walker *et al.*). Antinuclear antibodies and excess rheumatoid factor may be found; serum IgM values are high. Lymphocyte transformation may be induced *in vitro* by incubation of patient's lymphocytes with autologous liver. Thus a serologic overlap with chronic active hepatitis exists although the clinical picture of primary biliary cirrhosis is, in most instances, characteristic. The biochemical alterations result from regurgitation of bile through the bile ducts with jaundice appearing when the liver cells are no longer capable of excreting regurgitated bilirubin in a compensatory fashion. Eventually the bile ductules also become destroyed; this is associated with fibrosis and leads to intrahepatic obstructive jaundice. In later stages cirrhosis develops, giving its name to the disorder. Here histologic characteristics may not permit identification of the diease. This has raised arguments about existence of the entity so long as the study has been based on autopsy material only.

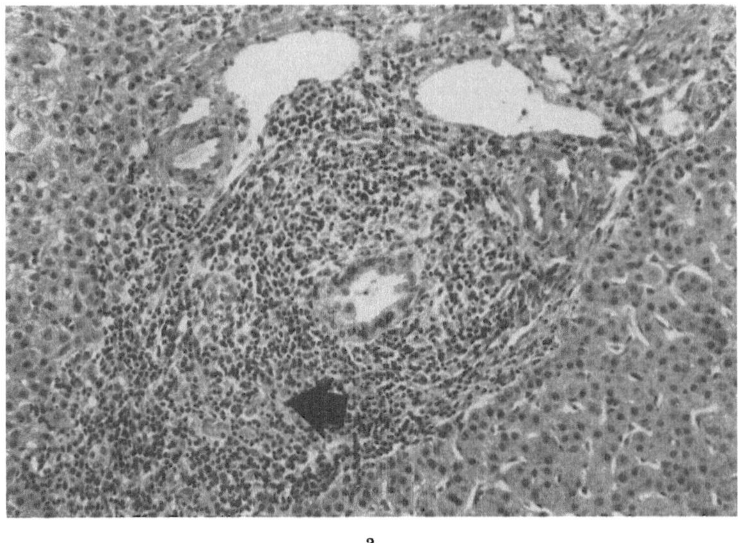

a

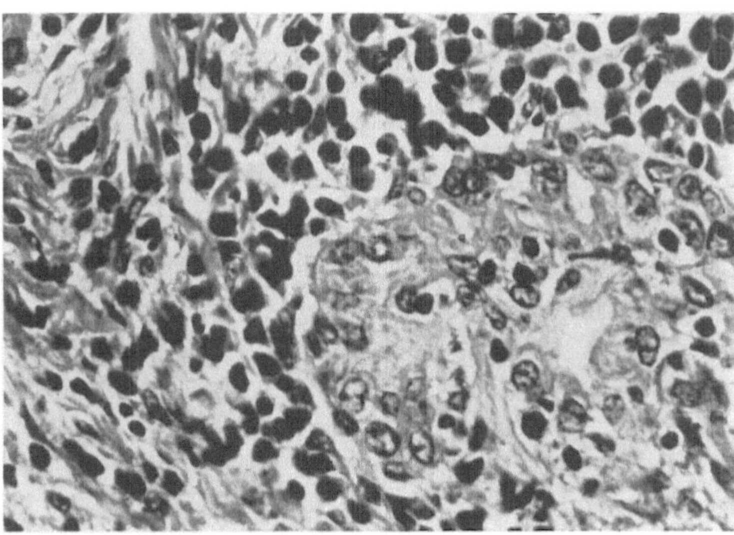

b

Fig. 6. a Early stages of primary biliary cirrhosis (chronic nonsuppurative destructive cholangitis), with marked accumulation of inflammatory cells around bile duct which shows alteration of the epithelium and infiltration of the wall. The portal tract is enlarged; a granuloma-like accumulation of macrophages can be seen (arrow) (hematoxylin and eosin, × 60). b The mononuclear cells around the bile duct are lymphocytes, plasma cells, histiocytes and fibroblasts. The epithelium of a bile duct is altered and infiltrated by inflammatory cells (hematoxylin and eosin, × 400). c Hepatocytes are normal while in the sinusoids macrophages and plasma cells accumulate (hematoxylin and eosin, × 250)

The hypothesis can be offered that diseases of the bile ducts lead to exposure of biliary material to lymphoid tissue, and that the resulting sensitization induces sustained destruction of the cells forming this biliary material by antibodies or by

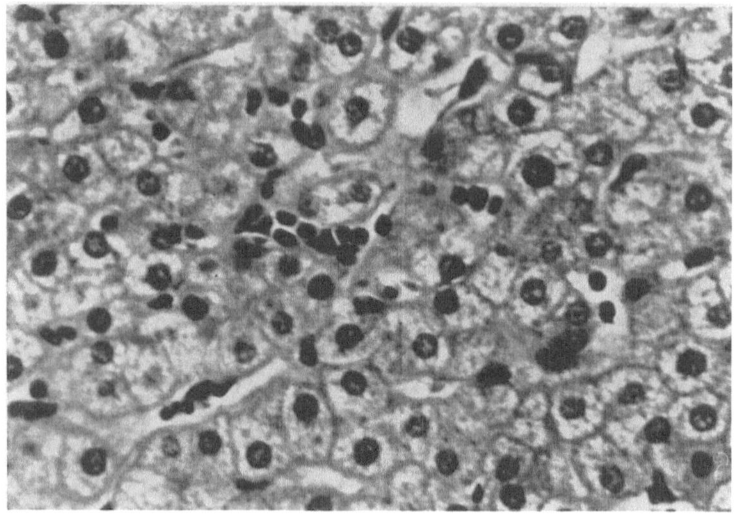

Fig. 6 c

Table 4. *Immunohistochemical and serologic findings in primary biliary cirrhosis*

	Investigators
High levels of IgM	Feizi Paronetto *et al.* (1964 b)
High titers of rheumatoid factors	Doniach *et al.* Paronetto *et al.* (1964 b)
Antimitochondrial antibodies	Walker *et al.* Doniach *et al.* Paronetto *et al.* (1967) Kantor and Klatskin
Antinuclear antibodies	Doniach *et al.* Paronetto *et al.* (1964 b)
Antismooth muscle antibodies	Doniach *et al.*
Antiductular cell antibodies	Paronetto *et al.* (1964 b)
Complement fixing non-liver specific antibodies	Walker *et al.*
Lymphocyte transformation with autologous liver	Tobias *et al.*, Warnatz (1969)
IgM in plasma cells of liver	Paronetto *et al.* (1964 b)
γ globulin and complement in bile duct	Paronetto and Popper (1968)

cell-bound immunity. However, this idea of autoaggression still requires confirmation.

Some drug-induced liver injuries are predictable effects of drugs known to be hepatotoxic, for instance, agents for cancer therapy and immunosuppression. In such injuries, a lesion develops in any patient receiving a sufficient dose of the drug. Other injuries of interest here are either cholestatic or hepatitic reactions in

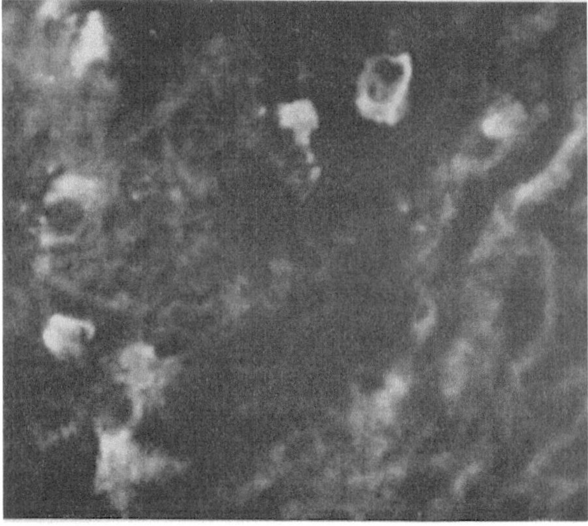

Fig. 7. Liver of a patient with primary biliary cirrhosis. Few plasma cells around a bile duct contain IgM (fluoresceinated anti-IgM, $\times$ 250)

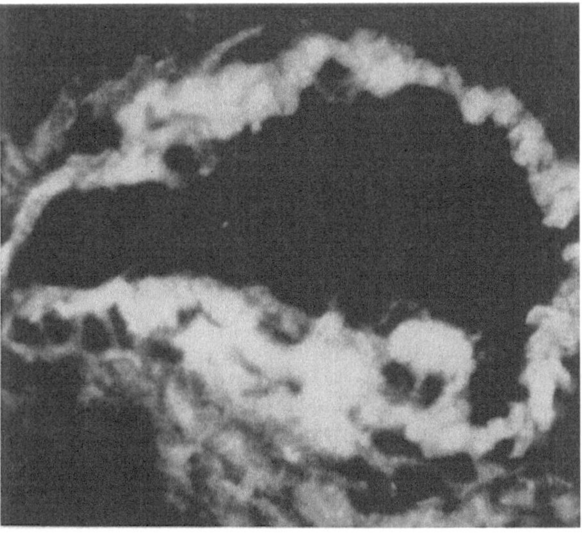

Fig. 8. Liver of a patient in the early stages of primary biliary cirrhosis. A bile duct and peribiliary tissue contain complement. γ globulin is localized in the same area (fluoresceinated antibeta$_{1c}$ antiserum, $\times$ 250)

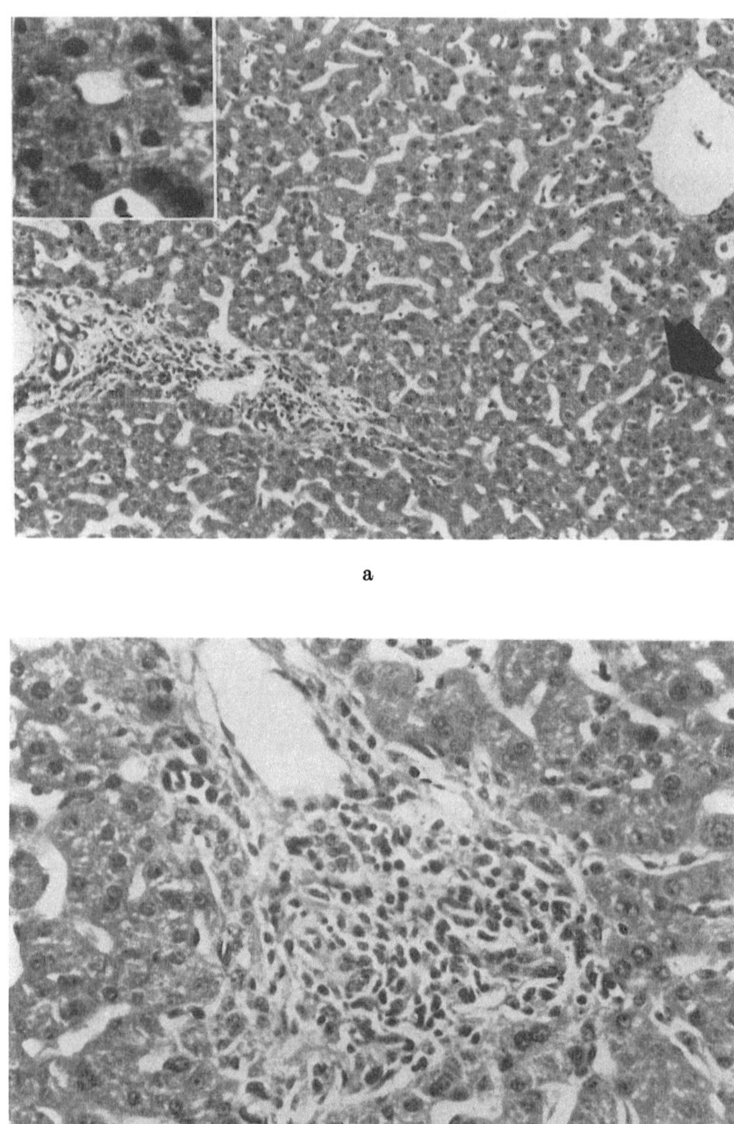

a

b

Fig. 9. a Cholestatic hepatitis following administration of an contraceptive drug. Intralobular focal necrosis (arrow) and portal inflammation (hematoxylin and eosin, × 250). Centrolobular cholestasis with bile plugs is noted (see insert, × 500). b The mononuclear inflammatory reaction is mainly around bile ducts and is composed of lymphocytes, eosinophils, histiocytes, and a few plasma cells (hematoxylin and eosin, × 250). c Biopsy of a patient with jaundice following repeated exposure to halothane. Note similarity with viral hepatitis such as spotty necrosis, eosinophilic bodies (straight arrow), portal tract inflammation and phlebitis around portal vein (curved arrow) (hematoxylin and eosin, × 100). d Fatal submassive necrosis in patient after third exposure to halothane anesthesia (hematoxylin and eosin, × 60)

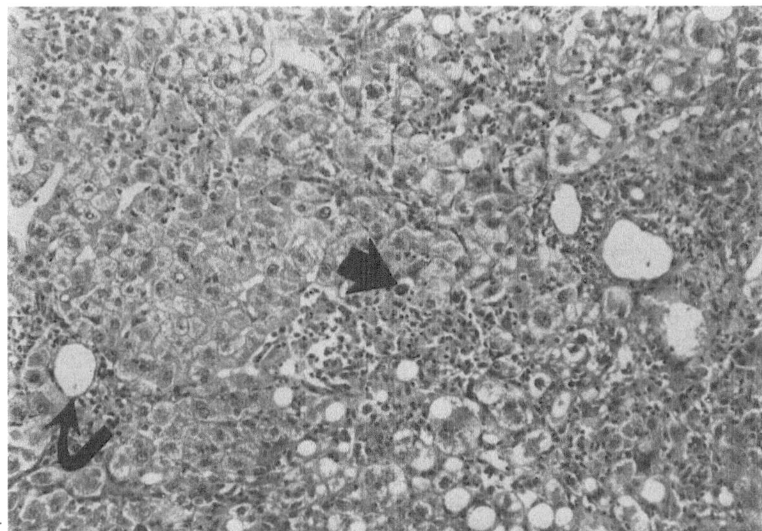

Fig. 9 c

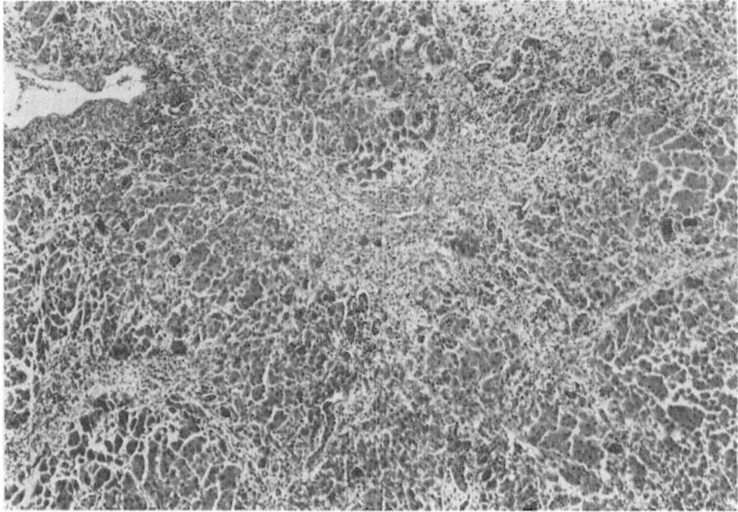

Fig. 9 d

a few persons exposed to the drug, usually without clear dose dependency (Popper *et al.*). Many of these drugs, at least those of the cholestatic group, regularly produce a mild cholestasis recognizable by electron microscopy or by biochemical techniques. Exacerbation to clinical jaundice may in some instances result from genetically determined metabolic alterations. In others immunologic reactions to the drug may occur. Several facts can be listed which favor this hypothesis:

1. The histologic picture, especially portal infiltration by eosinophils and plasma cells or granuloma formation.

2. Clinical allergic manifestations such as skin rashes or eosinophilia.

3. The onset or aggravation of the lesion after repeated drug administration, for instance after halothane.

4. The reported success of desensitization measures.

5. The presence of antimitochondrial antibodies, at least in chlorpromazine and halothane-induced lesions, in contrast to viral hepatitis which presents a similar picture otherwise (Rodriguez *et al.*) (Fig. 9). In a few instances the lymphocyte transformation test was positive with autologous liver or with the drug in question (Paronetto, unpublished observations). A haptene role of the drug has not been proven. Those drugs incriminated have all induced hypertrophy of smooth endoplasmic reticulum and increased the activity of drug-handling enzymes. These changes may be associated with the transformation of drugs to haptenes (Remmer).

A review of the observations pertaining to autoimmunity in liver disease is stimulating, complex but also inconclusive and indeed confusing. Some facts, such as self-perpetuation and its dependence upon mesenchymal activation secondary to liver cell injury, appear established. The role of its fibroblastic components in transition to cirrhosis has been established. Whether or not the activation of the lymphoid and plasma cellular component is an epiphenomenon with the hepatic inflammation a reaction similar to that found in the regional lymph nodes and spleen, or the demonstrated immune reactions cause hepatocellular injury is not established. Even less clear is whether an immunologic reaction can initiate liver disease. The frequency of immunologic reactions in a group of diseases suggests a pathogenetic role beyond nonspecific mesenchymal stimulation. However, it is not yet decided whether a nonautoimmune process with a preferential deposition of circulating antigen/antibody complexes is important, or if autoaggression from specific circulating antibody or cell-bound immunity occurs. In drug-induced liver injury, haptene formation is a hypothetical possibility. In chronic aggressive hepatitis delayed hypersensitivity is a challenge. In primary biliary cirrhosis an autoaggressive attack related to biliary antigens seems to make sense. As of today, however, the immunologic reactions, both serologic and morphologic, are more important in the delineation and diagnosis of liver diseases than in clarifying the pathogenesis.

References

Andrade, Z., F. Paronetto, and H. Popper: Immunocytochemical studies on schistosomiasis. Amer. J. Path. **39**, 589—598 (1961).

Asherson, G. L., and D. C. Dumonde: Autoantibody production in rabbits. II. Organ-specific autoantibody in rabbits injected with rat tissue. Immunology **3**, 19—29 (1963).

Atwater, E. C., and R. F. Jacox: The latex-fixation test in patients with liver disease. Ann. intern. Med. **58**, 419—425 (1963).

Badin, J., C. Lévy et M. Cachin: Fréquence et signification des réactions de Waaler-Rose et des tests au latex positifs dans les maladies du foie. Rev. int. Hépat. **13**, 655—667 (1963).

Bartholomew, L. G., A. B. Hagedorn, J. C. Cain, and A. H. Baggenstoss: Hepatitis and cirrhosis in women with positive clot test for lupus erythematosus. New Engl. J. Med. **259**, 947—956 (1958).

Bauer, H., F. Paronetto, R. F. Porro, A. Einheber, and H. Popper: The influence of the microbial flora on liver injury and associated gamma globulin elevation. A study in germfree rats treated with 3'-methyl-4-dimethylaminoazobenzene. Lab. Invest. **16**, 847—857 (1967).

Berg, P. A., D. Doniach, and T. M. Roitt: Mitochondrial antibodies in primary biliary cirrhosis I. Localization of the antigen to mitochondrial membranes. J. exp. Med. **126**, 277—290. (1967).

Bonomo, L., J. Lo Spalluto, and M. Ziff: Anti-gamma globulin factors in liver disease. Arthr. and Rheum. **6**, 104—114 (1963).

Cherrick, G. R., L. Pothier, J. J. Dufour, and S. Sherlock: Immunologic response to tetanus toxoid inoculation in patients with hepatic cirrhosis. New Engl. J. Med. **261**, 340—342 (1959).

De Groote, J., V. J. Desmet, P. Gedik, G. Korb, H. Popper, H. Poulsen, P. J. Scheur, M. Schmid, H. Thaler, and E. Uehlinger: A classification of chronic hepatitis. Lancet **1968 II**, 626—628.

Dóbiás, G. Y., and M. Balzás: Studies of the pathogenetic role of humoral antibodies reacting with subcellular organ antigens. I. Active immunization of rabbits with rat-organ antigens. Immunology **12**, 373—387 (1967).

Doniach, D., I. M. Roitt, J. G. Walker, and S. Sherlock: Tissue antibodies in primary biliary cirrhosis, active chronic (lupoid) hepatitis, cryptogenic cirrhosis and other liver diseases, and their clinical implications. Clin. exp. Immunol. **1**, 237—262 (1966).

Dorner, M. M., E. J. Simon, and P. A. Miescher: Studies on a liver specific antigen. Fed. Proc. **21**, 43 (1962).

Dresner, E., and P. Trombly: The latex-fixation reaction in nonrheumatic diseases. New Engl. J. Med. **261**, 981—988 (1959).

Elling, P., and V. Faber: Antinuclear antibodies in infectious mononucleosis. Lancet **1968 II**, 918—919.

Emetarom, N., D. Nelken, and J. H. Boss: Organ specific antigens in rat liver. Israel J. med. Sci. **3**, 809—813 (1967).

Engelhardt, M. V., N. T. Khramkova, and Z. A. Postnikova: Antigenic structure of mouse hepatomas. IV. Study of the liver organospecific antigen in the liver and hepatomas with fluorescent antibodies. Neoplasma (Bratisl.) **10**, 133—142 (1963).

Feizi, T.: Immunoglobulins in chronic liver disease. Gut **9**, 193—198 (1968).

Gocke, D. J., R. Preisig, T. Q. Morris, D. C. McKay, and S. E. Bradley: Experimental viral hepatitis in the dog: Production of persistent disease in partially immune animals. J. clin. Invest. **46**, 1506—1517 (1967).

Havens, W. P., Jr., R. M. Myerson, and J. Klatchko: Production of tetanus antitoxin by patients with hepatic cirrhosis. New Engl. J. Med. **257**, 637—643 (1957).

—, J. M. Shaffer, and C. J. Hopke Jr.: Production of antibody by patients with chronic hepatic disease. J. Immunol. **67**, 347—356 (1951).

Johnson, G. D., E. J. Holoborow, and L. E. Glynn. Antibody to smooth muscle in patients with liver disease. Lancet **1965 II**, 878—879.

— — — Antibody to liver in lupoid hepatitis. Lancet **1966 II**, 416—418.

Kantor, F. S., and G. Klatskin: Serological diagnosis of primary biliary cirrhosis: A potential clue to pathogenesis. Trans. Ass. Amer. Phycns. **80**, 267—274 (1967).

Kössling, F. K., and K. H. Meyer zum Büschenfelde: Zur Induktion einer aktiven chronischen Hepatitis durch heterologe, lösliche Leberproteine. Virchows Arch. Path. Anat. **345**, 365—376 (1968).

Klion, F. M., and F. Schaffner: Ultrastructural features of canine hepatic auxiliary transplant rejection. Exp. molec. Path. **6**, 361—369 (1967).

Lundkvist, U., G. C. Goeringer, and P. Perlman: Immunochemical characterization of parenchymal and reticuloendothelial cells of rat liver. Exp. molec. Path. **5**, 427—442 (1966).

Mackay, I. R., L. I. Taft, and D. C. Cowling: Lupoid hepatitis. Lancet **1956 II**, 1323—1326.

Meyer zum Büschenfelde, K. H.: Untersuchungen über die immunobiologische Bedeutung löslicher Leberproteine. Z. ges. exp. Med. **145** 131—163 (1968).

Milgrom, F., Z. Maide-Tuggac, and E. Witebsky: Organ-specific antigens of liver, testicle and pituitary. J. Immunol. **94**, 157—163 (1965).

Nairn, R. C., H. G. Richmond, M. G. McEntegart, and J. E. Fothergill. Immunological differences between normal and malignant cells. Brit. med. J. **1960 II**, 1335—1340.

Paronetto, F.: Immune reactions and hepatic alterations in guinea pigs sensitized with altered hepatic proteins. In: Miescher, P. A., and P. Grabar (Eds.). Immunopathology, Vth International Symposium, pp 122—143. Punta Ala. New York: Grune and Stratton Inc. 1967.

—, and H. Popper: Enhanced antibody formation in experimental acute and chronic liver injury produced by carbon tetrachloride or allyl alcohol. Proc. Soc. exp. Biol. (N. Y.) 115, 1060—1064 (1964).

— — Aggravation of hepatic lesions in mice by *in vivo* localization of immune complexes (Auer hepatitis). Amer. J. Path. 47, 549—563 (1965).

— — Chronic liver injury induced by immunologic reactions; cirrhosis following immunization with heterologous sera. Amer. J. Path. 49, 1087—1101 (1966).

— — Hetero-iso-and autoimmune phenomena in the liver. In: Miescher, P. A., and H. J. Muller-Eberhard (Eds.), Textbook of Immunopathology. New York: Grune and Stratton 1968, 563—583.

—, E. Rubin, and H. Popper: Local formation of γ-globulin in the diseased liver and its relation to hepatic necrosis. Lab. Invest. 11, 150—158 (1962 a).

—, F. Schaffner, R. D. Mutter, J. C. Kniffen and H. Popper: Circulating antibodies to bile ductular cells in various liver diseases. J. Amer. med. Ass. 187, 503—506 (1964 a).

— —, and H. Popper: Immunocytochemical and serologic observations in primary biliary cirrhosis. New Engl. J. Med. 271, 1123—1128 (1964 b).

— — — Antibodies to cytoplasmic antigens in primary biliary cirrhosis and chronic active hepatitis. J. Lab. clin. Med. 69, 979—988 (1967).

—, N. Woolf, D. Koffler, and H. Popper: Response of the liver to soluble antigen-antibody complexes. Gastroenterology 43, 539—546 (1962 b).

Pernis, B., and F. Paronetto: The adjuvant effect of silica (tridimyte) on antibody production. Proc. Soc. exp. Biol. (N. Y.) 110, 390—392 (1962).

Pinckard, R. N., and D. M. Weir: Antibodies against the mitochondrial fraction of liver after toxic liver damage in rats. Clin. exp. Immunol. 1, 33—43 (1966).

Popper, H., E. Rubin, D. Gardiol, F. Schaffner, and F. Paronetto: Drug-induced liver disease. A penalty for progress. Arch. intern. Med. 115, 128—136 (1965).

Renmar, H.: III Leber symposium in Vulpera. Schweiz. (in press).

Rodriguez, M., F. Paronetto, F. Schaffner, and H. Popper: Antimitochondrial antibodies in jaundice following drug administration. J. Amer. med. Ass. 208, 148—150 (1969).

Rubin, E., F. Schaffner, and H. Popper: Primary biliary cirrhosis. Chronic nonsuppurative destructive cholangitis. Amer. J. Path. 46, 387—407 (1965).

Sargent, A. U., J. Myers, B. Rose, and M. Richter: Organ and species specificity of rat hepatocellular antigens. Immunology 10, 199—210 (1966).

Scheiffarth, F., H. Warnatz, and K. Meyer: Studies concerning the importance of mononuclear cells in experimental hepatitis. J. Immunol. 98, 396—401 (1967).

Tobias, H., A. F. Safran, and F. Schaffner: Lymphocyte stimulation and chronic liver disease. Lancet 1967 I, 193—195.

Vogt, P.: Distribution of tissue-specific antigens in centrifugal fractions of rat liver. Nature (Lond.) 182, 1807—1808 (1968).

Walker, G., and D. Doniach: Antibodies and immunoglobulins in liver disease. Gut 9, 266 to 269 (1968).

— —, I. M. Roitt, and S. Sherlock: Serological tests in diagnosis of primary biliary cirrhosis. Lancet 1965 I, 827—831.

Warnatz, H.: Das Phänomen der Lymphocytentransformation in der Pathogenese und Diagnostik von Autoimmunerkrankungen. Z. ges. exp. Med. 149, 64—90 (1969).

Weiler, E.: Die Änderung der serologischen Organspezifität beim Buttergelb-Tumor der Ratte in Vergleich zu normaler Leber. Z. Naturforsch. 7b, 324—326 (1952).

Whitbeck, E. G., and L. T. Rosenberg: Antigenic properties of microsomes from guinea pig spleen, liver and lymph nodes. Immunology 7, 363—374 (1964).

Whittingham, S., J. Irwin, I. I. Mackay, and M. Smalley: Smooth muscle auto-antibody in "autoimmune" hepatitis. Gastroenterology 51, 499—505 (1966).

Yoon, D. S., B. S. Shim, and T. S. Kil: Bile specific protein component in human hepatic bile. J. Lab. clin. Med. 67, 640—649 (1966).

Zlotnick, A., and G. P. Rodnan: Immunoelectrophoresis of serum in "lupoid" hepatitis. Proc. Soc. exp. Biol. (N. Y.) **109**, 742—746 (1962).

Prof. Dr. H. Popper
Mount Sinai School of Medicine
of the City University of New York,
Fifth Avenue and 100th Street,
New York, N.Y. 10029, U.S.A.

Discussion

GRUNDMANN (Wuppertal): I thank you very much for your excellent review. I have two questions: — Are the plasma cells you find between the epithelial cells probable invaders or do you believe they arise locally ? — Concerning the liver necroses after halothane a pressing question is whether these patterns, corresponding to an acute yellow atrophy of the liver, are caused by the drug alone or whether a virus infection is additionally involved ?

POPPER (New York): To decide the origin of a cell is always very difficult. We did electron microscopic studies of the liver, and especially in chronic liver disease were able to distinguish several kinds of mesenchymal cell. There are the endothelial cells which are situated on the internal surface of the sinusoids. Also the Kupffer cells, which are electron microscopically characterized by their large lysosomes, are situated there. Not on the internal surface, but between the liver cells, are other cells which formerly were also considered to be Kupffer cells, these are plasma cells and lipocytes which are probably precursors of the fibroblasts. Both cell types can be electron microscopically well identified. — To the second question: The virus of virus hepatitis has not been cultured and no specific etiologic laboratory test is available. The histologic appearance of viral hepatitis is identical with the hepatitis developing in a few persons exposed to halothane or to some monoamine oxidase inhibitors. I wonder whether Dr. Deicher has found differences in serum macroglobulin levels between viral and drug-induced hepatitis.

DEICHER (Hannover): We have not yet had a chance to examine cases of acute drug hepatitis. In obstructive (cholostatic) drug hepatoses, we have not seen any significant immunoglobulin reactions. In a case of acute intoxication by an organic lacquer solvent, which was at first diagnosed as viral hepatitis on clinical reasons, the missing increase of IgM or of any other immunoglobulin in the serum, was one lead to the correct diagnosis.

POPPER (New York): It may be that in viral hepatitis peculiar immunologic factors have a pathogenetic role. Possibly a product of virus-host cell interaction may damage the liver without the virus ever being in the hepatocytes. When we described the first cases of hepatitis induced by monoamine oxidase inhibitors, we considered the possibility of an activation of a preexisting infectious or so-called serum hepatitis. Despite the persisting obscurity of the etiology of viral hepatitis, we do not believe this any more.

VORLAENDER (Aachen): In addition to the gammaglobulin determinations we have found a serological reaction to be useful for the clinical clarification of hepatic changes. We use saline suspensions of healthy livers and then of hepatitic livers. Digestion by trypsin is carefully induced in the suspensions, thereafter they are centrifuged and the supernatant is used as an antigen. In chronic active hepatitis the titres are seen to rise with increasing activity. With the transformation to fibrosis the titers subside. At the same time the 7S-globulins increase. In primary biliary cirrhosis the titres are more persistent, higher and remain raised when the 19S-globulins increase. Simultaneously, the rheumatoid factors become positive. A question arises from the observations on a 40-year-old male patient with a history of numerous infections, among them those by streptococci. Later he had acute rheumatic fever, thereafter an acute glomerulonephritis, then an acquired heamolytic anaemia of the warm auto-antibody type, and eventually chronic progressive interstitial hepatitis passing into cirrhosis. The patient died in hepatic coma. Histological examination post mortem revealed massive plasma cell infiltrations in all parts of the reticulo-endothelial system. Is it possible that a chronic liver damage can be caused by the stimulation of primarily extra-hepatic antigen-antibody complexes instead of a hepatic immune process ?

POPPER (New York): Experimental studies confirmed such a mechanism. In mice which have been mildly damaged by carbon tetrachloride it is possible to aggravate the necroses by preceding sensitization with bovine serum albumin. In this experiment, damaged liver cells bind antigen antibody complexes; they then take up complement and this causes a cytotoxic reaction. One may even go farther: when antigen antibody complexes are injected into animals with pre-existent liver lesions, necroses occur in one third of them. In the other two thirds which do not develop necroses, the antigen-antibody complexes are taken up by the Kupffer cells. This is probably the mechanism by which the Kupffer cells protect the liver parenchyma from immunologic injury. To produce larger necroses by the injection of antigen-antibody complexes, paralysis of the Kupffer cells is probably a requisite. In those cases in which a progressive hepatitis was preceded by many infections, probably a blockade or paralysis of the Kupffer cells exists.

BOCK (Tübingen): When secondarily the plasma-cell elements are very substantially increased in the reticulo-endothelial system, is this possibly an answer to the blockade of the Kupffer cells ?

POPPER (New York): That cannot be definitely said.

ROITT (London): In primary biliary cirrhosis there is a very high incidence of mitochondrial antibodies. If you look at other situations where liver damage has been caused, such as in extra-hepatic biliary obstruction or in viral hepatitis or in alcoholic cirrhosis, these antibodies are very rarely present Dr. Berg has established that the antibodies in biliary cirrhosis are in fact directed against the mitochondria, especially against the inner mitochondrial membrane. There is an interesting analogy in syphilis where the antibodies giving the WR test react with cardiolipin, which in fact is an inner mitochondrial membrane component. Drs. Doniach and Walker have been looking at biopsies from patients without overt liver disease but who have mitochondrial antibodies. They have found histological changes which they interpret as being early autoimmune hepatitis changes. I wonder whether it would be of value to look at the electron microscope level at biopsies from these types of individuals. Can one perhaps see evidence of some organism or abnormality in the mitochondria ?

POPPER (New York): Our cytologic methods for the study of the ultrastructure of the mitochondria in tissue sections are too poor to answer this, of course, crucial question.

RIETHMÜLLER (Tübingen): On which day after halothane exposition could you observe lymphocyte transformation by halothane in vitro ?

POPPER (New York): Are all of you acquainted with the halothane induced hepatic hypersensitivity reaction characterized by fever spike or bilirubinuria and sometimes jaundice ? If it appears after the first halothane anesthesia, we usually see it on the tenth day. After repeated anesthesia, it appears earlier and after the third halothane exposure an acute fatal liver atrophy may develop within one day after the operation. If after a halothane exposure fever or bilirubinemia are observed, halothane should no more be administered again. Lymphocyte transformation was studied on the 7th to 10th day after the operation.

DE WECK (Berne): The liver plays eventually an essential role in the induction of immunological tolerance. If, for example, a chemical antigen is injected into a mesenteric vein, tolerance can be produced with substantially smaller doses than are necessary if the antigen is injected into the greater circulation. The induction of immunological tolerance in dogs by injecting dinitrochlorobenzene into the mesenteric veins has also been reported. The same dose however fails to produce tolerance when a porto-caval shunt is present.

RIETHMÜLLER (Tübingen): I would like to refer to Calne's observations [Proc. Transplan. Soc. 1 (1968) (in press)] that liver tissue per se has an immunosuppressive activity in pigs. Thus, the simultaneous transplantation of liver can prevent the rejection of a grafted kidney.

Bayer-Symposium I, 234—237 (1969)

Cellular Immune Reactions in Experimental Hepatitis

H. WARNATZ

With 1 Figure

It is now generally agreed that circulating antibodies do not play a significant role in the pathogenesis of chronic liver diseases in men. In rabbits the formation of circulating antibodies against cytoplasmic, mitochondrial and nuclear antigens

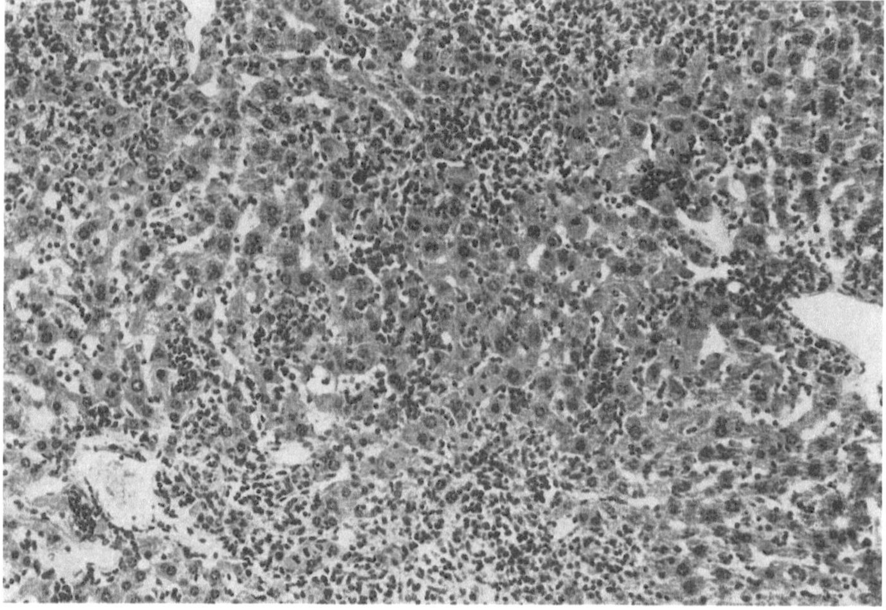

Fig. 1. Histological section of the liver of a C57Bl mouse suffering from experimental hepatitis

of liver tissue could be produced by active sensitization [2, 6]. These antibodies, however, have no pathogenetic effect on the liver as we could demonstrate by injection of great amounts of immune serum.

In the experimental hepatitis of the mouse the importance of lymphocytes for the pathogenesis of the disease could be demonstrated [1, 3—5]. In C57Bl mice we were able to induce an experimental hepatitis by intramuscular injection of homologous liver extract mixed with Freund's adjuvant over 2 to 3 months. For the sensitization we used a whole liver extract mixed with Freund's adjuvant in a ratio of 1:1. Controls were injected with Freund's adjuvant alone or were untreated animals. 72% of sensitized mice showed after 12 weeks liver injury which resembled morphologically the human chronic hepatitis. This experimental hepatitis, however, was in no case progressive; after ceasing the sensitization the liver changes disappeared during about 2 months. In Freund's adjuvant treated

Table 1. *Morphologic examination of the livers of the recipients after transfer of lymphocytes from isologous C57 Bl mice sensitized to liver extract of AKR mice*

Intervals after cell transfer	No. examined	No. showing histological liver lesions		
		∅	+	++
3	23	12	9	2
6	30	14	13	3
9	21	13	7	1
12	14	9	5	
15	15	9	6	
21	13	11	2	

Table 2. *Results of the histological investigation of the liver of parabiontic mice. The severity of morphological liver injury was listed as follows: ∅ normal histology of the liver; + moderate infiltration of the periportal fields with mononuclear cells and increase of Kupffer cells; ++ intensive infiltration of the periportal fields and intensive increase in Kupffer cells, as well as necrosis of liver parenchyma cells*

a) Parabiosis of sensitized mice with normal isologous mice

Day after operation	Liver changes in					
	sensitized mice			normal mice		
	∅	+	++	∅	+	++
5.	2	5	2	5	2	2
10.	0	6	3	1	6	2
15. or longer	3	2	0	1	4	0

b) Parabiosis of normal control mice

Day after operation	Liver changes in the					
	first parabiont			second parabiont		
	∅	+	++	∅	+	++
5.	4	0	0	3	1	0
10.	5	0	0	5	0	0
15. or longer	4	0	0	4	0	0

animals in 27% a slight liver injury was produced whereas no untreated mice showed histological changes of the liver (Fig. 1).

This experimental hepatitis could be transferred by intravenous injection of lymphocytes of the diseased mice to normal isologous animals, s. Table 1.

More than 50% of the recipients showed an infiltration of the periportal fields, an increase in Kupffer cells as well as localized liver cell necrosis.

More severe liver injury was induced if normal and liver diseased mice were united by parabiosis (Table 2).

By transfer of ^{3}H-thymidine labelled cells of mice with experimental hepatitis we could demonstrate that most of the cells are found in the spleen and lymph nodes of the recipients and only very seldom in the liver. About 0.1 to 0.3% of

Table 3. *Distribution of histological liver damage in the thymectomized animals and in the non-thymectomized controls after sensitization with homologous liver extract mixed with Freunds adjuvant (FA), with Freunds adjuvant alone or with liver extract alone*

Animals	Antigen	Histological liver damage		
		∅	+	++
Thymectomized mice	homologous liver + FA	24	16	13
	FA alone	15	3	0
	homologous liver	12	1	0
Non-thymectomized mice	homologous liver + FA	13	4	20
	FA alone	14	7	0
	homologous liver	14	1	0

Table 4. *Results of the lymphocyte transformation test in mice with experimental hepatitis. Mean values and standard deviation of the transformation rates in percent of the lymphocyte cultures without any added substance (N-culture), cultures with added isologous liver extract (L-culture), cultures with added isologous kidney extract (R-culture) and cultures with added phytohemagglutinin (P-culture). The underlined value of the L-culture is significantly different (p = 0.02) from the value of the N-culture*

	Percent labelled cells	
	sensitized mice [22]	with Freund's adjuvant treated mice [24]
N-culture	6.30 ± 1.31	6.92 ± 1.18
L-culture	19.00 ± 9.76	5.92 ± 1.13
R-culture	7.45 ± 3.49	6.18 ± 1.86
P-culture	22.20 ± 18.62	22.61 ± 16.17

mononuclear cells in the liver were labelled, i.e. lymphocytes of the sensitized donor.

In experiments with thymectomized mice we intended to investigate if in such animals a liver damage can be produced after sensitization with homologous liver extract mixed with Freund's adjuvant. Neonatally thymetomized mice were sensitized as described above. The histological findings in the liver of the thymectomized mice are listed in Table 3.

In the thymectomized mice a slight increase of Kupffer cells and of mononuclear cells in the periportal fields was observed in 16, liver cell necrosis in 13 out of 53 animals. The intensity and the frequency of these liver changes, however, were lower in thymectomized animals than in control animals of the same age.

In studies with the lymphocyte transformation test lymph node lymphocytes of mice with experimental hepatitis were cultured with isologous normal liver extract for 5 days. 24 h before harvesting 10 µC ^{3}H-thymidine were added; the transformed cells were detected by autoradiography. The results are shown in Table 4.

The transformation rate in experimental hepatitis was significantly increased after addition of liver extract to the tissue culture medium.

In conclusion the experiments demonstrate that the cellular immunity plays an important role in the pathogenesis of experimental hepatitis.

References

1. Scheiffarth, F., H. Warnatz, and K. Mayer: Studies concerning the importance of mono-nuclear cells in the development of experimental hepatitis. J. Immunol. **98**, 396 (1967).
— — u. W. Niederer: Tierexperimentelle Untersuchungen zur Pathogenese der chronischen Hepatitis. I. Morphologische Studien an der Leber nach Sensibilisierung mit homologen Leberzellfraktionen. Virchows Arch. path. Anat. **339**, 358 (1965).
2. — —, and H. J. Schmidt: Immunological studies on the development of experimental hepatitis in thymectomized mice. Int. Arch. Allergy **32**, 308—317 (1967).
3. Warnatz, H., F. Scheiffarth und E. Liebelt: Studien zur Übertragbarkeit der experimentellen Hepatitis im Parabioseversuch. Z. Immun-Forsch. **136**, 60—67 (1968).
4. — —, F. Wolf, and J. H. Schmidt: Autoradiographic experiments concerning the importance of mononuclear cells in experimental hepatitis. J. Immunol. **98**, 402 (1967).
5. — — u. G. Schwarz: Tierexperimentelle Untersuchungen zur Pathogenese der chronischen Hepatitis. II. Serologische Studien nach Sensibilisierung mit homologen Leberzellfraktionen. Virchows Arch. path. Anat. **339**, 363 (1965).

Priv.-Doz. Dr. H. Warnatz
Abteilung für klinische Immunologie des
Universitäts-Krankenhauses Erlangen-Nürnberg,
852 Erlangen, Krankenhausstraße 12

Bayer-Symposium I, 238—244 (1969)

Quantitative Serum Immunoglobulin Determinations in Active Chronic Hepatitis and Idiopathic Cirrhosis[1]

H. Deicher, P. Otto, and E. Gleichmann

With 3 Figures

A substantial increase in the serum gamma globulins is commonly observed in many types of chronic inflammatory diseases of the liver, and it is associated with an increased turnover rate (Popper and Schaffner; Cohen). Among the many different serum determinations available from the modern clinical laboratory, the serum gamma globulin level constitutes the only variale correlating roughly to the degree of mesenchymal inflammatory reaction in the liver (Emmrich and Petzold; Popper and Schaffner; Takatsuki; Waldstein *et al.*). However, the electrophoretically separated gamma globulin fraction contains only part of the total serum immunoglobulins (Ig), while some of the smaller immunoglobulin classes migrate as beta globulins, or with intermediate beta-gamma-mobility (Heremans). The participation of different immunoglobulin classes in the hypergammaglobulinemia of different types of chronic inflammatory liver disorders was observed first using immunoelectrophoretic techniques (Bargob *et al.*; Hartmann *et al.*; Heremans; Scheidegger and Zahnd). In recent years, a number of workers have used quantitative immunodiffusion methods (Mancini *et al.*) in an attempt to determine quantitative changes of individual immunoglobulins in liver disease (Fahey; Feizi; Gleichmann and Deicher, 1968a, b; Hobbs, 1967; Lee; McKelvey *et al.*; Paronetto *et al.*, 1964; Tomasi). These investigations have resulted in recognizing certain typical immunoglobulin "constellations" for different types of inflammatory liver disorders, some of which may have diagnostic value. These observations, on the other hand, pose important questions as to the reasons for the different reaction patterns found. The investigations reported in this paper were undertaken in an attempt to further substanciate earlier observations by several laboratories (Fahey; Gleichmann and Deicher 1968b; Hobbs, 1967; Tomasi) on the almost exclusive increase of immunoglobulin G (IgG) in chronic active hepatitis and in idiopathic cirrhosis, only accompanied by an insignificant rise of immunoglobulin M (IgM) and nearly or definitely normal serum levels of immunoglobulin A (IgA). Serum immunoglobulin values were determined using Mancini's single radial immunodiffusion technique, and results were calculated as milligrams per milliliter of serum (mg/ml). The sum of IgG, IgM, and IgA was called total Ig thus not regarding IgD and IgE levels. Normal values and details of the techniques have been described in an earlier publication (Gleichmann and Deicher, 1968a). Antinuclear factors in serum were measured by a antiglobulin consumption tech-

---

[1] Supported by a grant from the Deutsche Forschungsgemeinschaft.

nique (Deicher). All patients studied hat at least one liver biopsy, and necropsy reports were available in a few cases[2].

Among the different hepatic disorders the typical so-called immunological sequence (Fitch and Wissler) of IgM- and IgG-rise and decrease has been observed in acute hepatitis (Gleichmann and Deicher, 1968). In cases of chronic inflammatory disorders on a toxic basis (i.e., mostly chronic ethanol abuse), a particular rise of IgA, together with varying degrees of raised IgG levels, have been described (Gleichmann and Deicher, 1968b; Hobbs, 1967; Lee; Tomasi; Wilson *et al.*), and a good correlation has been found between the intensity of the

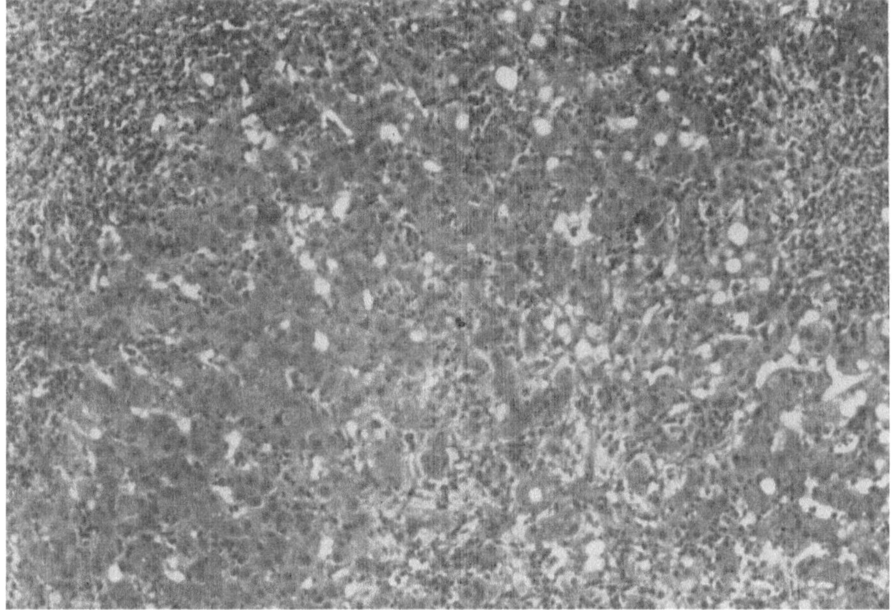

Fig. 1. Severe active chronic hepatitis showing the aggresive inflammatory lesion in the liver
(HE, × 100)

inflammatory reaction in the liver tissues, and the degree of serum immunoglobulin elevation (Gleichmann and Deicher, 1968b; Gleichmann *et al.*). An somewhat similar pattern has been observed in intrahepatic cholangitis, in contrast to uncomplicated mechanical bile obstruction where normal Ig values are the rule (Gleichmann and Deicher, 1968b). In primary biliary cirrhosis, a marked increase of IgM has been found (Hobbs, 1967). Clinical observation indicate that both the absolute level, and the relation of the different Ig to each other are useful parameters. A quotient IgG/IgA has been proposed by Tomasi as an indicator for the relative rise of these two Ig. Although the validity of the quantitative Ig determinations for the evaluation of the individual case has been questioned by some, the majority of workers agree that the exact quantitation of serum Ig is a useful additional tool for the clinician.

---

[2] The authors wish to thank Professor Dr. W. Wepler, Kassel, for the histological evaluation.

An immunopathological etiology has been implicated for another chronic inflammatory hepatic disorder now called active chronic hepatitis (Mackay *et al.*, 1965; Popper *et al.*, 1965). This disease entity was first described by Waldenström in 1950, and has since been designated as chronic liver disease in young women (Bearn *et al.*), active chronic viral hepatitis (Joske and King), active juvenile cirrhosis (Read *et al.*), lupoid hepatitis (Mackay *et al.*, 1956), idiopathic cirrhosis of menopausal women (Martini and Dölle), or progressive hypergammaglobulinemic hepatitis (Miescher *et al.*). It is now generally agreed that these different descriptions cover one and the same disease in different age groups and in different stages

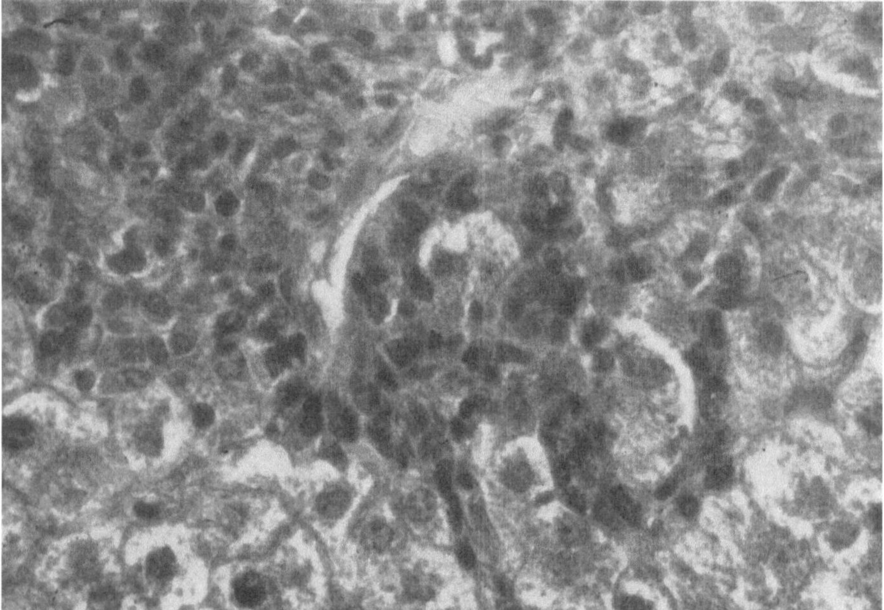

Fig. 2. Active chronic hepatitis. Larger magnification of the border between portal inflammation, and liver parenchyme. Intimate contact between inflammatory cells, and liver cells (piecemeal necrosis) is seen (HE, × 250)

of development (Schmid). The clinical syndrome in these predominantly female patients varies considerably, and sighns often appear late. Many patients have associated systemic symptoms such as arthritis, skin rashes, pleural effusion, colitis, and different hematological abnormalities. The histological features of this disease entity have recently been described as chronic aggressive hepatitis (de Groote *et al.*), characterized by an intensive inflammatory portal infiltration spilling into the parenchyma, with piecemeal necrosis and rosette formation, and subsequent fibrosis proceeding to a postnecrotic type cirrhosis of the liver (Figs. 1, 2). Several types of tissue antibodies can be found in the serum of a rather high percentage of patients, but the relation of such antibodies to the clinical disease is still largely a matter of conjecture (Mackay *et al.*, 1956, 1965; MacLachlan *et al.*). Among these antibodies, antinuclear factors (ANF) have found particular attention; a correlation between ANF titers and serum gamma globulin levels has been noted by Doniach *et al.*

The group of 30 patients observed to-date in our department consists of 27 women and 3 men. The hepatitis group comprises 20 women and 1 man, 10 of them showing a positive ANF reaction. 9 patients presented a fully developed idiopathic cirrhosis when first referred to the hospital. A consistent serum Ig pattern has been observed in these patients, characterized by a pronounced increase of IgG and a normal, or nearly normal IgA. Only 1 patient had a serum IgA above 5 mg/ml. The IgM values usually exceeded the normal range, but a consistent pattern could not be found. The average values obtained from this group of patients at the time of admission are given in Table 1. Of particular interest is the finding of an identical Ig pattern in active chronic hepatitis, and in "idiopathic" cirrhosis, favouring the view that these two clinical conditions have a common etiology (Feizi; Gleichmann and Deicher, 1968b). The group of patients with positive ANF showed the highest IgG levels, but their clinical status differed but little from the ANF negative group. Serial Ig determinations in the sera of these

Table 1. *Serum immunoglobulin levels in active chronic hepatitis and "idiopathic" cirrhosis*

Immunoglobulin mg/ml	Normal range[b]	Active chronic hepatitis (ANF +)	Active chronic hepatitis (ANF —)	"Idiopathic" cirrhosis
IgG	11.8 ± 2.3	43.0 ± 15.1	32.0 ± 12.2	31.0 ± 10.3
IgA	2.4 ± 1.4	2.9 ± 1.4	3.0 ± 1.9	3.6 ± 1.2
IgM	1.5 ± 0.7	3.0 ± 1.3	3.3 ± 2.1	2.8 ± 2.3
Total Ig[a]	15.7 ± 3.0	48.7 ± 15.5	38.3 ± 13.8	37.4 ± 10.3
IgG/IgA	5.6 ± 2.0	13.8 ± 7.1	13.5 ± 7.6	9.3 ± 4.4
n	100/150	10	11	9

[a] Total Ig = Sum of IgG, IgA, and IgM not regarding IgD and IgE.
[b] From E. Gleichmann, and H. Deicher: Klin. Wschr. 46, 171 (1968).

patients have shown that this particular Ig pattern is a consistent feature of this disease (Fig. 3). Exacerbations have been accompanied by a sole rise of IgG in these cases, in sharp contrast to the conjoint increase of IgG and IgA in alcoholic liver disease (Gleichmann and Deicher, 1968b). The IgG level fell during remission periods, and this was accompanied by an improvement of the histological picture. A study on 84 consecutive liver biopsies (Gleichmann *et al.*) has clearly established that a statistically significant correlation exists between the degree of inflammatory infiltration in the liver, and the IgG level found in the serum. Little of no correlation was found between the degree of fibrosis, and Ig values in the serum. A similar study relating serum IgA levels and severity of alcoholic cirrhosis has recently been published by Wilson *et al.*

Although these results are of interest for the clinician, their interpretation in nosological terms appears to be difficult at present. The production of Ig protein in the inflamed liver has been reported (Paronetto *et al.*, 1962). Certainly the different tissue antibodies mentioned above constitute only a negligible fraction of total serum Ig (Holman and Deicher), and this probably also applies for the antibody to liver protein recently described by Meyer zum Büschenfelde. During longer observation periods we have found that the rise of IgG accompanying exacerbation periods of active chronic hepatitis is a sequel rather than a precursor

     H. Deicher, P. Otto, and E. Gleichmann

of the inflammatory damage to the liver parenchyme; this certainly argues against a direct relation between Ig of any sort and the tissue lesion. Also, a direct cytotoxic reaction of patients' lymphocytes in culture (Warnatz *et al.*) towards autologous liver tissue has not been confirmed by others (Rössler and Havemann). Thus any autoimmune concept of this type of liver disease cannot be based on firm grounds at present, and the self perpetuation mechanism proposed by Popper may be a more likely pathogenetic mechanism. Hobbs has viewed the particular type of the Ig pattern observed in active chronic hepatitis as an abnormal immune response, in contrast to the "normal" response of all Ig fractions in some other types of chronic liver inflammation. Most cases of systemic lupus erythematosus

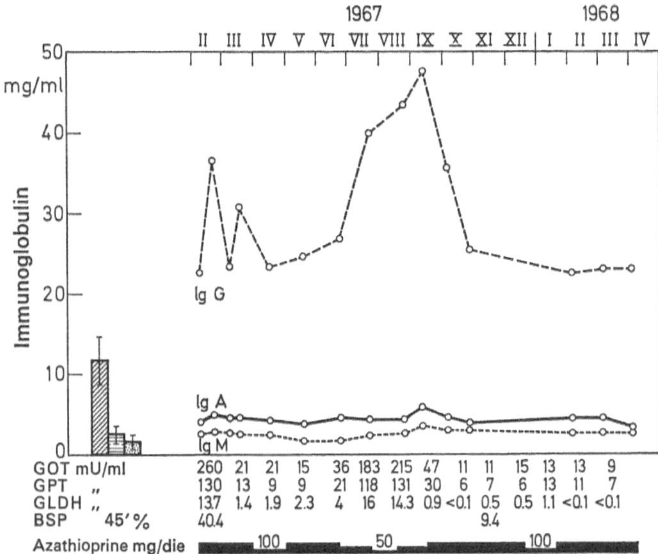

Fig. 3. Immunoglobulin levels of a case of active chronic hepatitis during a sixteen months observation period. Exacerbation periods, indicated by markedly elevated serum transaminase values, are accompanied by a substantial increase of serum IgG. In contrast, IgA and IgM show no reaction at all. IgG; IgA; IgM

show a serum Ig picture very similar to that observed in active chronic hepatitis, and systematic lupus is commonly taken as the best example of an autoimmune disorder (Deicher and Krull).

The peculiar Ig reaction so regularly seen in active chronic hepatitis may at present be interpreted as an unusual and somehow abnormal reaction of the immune system, to an unknown antigenic stimulus possibly connected to the body's own tissues. However, this reaction pattern adds little to our understanding of the diseases process, and should thus be used as a diagnostic tool rather then interpreted in "autoimmune" terms.

References

Bargob, I., H. Cleve u. F. Hartmann: Immunelektrophoretische Serumuntersuchungen bei Lebererkrankungen. Dtsch. Arch. klin. Med. **204**, 708 (1958).
Bearn, A. G., H. G. Kunkel, and R. J. Slater: The problem of chronic liver disease in young women. Amer. J. Med. **21**, 3 (1956).

Bonomo, L., and U. Gillardi: Broad-band hypergammaglobulinemia and chronic liver disease. II. Immunoglobulin levels in liver cirrhosis. Acta hepato-splenol. (Stuttg.) 14, 152 (1967).

Cohen, S.: γ-globulin metabolism. Brit. med. Bull. 19, 206 (1963).

Deicher, H.: Der Antiglobulin-Konsumptiontest in der Diagnostik des Lupus erathematodes visceralis. Laboratoriumsblätter 1967, 74.

—, and P. Krull: Unpublished observations.

Doniach, D., I. M. Roitt, J. G. Walker, and S. Sherlock: Tissue antibodies in primary biliarly cirrhosis, active chronic (lupoid) hepatitis, crytogenic cirrhosis and other liver disease and their clinical implications. Clin. exp. Immunol. 1, 237 (1966).

Emmrich, R., u. H. Petzold: Das Bluteiweißbild bei chronischen interstitiellen Entzündungen der Leber. Dtsch. Arch. klin. Med. 202, 303 (1955).

Fahey, J. L.: Antibodies and immunoglobulins. II. Normal development and changes in disease. J. Amer. med. Ass. 194, 255 (1965).

Feizi, T.: Immunoglobulins in chronic liver disease. Gut 9, 193 (1968).

Fitch, F. W., and R. W. Wissler: The histology of antibody production. In: Samter, M., and H. L. Alexander, Immunological diseases. Boston: Little, Brown & Co. 1965.

Gleichmann, E., u. H. Deicher: Quantitative Immunglobulinbestimmungen im Serum bei entzündlichen Leberkrankheiten. I. Normalwerte und Untersuchungen im Verlaufe der akuten Hepatitis. Klin. Wschr. 46, 171 (1968a).

— — Quantitative Immunglobulinbestimmungen im Serum bei entzündlichen Leberkrankheiten. II. Chronisch entzündliche Lebererkrankungen. Klin. Wschr. 46, 793 (1968b).

—, W. Wepler und H. Deicher: Quantitative Immunglobulinbestimmungen im Serum bei entzündlichen Leberkrankheiten. III. Korrelation zur Entzündungsreaktion im histologischen Bild. Acta hepato-splenolog. (Im Druck).

De Groote, J., V. J. Desmet, P. Gedigk, G. Korb, H. Popper, H. Poulsen, P. J. Scheuer, M. Schmid, H. Thaler, E. Uehlinger, and W. Wepler: A classification of chronic hepatitis. Lancet 1968 II, 626.

Hartman, L., P. Burtin, P. Grabar et R. Fauvert: L'analyse immunoélectrophorétique des sérums de malades atteints d'affections hepatiques. C. R. Acad. Sci. (Paris) 243, 1937 (1956).

Heremans, J. F.: Les globulins sériques du système gamma. Leur nature et leur pathologie. Brüssel: Arscia 1960.

Hobbs, J. R.: Serum proteins in liver disease. Proc. roy. Soc. Med. 60, 1250 (1967).

—, and G. W. Hepner: Immunoglobulins and alimentary disease. Lancet 1968 II, 47.

Holmann, H. R., and H. Deicher: The reaction of the lupus erythematosus (L. E.) cell factor with desoxyribonucleoprotein of the cell nucleus. J. clin. Invest. 38, 2059 (1959).

Joske, R. A., and N. E. King: The "L. E." cell phenomenon in active chronic ciral hepatitis. Lancet 1955 II, 477.

Lee, F. I.: Immunoglobulins in viral hepatitis and active alcoholic liver disease. Lancet 1965 II, 1043.

Mackay, I. R., L. I. Taft, and D. C. Cowling: Lupoid hepatitis. Lancet 1956 II, 1323.

—, S. Weiden, and J. Hasker: Autoimmune hepatitis. Ann. N. Y. Acad. Sci. 124, 767 (1965).

— and B. Ungar: Treatment of active chronic hepatitis (lupoid hepatitis) with 6-mercaptopurin and azathioprine. Lancet 1964 I, 2339.

Maclachlan, M. J., G. P. Rodnan, W. M. Cooper, and R. H. Fennel: Chronic active ("lupoi") hepatitis. Clinical, serological and pathological studies of 20 patients. Ann. intern. Med. 62, 425 (1965).

Mancini, G., A. O. Carbonara, and J. F. Heremans: Immunochemical quantitation of antigens by single radial immunodiffusion. Immunochemistry 2, 235 (1965).

Martini, G. A., u. W. Dölle: Idiopathische Lebercirrhose bei Frauen in der Menopause. Klin. Wschr. 38, 13 (1960).

McKelvey, E. M., and J. L. Fahey: Immunoglobulin changes in disease: quantitation on the basis of heavy polypeptide chains, IgG (γG), IgA (γA), and IgM (γM), and of light polypeptide chains, type K (I), and type L (II). J. clin. Invest. 44, 1778 (1965).

Miescher, P. A., A. Braverman, and E. L. Amorosi: Progressive hypergammaglobulinämische Hepatitis. Dtsch. med. Wschr. 91, 1525 (1966).

Meyer zum Büschenfelde, K. H.: Untersuchungen über die immunbiologische Bedeutung löslicher Leberproteine. Verh. dtsch. Ges. inn. Med. 74 (1968) (im Druck).

Paronetto, F., E. Rubin, and H. Popper: Local formation of γ-globulin in the diseased liver, and its relation to hepatic necrosis. Lab. Invest. 11, 150 (1962).

—, F. Schaffner, and H. Popper: Immunocytochemical and serologic observations in primary biliary cirrhosis. New. Engl. J. Med. 271, 1123 (1964).

Popper, H., u. F. Schaffner: Die Leber, Struktur und Funktion. Stuttgart: Thieme 1961.

— Die chronische Hepatitis. Internist 7, 8 (1966).

Read, A. E., S. Sherlock, and C. V. Harrison: Active "juvenile" cirrhosis considered as part of an systemic disease and the effect of corticosteroid therapy. Gut 4, 378 (1963).

Rössler, R., u. K. Havemann: Untersuchungen zur Frage der Immunpathogenese chronischer Lebererkrankungen. Verh. dtsch. Ges. inn. Med. 74 (1968) (im Druck).

Saint, E. G., W. E. King, R. A. Joske, and E. S. Finckh: Aust. Ann. Med. 2, 113 (1953).

Scheidegger, J. J., et G. Zahnd: Etude immuno-électrophorétique et électrophorétique des protéins sériques dans certaines affections hépatiques. Helv. med. Acta 24, 499 (1957).

Schmid, M.: Die chronische Hepatitis. Berlin-Heidelberg-New York: Springer 1966.

Takatsuki, R.: Electrophoretic studies of blood serum proteins in hepatobiliary disease: IV. correlations between electrophoretic patterns of human serum proteins and histologic findings of the liver. Jap. Arch. Int. Med. 6, 345 (1959).

Tomasi, T. B.: Diseases of the liver. In Samter, M., and H. L. Alexander: Immunological diseases. Boston: Little, Brown & Co. 1965.

Waldenström, J.: Leber, Blutprotein und Nahrungseiweiß. Stoffwechselkrankheiten. Sonderband der XV. Tag. dtsch. Ges. Verdauungs- und Stoffwechselkrankh., Bad Kissingen, p. 8, 1950. Zit. nach Sherlock, S.: Waldenström's chronic active hepatitis. Acta med. scand. Suppl. 445, 426 (1966).

Waldstein, S. S., H. Popper, P. B. Szanto, and F. Steigmann: Liver cirrhosis. Relation between function and structure based on biopsy studies. Arch. intern. Med. 87, 844 (1951).

Walker, G., and D. Doniach: Antibodies and immunoglobulins in liver disease. Gut 9, 266 (1968).

Warnatz. H.: Das Phänomen der Lymphocytentransformation in der Pathogenese und Diagnostik von Autoimmunerkrankungen. Z. ges. exp. Med. (im Druck).

Wilson, I. D., G. R. Onstad, R. C. Williams, and J. B. Carey: Serum immunoglobulin changes in patients with alcoholic cirrhosis. Clin. Res. 15, 246 (1967).

Prof. Dr. H. Deicher
Medizinische Klinik der Medizinischen Hochschule Hannover im Krankenhaus Oststadt,
3 Hannover, Podbielskistraße 380

Discussion

HAMMER (Freiburg): Is it possible to demonstrate whether the IgA which you have found in increased amounts in your studies is a monomeric or a dimeric type with T-chain specificity? A second question concerns the multiplication of IgG globulin in liver damage: is this a monoclonal IgG and which gamma-G type is it?

BOCK (Tübingen): May I extend this question to IgM?

DEICHER (Hannover): Concerning the first question about IgA, this is under investigation in our laboratory. Answering the second question concerning IgG, we have no indication as yet that there is multiplication of a monoclonal type IgG in active chronic hepatitis. Some earlier investigators have reported "paraprotein-like" electrophoretic gamma globulin fractions in certain cases [Schmidt, F. W., u. E. Wildhirt: Klin. Wschr. 35, 1139 (1957)]. However, in the majority of cases, and certainly in all of ours, the IgG are of the polyclonal type. According to immunoelectrophoretic results, the IgM also arise as polyclonal type proteins, very similar to their appearance in any other infection.

Bayer-Symposium I, 245—250 (1969)

The Possible Role of Lipid Containing RNA Viruses for the Etiology of Autoimmune Diseases

R. DRZENIEK, and R. ROTT

With 1 Figure

The role of antibodies in the course of virus infections is not well understood. It can be said, however, that the elimination of infectious particles is not their only function. It was shown by Hotchin (1962) that in infections of mice with the virus of lymphocytic choriomenigitis the overt disease is an immediate sequela of the formation of specific antibodies. A similar mechanism, i.e. an antigen-antibody reaction as a trigger for a disease, is currently discussed for the chronic infections with neuropathogenic agents or "slow viruses" (Johnson, 1967). In these diseases complexes of antibodies and viral antigens are supposed to be formed at the surface of the cells of the central nervous system (CNS).

As far as known today all the viruses, which are thought to be responsible for those diseases belong into the group of lipid-containing viruses. The structure of the lipid-containing viruses is rather complex in contrast to those viruses which contain only nucleic acid and protein. They have a core consisting of a highly organized nucleoprotein which is enclosed by an envelope consisting of proteins, lipids and carbohydrates.

Data have been presented which are in favour of the idea that the lipids and carbohydrates of these viria are predominantly derived from cell-specific material (Knight, 1954; Kates et al., 1961; Ada and Gottschalk, 1956; Wecker, 1957; Frommhagen et al., 1958, 1959).

Recently it was demonstrated that not only cellular constituents of low molecular weight are incorporated into the viria. Specific cellular structures of high molecular weight like blood group A substance or Forssman antigen are incorporated into influenza viruses as shown by Springer and Schuster (1964). Similar results were obtained by Isacson and Koch (1965) using parainfluenza II viruses, which contained blood group B substance, when grown in rhesus monkey kidney cells, in which this antigen is present. About 40% of the virus particle can consist of host specific material as shown by serological means (Munk u. Schäfer, 1951).

We found that blood group substances, Forssman antigen, and mononucleosis antigens as well as specific carbohydrates could be demonstrated in NDV preparations only when these antigens were present in the cells which had been used to grow different NDV preparations (Drzeniek et al., 1966a).

These phenomena originally observed in myxoviruses hold also true, as far as known, for all other lipid containing RNA viruses. We investigated representatives of the arboviruses, the leucosis viruses, as well as additional myxoviruses (Rott *et al.*, 1966). The antigens under investigation were demonstrated by absorption of antisera with purified virus preparations. The sera used in these experiments were anti-Forssman-antigen sera prepared in rabbits by immunization with guinea pig kidney tissue, reconvalescent sera from mononucleosis patients, and commercially available blood group hyperimmune sera. In addition phytagglutinins were used as reagents for the demonstration of specific carbohydrates.

As already said, the presence of Forssman, mononucleosis and blood group antigens could only be made evident, when the very same antigens were constituents of the cells in which the virus investigated had been multiplied. When a

Table 1. *Antigenicity of lipid containing RNA viruses and of corresponding host cells*[a]

Host	Viruses or host cells	Antigens			
		Forssman	Mono-nucleosis	Blood group A	Blood group B
Chick embryo	Newcastle disease	+	+	+	—
	parainfluenza 1	+	+	+	—
	mumps	+	+	+	—
	influenza A2	+	+	+	—
	fowl plague	+	+	+	—
	Sindbis	+	+	+	—
	host cells	+	+	+	—
Duck embryo	Newcastle disease	—	—	—	—
	fowl plague	—	—	—	—
	host cells	—	—	—	—
Rhesus kidney	Newcastle disease	+	n. t.	—	+
	measles	+	—	—	+
	host cells	+	n. t.	—	+
Cercopithecus kidney	Newcastle disease	—	n. t.	+	+
	measles	—	—	+	+
	host cells	—	n. t.	+	+

+ present; — absent; n. t. not tested.

[a] For details see: R. Rott *et al.* (1966); R. Drzeniek (1968).

different host was used for viral multiplication only corresponding antigens were found. Table 1 shows that all the lipid-containing viruses, which had been grown in embryonated chicken eggs, incorporate Forssman, mononucleosis and blood group A antigens. When the same viruses were grown in embryonated duck eggs, these antigens were not found. This agrees with the failure to demonstrate these antigens in duck embryos. Viruses grown in embryonated duck eggs contain specific substances which could be demonstrated also in duck embryo tissue with the aid of phytagglutinins. E.g. such viruses contain L-fucose as well as other carbohydrates which react with extracts from ricinus communis.

Different blood group substances were demonstrable in NDV and measles virus, when these viruses had been grown in various monkey kidney cell strains, which possess different blood group specificities. For such experiments we made use of rhesus monkey kidney cells which contain blood group B antigens and african green monkey kidney cells which possess both A and B antigens. As can be seen in Table 1 only those antigens are incorporated into the virus particle which are also present in the tissue used for virus multiplication.

In all these experiments a single passage in a different host was sufficient to achieve a change in the pattern of the host specific antigen. In the course of these experiments the virus specific antigens as well as the biological properties of the viria remained unchanged. The observed changes in the antigenic activities must therefore be interpreted as a modification due to the incorporation of host specific antigens into the virion.

Such changes occur most likely with those structures which possess certain structural similarities. This would explain the ease with which these antigens are exchanged.

At this point the question arises whether the host specific antigens found in the various preparations are actually constituing components of the virus particles or whether they are contaminants derived from the various hosts. Therefore different procedures of purification of myxoviruses were investigated. Adsorption to and elution from erythrocytes, carrier-free electrophoresis, chromatography with different adsorbing media and gradient centrifugation were used (Rott *et al.*, 1966; Isacson and Koch, 1965; Munk and Schäfer, 1951). None of these procedures yielded virus particles free of host specific components. Furthermore, as already shown by Springer and Schuster (1964) for blood group A activity, we were also unable to separate the three mentioned antigens from virus specific surface constituents by ether treatment (Drzeniek *et al.*, 1966b). While the internal ribonucleic acid containing capsid did not contain any host-specific antigens these activities were found in the hemagglutinin portion to the same extent as in the whole virus. The hemagglutinin is one of the major components of the viral envelope.

Only after treatment with methanol virus specific material could be obtained which was free of host derived antigens from hemagglutinin or whole virus. Since with the same procedure the same antigens can be extracted from host cells, we must assume that these host specific antigens are bound to the viral envelope in the same manner as in the host cell.

It is therefore not surprising when it is generally assumed that the envelope of the lipid containing viruses is understood as a virus-specifically modified cellular membrane. Convincing evidence for this interpretation was presented by Choppin (1968). His electron microscopic investigations showed that the cellular membrane obtains the properties of the viral envelope whereever viral cores aggregate underneath the cellular membrane. This phenomenon is most probably responsible for the observation that erythrocytes are adsorbed to infected cells (hemadsorption, Vogel and Shelokov, 1957) as well as to isolated virus particles (hemagglutination, Hirst, 1941).

During the process of viral maturation not only virus specific substances are incorporated into the cellular membrane. At the same time the structure of the membrane is altered. In this manner preexisting but masked antigens can become exposed. If e.g. chicken erythrocytes are treated with neuraminidase, Forssman antigen can be demonstrated, while untreated chicken red blood cells cannot be agglutinated by anti-Forssman-antigen sera. Forssman antigen, however, is present in the surface of virus particles (Drzeniek *et al.*, 1966 a). On the basis of these observations it appears to be possible that lipid-containing viruses can induce the production of autoantibodies.

During virus multiplication in an infected organism virus particles appear which carry on their surface besides virus specific also host specific antigens. These particles are dissiminated throughout the infected host. Thereby other cells will be infected and antibody producing cells will be stimulated. The antibody formation is not only stimulated because viruses are spread throughout the organism, but more important is the role of these viruses as ideal carriers for material which is only weakly antigenic or has the properties of a hapten. On the virus surface virus specific or host specific substances are in very close vicinity. Thereby the specificity of an antigen may be altered in such a way that it is no longer recognized as being "self". A further possibility is that due to this close vicinity antigen specificities are formed which consist partly of host derived and partly of virus derived material. Antibodies formed against such complexes may well be able to react also with a constituent of these antigen complexes yet possibly with reduced avidity.

Besides this carrier effect the presence of lipids in the viral envelope might stimulate the production of antibodies versus host specific material. This effect would be comparable to the action of Freund's adjuvans. In this way it is conceivable that an existing tolerance can be overcome.

It is well known that the virus specific antibodies react with virus infected cells since these cells possess in their surface virus specific antigens. Similarly the postulated auto-antibodies could react with such cells. Those interactions may lead to an elimination or destruction of these cells which in turn results in a liberation of new antigen complexes. This mechanism may ultimately result in an escalation of immunological reactions which would manifest itself as specific pathological changes in a given organ. This hypothesis is depicted in Fig. 1.

Antigens which by themselves do not elicit antibody production can do so if incorporated into the surface of a lipid-containing virus (Lindemann and Klein, 1967). He found that with homogenates of Ehrlich ascites cells mice could not be immunized against a subsequent transplantation of the same cells. If however, he inoculated mice with influenza virus, or other lipid-containing RNA-viruses which had been grown in E. ascites cells these mice showed a measurable resistance against the corresponding tumor cells. When the same viruses were grown in other cells they had no effect.

The close similarity between the microscopic findings in post infectious mumps encephalitis and in experimentally induced allergic encephalomyelitis has been noted (Donahue, 1955). The post infectious mumps encephalitis can be clearly differentiated from the primary mumps meningoencephalitis. The latter disease may be an expression for cell damage induced by the multiplying virus, while the post infectious encephalitis may be a manifestation of the action of autoantibodies (Witebsky, 1967).

A similar mechanism may be responsible for the subacute sclerosing panencephalitis which is supposed to be due to a preceding infection with measles virus (Lennette *et al.*, 1968) and in mumps orchitis (Witebsky, 1967) which usually develops after the typical findings of the acute parotitis are already subsiding.

The aim of this presentation is to give a hypothesis which might explain the genesis of autoimmune diseases. We have attempted to demonstrate which consequences the interaction between lipid containing viruses, cells and antibodies may

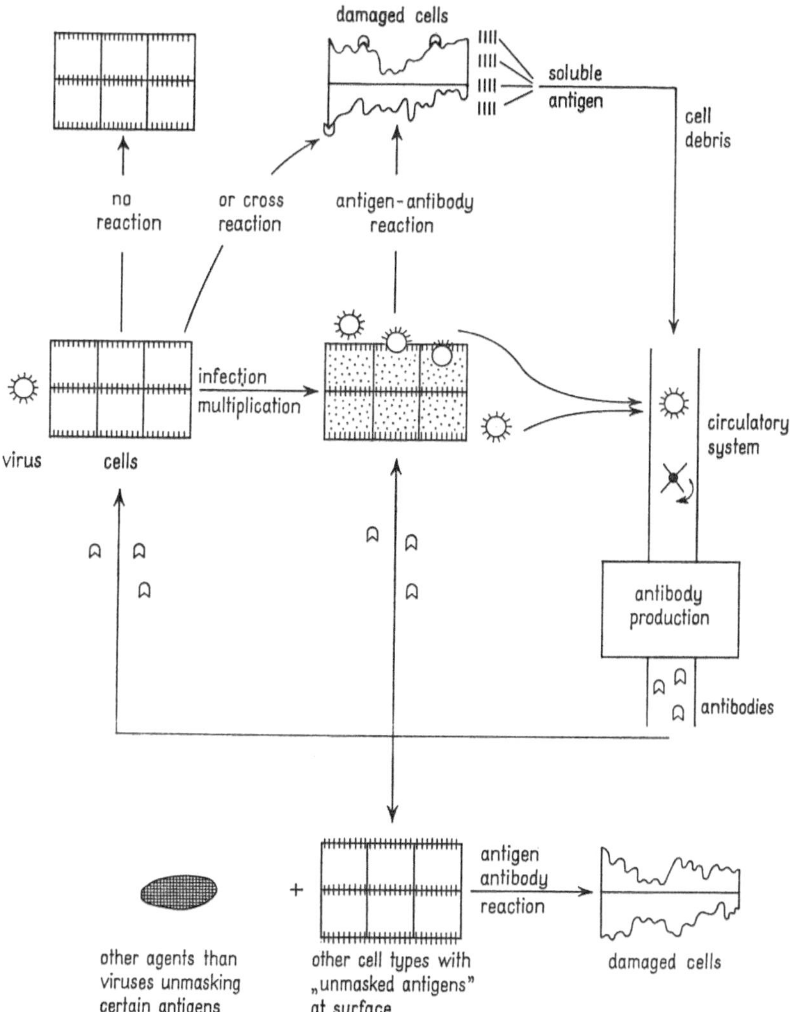

Fig. 1. Production of auto-antibodies after virus infection, a simplified scheme. (R. Drzeniek, and R. Rott, 1967)

have. Most important is that lipid-containing viruses of different groups may cause the same pathological reactions because they act by a similar principle.

References

Ada, G. L., and A. Gottschalk: Biochem. J. 62, 686 (1956).
Choppin, P. W.: First International Congress for Virology, 1968.
Donahue, W. L., F. D. Playfair, and L. Whitaker: J. Pediat. 47, 395 (1955).

Drzeniek, R.: Habilitation thesis, Giessen 1968.
—, and R. Rott: Int. Arch. Allergy (1967) (in press).
—, M. S. Saber, and R. Rott: Z. Naturforsch. **21b**, 254 (1966a).
—, E. Reichert, and R. Rott: Zbl. Vet.-Med. **12B**, 260 (1966b).
Frommhagen, L. H., N. K. Freeman, and C. A. Knight: Virology **5**, 173 (1958).
—, C. A. Knight, and N. K. Freeman: Virology **8**, 176 (1959).
Hirst, G. K.: Science **94**, 22 (1941).
Hotchin, J.: Cold Spr. Harb. Symp. quant. Biol. **27**, 479 (1962).
Isacson, P., and A. E. Koch: Virology **27**, 129 (1965).
Johnson, R. T.: Curr. Top. Microbiol. Immunol. **40**, 3 (1967).
Kates, M., A. C. Allison, D. A. J. Tyrell, and A. T. J. James: Biochim. biophys. Acta (Amst.)
    52, 455 (1961).
Knight, C. A.: Advanc. Virus Res. **2**, 153 (1954).
Lennette, E. H., R. L. Magoffin, and J. M. Freeman: Neurology (Minneap.) **18**, 21 (1968).
Lindenmann, J., u. P. A. Klein: J. exp. Med. **126**, 93 (1967).
Munk, K., u. W. Schäfer: Z. Naturforsch. **6b**, 372 (1951).
Rott, R., R. Drzeniek, M. S. Saber u. E. Reichert: Arch. ges. Virusforsch. **19**, 273 (1966).
Springer, G. F., u. R. Schuster: Klin. Wschr. **42**, 221 (1964).
Vogel, J., and A. Shelokov: Science **126**, 358 (1957).
Wecker, E.: Z. Naturforsch. **12b**, 208 (1957).
Witebsky, E.: In: Probleme der Verhütung von Viruserkrankungen. J. Ströder u. W. Henle
    (Ed.), Berlin-Heidelberg-New York: Springer 1967, p. 208.

Prof. Dr. R. Drzeniek
Institut für Virologie der Veterinärmedizinischen Fakultät der Universität
63 Gießen, Frankfurter Straße 87

Discussion

DEICHER (Hannover): We have observed a 16 year old female patient who after severe measles together with a recurrent urticaria, and half a year later showed the full blown picture of lupus erythematodes visceralis. Perhaps more clinical histories like this one are available. They would agree with the suggested hypothesis concerning the importance of RNA viruses in the aetiology of auto-immune diseases.

FISCHER (Hamburg): I would like to draw attention to the Thomsen-Friedenreich phenomenon, i.e. haemolytic disease in chronic infections in which the bacteria produce neuraminidase. This enzyme exposes the T receptors of the erythrocytes. As a result, blood transfusions can be followed by severe haemolysis. — I would also like to mention post-infectious thrombocytopenia as is observed, for example, after oral poliomyelitis vaccination. We have seen three such cases. It should be discussed whether the virus forms together with the thrombocytes a new antigen against which antibodies arise. This would be a similar process as in sedormit purpura in which the sedormit together with the thrombocytes represents a new antigen.

DRZENIEK (Gießen): We have only examined viruses which contain lipids; poliomyelitis virus does not belong to them. Nevertheless. I wish to stress the possibility that virus-specific antigens can be situated on the cell surface — probably in the form of certain complexes — and that this is the reason why cell destruction also takes place if the antibodies are not directed against the cell antigens but against the viral particles. Also, as is known, viruses can well multiply in various blood cells. I mention as an example the virus infections persisting in leucocytes.

KLEIN (Mainz): Does the Forssmann antigen interfere with a test like the Hirst test ? Is it known that some haemagglutination phenomena may suffer when the erythrocyte contains Forssmann antigen ?

DRZENIEK (Gießen): The antibodies against host-specific components do not interfere with the haemagglutination inhibition test when relatively high dilutions of antisera are used. In the case of high antiserum concentrations the agglutination between erythrocytes and myxoviruses is also inhibited by antibodies against cell-specific components [Knight, C. A.: J. exp. Med. 80, 83 (1944)].

KLEIN (Mainz): Should one assume that the antigenic sites involved into the reaction are located near the spikes ?

DRZENIEK (Gießen): We do not yet exactly know where on the viral surface the cell-specific antigens are situated. Our electron-microscopic examinations of myxoviruses suggest that the spikes consist of haemagglutinin and that the neuraminidase is situated at the ends of the spikes. The cell-specific antigens are very probably situated between these spikes.

WESTPHAL (Freiburg): In this connection the following question is interesting: — is a virus conjugate able to break tolerance ? Several pilot experiments exist on this score. It is possible for example to produce tolerance with serum protein in a foreign animal for the duration of its life time. If the tolerance is broken with azodyes or tyrosine, first the tyrosine specificity and gradually the carrier specificity emerges. The same may be assumed with regard to the model that has been discussed here: maybe that initially the viral antibody is demonstrable and the auto-antibody against the cell occurs later. A virus leaving a cell carries very different cellular components. It is possible that in certain circumstances it is completely covered by cellular components. In this case it does not show any antigenic action in the way of viral antigenicity. Only when in the course of time the cover is removed, a quiescent virus after a long period of interference suddenly becomes again antigenic. Is anything known about the time of the appearance of antibodies relative to the carrier ?

DRZENIEK (Gießen): For the various RNA viruses which contain lipid we know different relations between virus-specific and host-specific components. The leucosis viruses have on their surface mostly host-specific components and therefore antibodies against the virus can hardly be obtained [Eckert, E. A., R. Rott, and W. Schäfer: Virology 24, 426 (1964)]. The myxoviruses, on the other hand, have on their surface host-specific and virus-specific components side by side. Gradual shifts are encountered. — The other question, whether virus-specific antigens occur first and secondary cell-specific antigens subsequently, has not yet been studied in detail.

WESTPHAL (Freiburg): The observations in Japan with rabies vaccine certainly also belong in this place. The vaccine had been produced on monkey kidney cells.

After vaccination several people became ill with encephalitis and showed pictures
as in disseminated sclerosis.

RICKEN (Bonn): I would like to refer to a disease in which the mechanism you
have described is highly probable, that is post-infectious mumps-tracheitis or
pancreatitis. Preliminary investigantions carried out together with Prof. Witebsky/
Buffalo show that mumps sera may contain precipitating antibodies against
human testis.

DRZENIEK (Gießen): Such investigations are very important. Working with
viruses one has always to differentiate between antibodies directed against the
virus-specific components and those directed against the cell-specific components.
Only in the latter case would it be possible to speak of an auto-immune disease.

Bayer-Symposium I, 253—257 (1969)

Humoral Antibodies in Older Humans

(Preliminary Communication)

H. G. SCHWICK, and W. BECKER

With 3 Figures

Two years ago we worked together with Haferkamp and Schlettwein-Gsell in examining the immunoglobulin content and certain antibody activities in the serum of young and old humans. In these studies, a comparison of the two extreme

Table 1. *Immunoglobulins in old and young blood donors*

Group of age	n	IgG[a]	s	IgA[a]	s	IgM[a]	s	IgD[a]
20—30 years	100	1250	268	214	96	206	107	100%[b]
♀	44	1221	258	232	111	166	82	
♂	56	1273	275	200	80	238	113	
55—65 years	86	1297	334	259	107	158	84	66%[b]
♀	62	1323	332	264	108	159	86	
♂	24	1235	334	246	104	156	81	
Significant differences:		none		between the groups of age		between the groups of age and sex (20—30 years)		

[a] Arithmetric mean value in mg/100 ml.
[b] Referred to a relative-standard.

age groups showed that a marked increase in immunoglobulins, especially IgG- and IgA-globulin, is demonstrable in the serum of older persons, whereas certain antibody activities found in all sera are clearly decreased [1, 2].

We have continued these examinations with sera from a total of 186 younger and older persons; the one group was aged 20 to 30 years the other aged 55 to 65 years. Study was made of the immunoglobulins IgG, IgA and IgM, as well as IgD, using the radial immunodiffusion method [3] with Partigen plates. For IgD-globulin, only relative values can be given, since no pure IgD standard protein was available.

References to the literature in regard to the methods used for various antibody determinations will be given in the individual tables.

The results of immunoglobulin determination (Table 1) show no differences between the young and the old group in regard to IgG-globulin content. With IgA-globulin, however, there is a difference between the two groups: The older persons we examined had a significantly higher γA-globulin level than did the younger ones. With regard to IgM-globulin, we confirmed the finding already made by other authors [4—7] and ourselves [3], namely that IgM-globulin content is higher in women than in men. However, this could be demonstrated only in the younger group. Furthermore, the older group showed a significantly lower IgM-globulin content.

Agglutinating antibodies against various bacteria were decreased without exception in the older persons; in certain cases this was statistically significant (Fig. 1).

Of the bacterial-toxin antibodies which we examined (Fig. 2), the tetanus-toxin antibody behaved in a manner similar to the bacterial antibodies, whereas

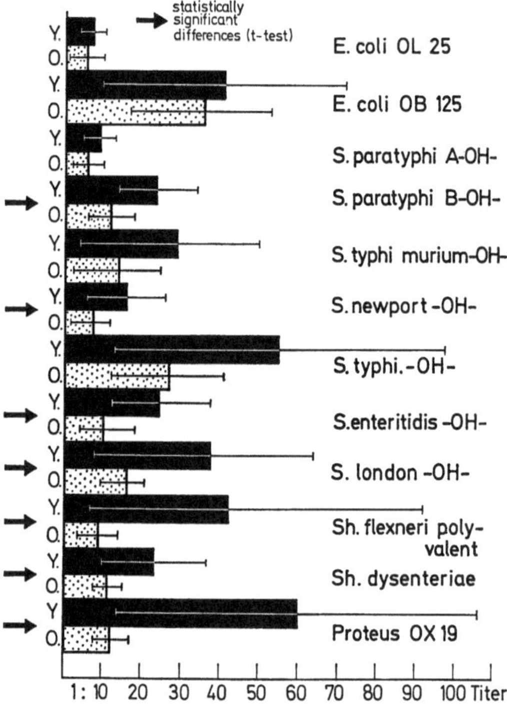

Fig. 1. Bacterial agglutinating antibodies in old (55 to 65 years) and young (20 to 30 years) blood donors

diphtheria and streptolysin antibodies were slightly increased, and staphylolysin antibodies showed no difference.

Study of anti-virus antibodies showed a significant decrease in the serum of older persons in practically every case (Fig. 3).

In summary, it can thus be said that almost all of the antibody activities we examined were decreased in the serum of persons between 55 and 65 years of age in comparison with that of persons aged 20 to 30 years.

So far, there have been only few examinations of the antibody level in older persons. Certain authors have reported that the anti-streptolysin [14—17] and anti-staphylolysin [18] titer is markedly lower in persons over 66 years old; this agrees with the findings which we obtained together with Haferkamp [1, 2]. The decrease in isoagglutinin titer in the serum of older people, as demonstrated by

various authors, is particularly impressive [19—21]. There are also few comparative examinations of antibody conditions after active immunization of younger
and older persons. However, Hertel [22] demonstrated as early as 1940 that persons over 65 years of age form less antibody against animal protein than do
younger persons.

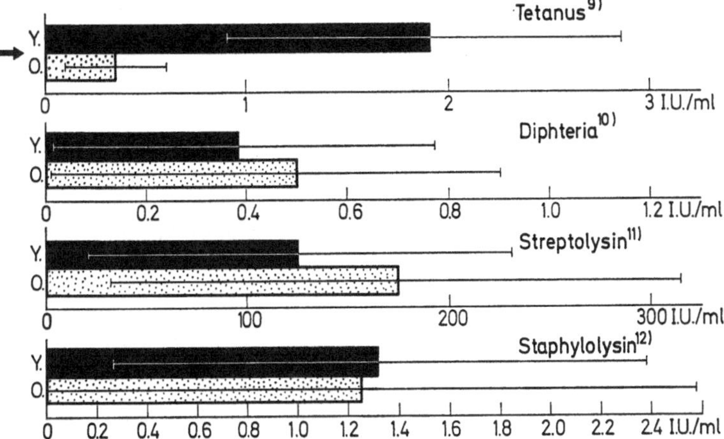

Fig. 2. Toxin-antibodies in old (55 to 65 years) and young (20 to 30 years) blood donors

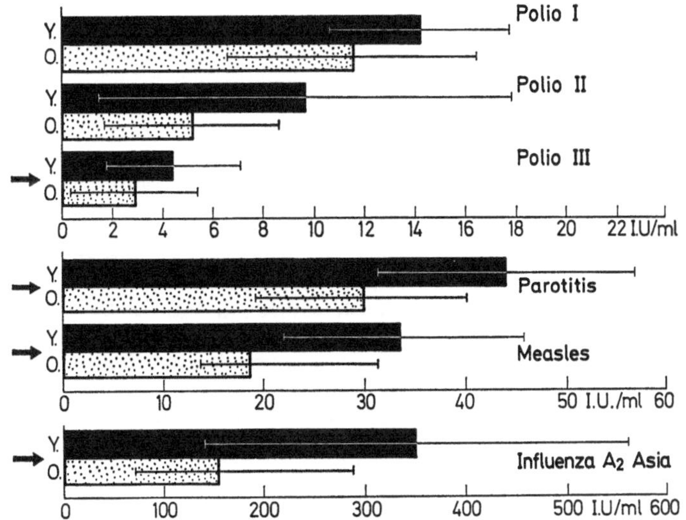

Fig. 3. Virus-antibodies in old (55 to 65 years) and young (20 to 30 years) blood donors

In contrast to the decrease in antibodies against exogenous antigens in the
serum of older persons, the findings reported of late reveal an increase in auto-
antibody activities in older persons [23, 24]. Finally, in this connection and also in
connection with the increase in immunoglobulin proteins in older persons, the increase in M-components, i.e. monoclonal immunoglobulins in the serum of older
people, must be pointed out [25].

The decrease in antibodies in the serum of older persons can be used to help explain their greater susceptibility to infections. As to the question of the cause of this decrease in antibody activities in the serum of older people, there are some points which must be discussed: a possible direct connection between the increase in antibodies against endogenous antigens (loss of tolerance?), and perhaps also the increase in monoclonal immunoglobulin, as well as a decrease in thymus function [26].

We are much obliged to: Dr. L. Körner, Dr. H. Kindt, Dr. R. Mauler Behringwerke AG. and their coworkers for antibody-estimations.

References

1. Haferkamp, O., D. Schlettwein-Gsell, H. G. Schwick und K. Störiko: Serumproteine im hohen Lebensalter unter besonderer Berücksichtigung der Immunglobuline und Antikörper. Klin. Wschr. **44**, 725 (1966).
2. — — — — Serum protein in an aging population with particular reference to evalution of immune globulins and antibodies. Gerontologia (Basel) **12**, 30 (1966).
3. Becker, W., W. Rapp, H. G. Schwick und K. Störiko: Methoden zur quantitativen Bestimmung von Plasmaproteinen durch Immunpräzipitation. Z. klin. Chem. **6**, 113 (1968).
4. Lichtman, M. A., J. H. Vaughan, and C. G. Hames: The distribution of serum immuno-globulins, anti-γG-globulins ("rheumatoid factors") and antinuclear antibodies in white and negro subjects in Evans County, Georgia. Arthr. and Rheum. **10**, 204 (1967).
5. Crabbé, P. A., and J. F. Heremans: Lack of gamma A-immunoglobulin in serum of patients with steatorrhoea. Gut **7**, 119 (1966).
6. Jensen, K. B.: Immunochemical determination of serum concentrations of albumin, IgG and IgM. Proc. 14th. Coll. Protides biol. Fluids 677 (1967). Brügge 1966.
7. Norberg, R.: The immunoglobulin content of normal serum. Acta med. scand. **181**, 485 (1967).
8. Kabat, E. A., and M. M. Mayer: Experimental immunochemistry, 2. Ed. 1961, p. 99. Springfield, Ill., USA: Charles C. Thomas Publ.
9. Eissner, G.: The biological assay of tetanus antitoxin. WHO/BS/SR/22 v. 3. 10. 1957.
10. Schmidt, H.: Die Basis der Auswertung von Toxinen und Antitoxinen, p. 22—23. Jena: Fischer 1931.
11. Schultze, H. E., G. Schwick und H. Vasters: Nachweis von Anti-Streptolysin O mit stabilem Trockenantigen. Ärztl. Wschr. **9**, 324 (1954).
12. Harter, F., H. G. Schwick und K. Störiko: Nachweis von Anti-Staphylokokken-α-Hämo-lysin mit stabilem Trockenantigen. Klin. Wschr. **43**, 1114 (1965).
13. Fiset, P.: Serological techniques. In: Techniques in experimental virology. R. J. C. Harris, Ed. London-New York: Acad. Press. 1964.
14. Rantz, L. A., J. M. di Caprio, and A. Randall: Antistreptolysin O and antihyaluronidase titers in health and various diseases. Amer. J. med. Sci. **224**, 194 (1952).
15. Köhler, W.: Der Antistreptolysin-Normaltiter in NO-Deutschland; Untersuchungen an 600 Personen. Z. Immun.-Forsch. **115**, 145 (1958).
16. Seifert, H.: Antistreptolysintiter und Lebensalter. Z. ges. inn. Med. **14**, 641 (1959).
17. Wildführ, G.: Altern und Immunitätslage. Z. ges. Hyg. **5**, 317 (1951).
18. Brzezinski, S.: Untersuchungen über die normalen Antistaphylolysine des menschlichen Serums. Schweiz. Z. Path. **2**, 18 (1939).
19. Thomsen, O., u. K. Kettel: Die Stärke der menschlichen Isoagglutinine und entsprechenden Blutkörperchenrezeptoren in verschiedenen Lebensaltern. Z. Immun.-Forsch. **63**, 67 (1929).
20. Prokop, O., u. G. Uhlenbruck: Lehrbuch der menschlichen Blut- und Serumgruppen, S. 27. Edition Leipzig 1963.
21. Mollison, P. L.: Blood transfusion in clinical medicine, p. 248. Oxford/Edinburgh: Blackwell Scientific Publ. 1967.

22. Hertel, H.: Das Verhalten der Präzipitation in den verschiedenen Altersstufen. Z. Alterns-
    forsch. **2**, 125 (1940).
23. Whittingham, S.: Autoantibodies and ageing. Proc. of the Haematol. Soc. of Australia —
    Sydney, May 1968.
24. Rowley, M. J., H. Buchanan, and I. R. Mackay: Reciprocal change with age in antibody
    to extrinsic and intrinsic antigens. Lancet **1968**, 24.
25. Hallén, J.: Frequency of "abnormal" serum globulins (M-components) in the aged. Act.
    med. scand. **173**, fasc. 6, 737 (1963).
26. Miller, J. F. A. P., and D. Osoba: Current concepts of the immunological function of the
    thymus. Physiol. Rev. **47**, 437 (1967).

Dr. H. G. Schwick
Behringwerke AG, 355 Marburg/Lahn

Discussion

FISCHER (Hamburg): Is the decrease of IgM with age parallel to the decrease of
the iso-antibodies anti-A and anti-B ? Are you still of the opinion that the excess
of IgM parallel with the decrease of antibody formation is due to an uncoined
IgM ?

SCHWICK (Marburg): That cannot be derived from the findings.

Bayer-Symposium I, 258—262 (1969)

Experimental Glomerulonephritis in Unresponsive Rabbits after Termination of Immunologic Tolerance

D. K. HAMMER

In recent studies, anti-glomerular basement membrane antibodies (anti-GBM) have been implicated as causative agent in the pathogenesis of certain human glomerulonephritides [1]. This conclusion was based on the observation that anti-GBM antibodies are present in the kidneys of all cases of Goodpasture's syndrome and one-half of the cases of human subacute glomerulonephritis so far examined. Glomerulonephritis can be passively transferred with anti-GBM antibodies, eluted from nephritic human kidneys.

Concerning the action of autoantibodies to GBM antigens, much of the information however is based on the experience with heterologous anti-GBM antibodies. Thus the Masugi model provides an excellent approach to elucidate the various immunological components involved in the pathogenesis of experimental glomerulonephritis [2].

Previous observations support the concept that

1. heterologous anti-GBM antibodies injected into recipients do produce immediate structural and functional damage of the kidney (*heterologous phase.*)

2. superimposed upon this initial immunological insult by heterologous anti-GBM antibodies, there is a specific immunological response of the recipient to the heterologous γ-globulin fixed in the glomerular capillary wall resulting in a progressive renal injury (*autologous phase*).

It was considered, therefore, that the autologous phase might be inhibited by rendering rabbits tolerant to the γ-globulin fraction of the heterologous anti-GBM antibody. Furthermore, on the basis of acquired tolerance it was postulated, that the termination of tolerance to the heterologous anti-GBM antibody might reactivate the nephritic state.

The anti-GBM antibody was obtained from sheep (SARB) by injecting preparations of rabbit GBM.

Tolerance in rabbits was induced within the first 12 h of birth by subcutaneous injection of 100 mg sheep γ-globulin (SγG) and subsequent injections during the next 5 days totalling 500 mg.

Rabbits at 3 months of age were injected intravenously with 20 mg of ^{131}I-labelled SγG to show failure of immune elimination as an index of a tolerant state. The breakdown of tolerance was obtained in rabbits by injection of 25 mg of an azo-SγG in complete Freund's adjuvant or by a p-tyrosyl-SγG p-Tyr-SγG [3]. The latter preparation was made by the reaction of the protein with the appropriate N-carboxy-L-tyrosyl anhydride. The second preparation were diazonium derivatives of the p-arsenilic and p-sulfanilic acid (A-S-SγG) prepared in HCl with $NaNO_2$ and coupled to protein [4]. Equal molar amounts of each derivative were added so that the total molar quantities were the same as when only one of the derivatives were coupled to a protein. The azoprotein contained 16.9 azogroups per molecule of protein. For breaking tolerance 25 mg of each preparation in complete Freund's adjuvant were given once a week for 3 weeks, and 3 additional intravenous injections with the native component, i.e. native $S\gamma G$. On the other hand, p-Tyr-$S\gamma G$ were also used to break the tolerant state by the same procedure mentioned above. The antibody analysis after termination of tolerance was done by employing ammonium sulfate technique of FARR utilizing iodinated antigens.

23 normal rabbits injected with 4.7 mg N/kg of a purified $I\gamma G$ fraction of the anti-GBM antibody (SARB) developed proteinuria detectable within 2 h and resulted in an initial 24 h urinary protein of 2167 mg-% (Table 1). The proteinuria in these rabbits remained during a subsequent 24 weeks observation period. 27 rabbits in a tolerant state however given the same amount of SARB developed the initial step of the disease. Heterologous $S\gamma G$ was fixed to the basement membrane and in the presence of complement renal injury was obtained. 5 to 7 days

Table 1. *Effect of SARB-IγG[a] on normal rabbits and rabbits injected with SγG at birth*

Group	No of rabbits	SARB-γG injected mg N/kg	Ave. proteinuria mg-%/24 h Days				
			1	5	7	28	56
Normal	23	4.7[b]	2167	264	840	567	430
Tolerant	27	4.7	1434	—	—	—	—

[a] SARB-IγG = IγG-globulin of sheep anti-rabbit GBM serum.
[b] A single dose was given intravenously.

after injection the proteinuria disappeared and the rabbits became clinically and functionally normal.

As demonstrable by fluorescent antibody technique in normal and tolerant rabbits, SγG was found concentrated and fixed to the glomerular capillary wall and persisted throughout the period of observation.

In normal rabbits host γ-globulins began to concentrate similarly within 5 to 6 days after injection of SARB and increased within the next several weeks roughly in proportion to the degree of renal injury.

27 rabbits injected with SγG at birth and checked for tolerance produced the initial but failed to develop the autologous phase of glomerulonephritis after injection with 4.7 mg N/kg SARB. Tolerant rabbits also failed at any time to show host γ-globulin concentrated in the glomeruli, when observed with fluorescent antibody technique. The failure to show secondary proteinuria was related to the inability to form anti-SγG antibodies. Therefore it was reasoned that restoration of the specific immunological reactivity of tolerant rabbits would precipitate a proteinuria.

Further experiments were concerned with this immune response elicited by p-Tyr-SγG or SγG respectively in rabbits made tolerant to SγG and injected with SARB.

9 to 17 tolerant rabbits which failed to produce the autologous phase developed proteinuria after immunization with p-Tyr-SγG (Table 2). Only 3 of 16 tolerant controls immunized with native SγG had a mild proteinuria and focal glomerular changes when autopsied at different time intervalls after initial immunization. As anticipated all of the normal controls immunized with p-Tyr-SγG or native SγG reacted with a severe proteinuria and a progressing glomerulonephritis.

Table 2. *Proteinuria and fluorescent observations after production of antibody in normal and SγG-tolerant rabbits injected with p-tyrosyl-sheep-γ-globulin*[a]

Group	Treatment	Proteinuria/ No. rabbits	Glom. fixed autol. γG (No. positive/ No. studied)
Tolerant	p Tyr-SγG	9/17	12/17
	SγG	3/16	3/16
Normal	p Tyr-SγG	10/10	10/10
	SγG	9/9	9/9

[a] Injected once a week for 3 weeks with 25 mg p Tyr-SyG in complete Freund's adjuvant. 3 weeks after the third injection 20 mg SγG was given i.v.

Table 3. *Proteinuria and fluorescent observations after production of antibody in normal and SγG-tolerant rabbits injected with arsanil-sulfanil-SγG*[a]

Group	Treatment	Proteinuria/ No. rabbits	Glom. fixed autol. γG (No. positive/ No. studied)
Tolerant	A-S-SγG	18/33	24/33
	SγG	4/24	4/24
Normal	A-S-SγG	6/6	6/6
	SγG	5/5	5/5

[a] Arsanil-sulfanil-SγG containing 16.9 azo groups/molecule. Injected once a week with 25 mg Ars-Sulf-SγG in complete Freund's adjuvant, followed by an intravenous injection of 20 mg soluble SγG 4 weeks later.

After termination of tolerant state, all rabbits developing proteinuria showed fixation of host γ-globulin. In most cases pathologic changes progressed to a severe diffuse membranous glomerulonephritis with scarring and synechia.

Using A-S-SγG for immunization of tolerant rabbits, 18 of 33 developed proteinuria (Table 3). All of them had fixation of autologous γ-globulin to their glomerular capillary wall. Histopathologically, the rabbits exhibiting proteinuria showed glomerular changes and were capable of perpetuating renal disease.

Only 4 of 24 tolerant controls immunized with native SγG produced mild proteinuria and focal glomerular changes. However, 83% of tolerant rabbits immunized with native SγG failed to develop proteinuria and renal changes and the fixation of autologous γ-globulin to their glomerular capillary wall was lacking, It might be expected, that in tolerant rabbits injected with SARB and immunized with p-Tyr-SγG and A-S-SγG respectively exists a direct relationship between amount and affinity of antibody formed and the degree of renal disease.

In further experiments with tolerant rabbits a total of six injections of p-Tyr-SγG and A-S-SγG respectively caused termination of tolerant state. 27 of 50 rabbits responded usually after the third injection with the formation of antibodies capable of reacting with native SγG (Table 4).

Proteinuria was developed between 28 and 133 days after initial immunization and resulted in a 24 h urinary protein between 150 and 600 mg-% (Table 4). There

Table 4. *Effect of antibody response to p-Tyr-SγG and A-S-SγG in normal rabbits and rabbits tolerant to SγG on development of glomerulonephritis*[a]

Status at start of experiment	Treatment	Binding Ab to ^{131}I-SγG after injection						Proteinuria	
		1	2	3	4	5	6	started days	highest figures mg-%/ 24 h
Tolerant	p-Tyr-SγG	—	—	735	395	510	630	28	150
Tolerant	A-S-SγG	—	—	425	500	210	440	133	600
Tolerant	SγG	—	—	—	—	—	—	—	—
Normal	p-Tyr-SγG	64	75	73	1250	1830	2420	1	2000

[a] Binding capacity expressed as reciprocal of serum dilution at which 33% of ^{131}I-SγG was bound to globulin.

exists a good correlation between antibody response and the degree of glomerular lesions.

Normal rabbits subjected to the same immunization schedule usually produce higher quantities of antibodies and in relation to this proteinuria and renal changes are more severe (2000 mg-%).

Rabbits made tolerant to SγG produced antibodies capable of precipitating native SγG, when they were injected with A-S-SγG. Anti-SγG antibodies were purified from the sera of tolerant and of normal rabbits using SγG-cellulose derivatives as immunoadsorbent according to the method of Behrens *et al.* [5]. In competitive binding experiments with ^{131}I-SγG and ^{125}I-A-S-SγG, the anti-SγG antibodies bound A-S-SγG preferentially to native SγG.

Thus anti-SγG antibodies from previously tolerant rabbits always exhibited a higher binding affinity for A-S-SγG, the cross-reacting antigen used to terminate tolerance, than for native SγG. Normal rabbits however subjected to immunization with A-S-SγG produced anti-SγG antibodies which bound A-S-SγG only slightly better than SγG.

These observations support the following concept of the pathogenesis of experimental glomerulonephritis: 1. The immediate phase of nephritis is caused by interaction of heterologous antikidney antibody with GBM antigens. 2. The autologous phase however is produced by antibodies formed by the host against heterologous γ-globulin reacting with the foreign protein fixed to the basement membrane. 3. Rabbits made tolerant developed neither secondary or autologous phase nor an accumulation of host γ-globulin in the glomerulus. 4. This acquired tolerance is specific and in many respect resembles tolerance to self constituents. 5. The termination of tolerance by cross-reacting antigens resulted in the development of a morphologically and functionally complete secondary phase. This may be discussed in relation to autoimmunity. 6. After termination of tolerance the degree of injury is dependent upon the amount of antibodies formed and its affinity to the native determinants of heterologous γ-globulin. 7. Obviously, antibodies best adapted to the determinants of native SγG remained inhibited in the tolerant rabbit. Although a true termination of tolerance had not occurred, the immunization with cross-reacting antigens may be of importance to the genesis of autoimmune anti-GBM glomerulonephritis.

References

1. Lerner, R. A., and F. J. Dixon: J. Immunol. **100**, 1277 (1968).
2. Hammer, D. K., and F. J. Dixon: J. exp. Med. **117**, 1019—1034 (1962).
3. Schechter, J., and S. Bauminger: Immunochemistry **1**, 249—265 (1964).
4. Weigle, W. O.: J. exp. Med. **116**, 913—928 (1962).
5. Behrens, M. M., J. K. Imman, and W. E. Vannier: Arch. Biochem. **119**, 411 (1967).

Doz. Dr. D. Hammer
Max-Planck-Institut für Immunbiologie,
78 Freiburg-Zähringen, Stübeweg 51

Discussion

FISCHER (Hamburg): When the first reaction phase has taken place is it then possible to transfer antibodies also passively and how long does their attachment to the basal membrane last ?

HAMMER (Freiburg): In the rat it is after several months still possible to show the fixation of heterologous γ-globulin to the glomerular basement membrane. Immunizing rats against sheep gamma-globulin and passively transfering the antibody is also a possible mechanism for starting a nephritis in rats which had received anti-GBM-serum several months before.

FISCHER (Hamburg): Why does the antigen fixation only initially cause proteinuria and why does the proteinuria cease although the fixation persists for a prolonged period ?

HAMMER (Freiburg): The primary fixation is virtually only a kind of initial injury. Only the formation of the autologous antibody sustains the perpetual process. After some time the quantity of membrane-fixed antibody probably no longer suffices to maintain the nephritis.

ROTHER (Freiburg): A possible alternative pathway has recently been proposed by Dixon's group for some forms of human autoimmunization against kidney. Basalmembrane constituents, normally secluded in an immunogenic sense, may become accessible by some as yet unknown primary process such as an infection [Lerner et al.: J. exp. Med. **126**, 989 (1967)].

FISCHER (Freiburg): Do tolerant cells actually exist or is tolerance the elimination of certain clones ? Tolerant cells must have become tolerant against many determinants.

HAMMER (Freiburg): I imagine as the developmental mechanism of tolerance that all cells which have high affinity receptors disappear and only the cells with a relatively low affinity remain. In our case it is certainly conceivable that the receptors which have only weak affinity for the sheep gamma globulin react so that we are concerned with a kind of selectioning.

Bayer-Symposium I, 264—267 (1969)

From the Department of Immunology, Middlesex, Hospital Medical School, London, W. 1

The Long Acting Thyroid Stimulator (LATS) in Thyrotoxicosis

Ivan M. Roitt, and Deborah Doniach

For some time evidence has accumulated regarding the association of thyrotoxicosis with autoimmune phenomena. Varying degrees of the lymphadenoid changes characteristic of Hashimoto's disease are commonly observed in the glands of patients with thyrotoxicosis and a high incidence of antibodies to thyroglobulin and the thyroid cytoplasmic antigen can be demonstrated. In addition, 30% of patients have gastric parietal cell antibodies while the association with pernicious anaemia, a well established autoimmune disorder, is much greater than would be expected by chance. Furthermore, among the first degree relatives of patients with Hashimoto's disease there are many cases of hyperthyroidism. A notable advance in this field was provided by the work of Adams and Purves (1957) who established a new assay for pituitary TSH depending upon the release of radioisotope from the thyroid of guinea pigs prelabelled with ^{131}I. Whereas injection of TSH led to an increase in blood radioactivity reaching a maximum by 2 to 3 h, Adams and Purves found that the serum of patients with Graves' (Basedow's) disease caused a rise in blood ^{131}I which was maximal at 7 h or later. The assay was improved by McKenzie (1958) using mice. The active component has been termed the 'long acting thyroid stimulator' (LATS).

TSH and LATS both increase the uptake of ^{131}I by the thyroid and the level of serum protein bound ^{127}I and both cause hypertrophy of the acinar epithelial cells: nonetheless it is clear that they are distinct. Thus LATS can be demonstrated in hypophysectomized patients. LATS and TSH have different half-lives in vivo and this presumably is responsible for their different effects in the mouse assay. Furthermore they can be separated from each other by gel filtration. The biological effect of TSH can be neutralized by an antiserum raised against TSH but not by anti-immunoglobulin G; conversely LATS is unaffected by anti-TSH but can be completely inactivated by admixture with anti-IgG.

The Antibody Nature of LATS

The neutralizing effect of anti-IgG is consistent with the finding of LATS activity in purified IgG fractions obtained from patient's serum. Thyroid stimulating activity is associated with the $F(ab')_2$ fragment obtained by pepsin digestion and with the Fab but not Fc fragment resulting from papain cleavage. That the activity is an inherent property of the IgG molecule rather than a result of the binding of a hypothetical stimulator to IgG may be deduced from the finding that heavy chain preparations isolated by a modified technique were weak short acting thyroid stimulators, but recombination with complementary light chains restored potent long acting activity (Munro *et al.*, 1967).

LATS can be absorbed completely from the sera of thyrotoxic patients by homogenates of thyroid but not of other tissues (Kriss *et al.*, 1964; Sharard and Adams, 1965; Beall and Solomon, 1966; Dorrington *et al.*, 1966; El Kabir *et al.*, 1966) thereby demonstrating a high degree of organ specificity; LATS activity can be recovered from the thyroid homogenate by acid treatment under conditions known to cause dissociation of antigen-antibody complexes. It has also proved possible to produce a serum thyroid stimulator experimentally by immunization of animals with thyroid preparations. Collectively these studies may be taken to establish LATS as an antibody directed against the thyroid.

Attempts have been made to identify the antigen by absorption studies. All 'conventional' subcellular fractions prepared by differential centrifugation of thyroid homogenates can inhibit LATS to different extents. The inhibitor can even be recovered in the soluble 'cell sap' fraction (Berumen *et al.*, 1967; Benhamou-Glynn *et al.*, 1968) but is distinguishable from thyroglobulin (Beall *et al.*, 1968a). Microsomal preparations are effective inhibitors and subfractionation has indicated a degree of correlation with 5-nucleotidase activity considered to be a marker of the plasma cell membrane (Beall *et al.*, 1968b). Evidence for the cell membrane as the site of action of LATS has been obtained by simultaneously injecting LATS and ferritin: numerous vesicles containing ferritin marker were observed at the base of the cell within 15 min presumably formed by endocytosis of the surface membrane (Bradbury *et al.*, 1968). In a different context we have shown that anti-lymphocyte serum containing antibodies to surface antigens provokes endocytosis when added to cultures of lymphocytes (Greaves and Roitt, 1968).

LATS probably acts through stimulation of adenyl cyclase so generating adenosine 3′,5′-monophosphate (cyclic AMP). TSH, LATS and cyclic AMP all stimulate the uptake of ^{131}I by the mouse thyroid and these effects can be potentiated by theophylline, a phosphodiesterase inhibitor which prolongs the survival of cyclic AMP within the cell (McKenzie, 1968; Brown, Ensor and Munro, 1968). LATS and TSH may both combine with a specific receptor site on the surface membrane, conceivably a part of the adenyl cyclase molecule, and activate this enzyme by an allosteric effect.

The stimulation of a cell by antibody although unusual is not without precedent. For example anti-lymphocyte sera are often mitogenic for small lymphocytes and cause blast cell transformation. The lack of a cytotoxic effect of LATS on the thyroid could be explained by a small number of antigen molecules on the cell surface since two IgG molecules must be bound to antigen in close proximity to each other for complement fixation to occur. In this connection our preliminary studies have indicated that the amount of LATS which can be bound by a thyroid homogenate is small relative to the total IgG binding non-specifically; such considerations may account for the difficulties encountered in developing a radio-immunoassay for LATS.

Clinical Aspects of LATS

With the McKenzie assay up to 40% of sera from thyrotoxic patients show detectable levels of LATS; this can be increased to approximately 80% by using concentrated IgG preparations (Carneiro, Dorrington and Munro, 1966a) suggesting that insensitivity of the assay is responsible for the failure to detect LATS in many sera. One factor contributing to this lack of sensitivity could be a low cross-reactivity of the antibody with mouse thyroid due to the phylogenetic disparity between man and mouse.

High levels of LATS are frequently associated with pretibial myxoedema and a higher incidence is demonstrable in patients with severe eye signs. Although the level of LATS does not correlate well with the degree of clinical hyperthyroidism, Carneiro *et al.* (1966b) have found a significant correlation with rate of production of ^{131}I-labelled thyroxine per g of thyroid tissue.

The lack of suppression of thyroid ^{131}I uptake in thyrotoxic patients given high doses of tri-iodothyronine forms the basis of one of the important discriminating diagnostic tests for Graves' disease. In the light of our present knowledge we assume that LATS has a direct action on the thyroid independently of the pituitary-thyroid feedback mechanism and would therefore be unaffected by administration of tri-iodothyronine which acts by inhibiting TSH secretion.

The transient neonatal hyperthyroidism which is sometimes observed in the offspring of thyrotoxic mothers can also be readily understood. LATS, being an IgG molecule, crosses the placenta and stimulates the foetal thyroid. After birth the passively acquired maternal IgG is slowly catabolized and after 2 to 3 months the LATS level becomes too low to affect the thyroid significantly.

In conclusion, the hypothesis that LATS is a thyroid-specific antibody which gives rise to the hyperthyroidism of Graves' disease by stimulating the gland through combination with a cell-surface antigen, is supported by considerable evidence and adequately accounts for many facets of the disorder.

References

Adams, D. D., and H. D. Purves: Thyrotrophin assay by plasma ^{131}I measurements. Canad. J. Biochem. **35**, 993 (1957).

Beall, G. N., and D. H. Solomon: On the immunological nature of LATS. J. clin. Invest. **45**, 552 (1966).

—, D. Doniach, I. M. Roitt, and D. J. El Kabir: Inhibition of LATS by soluble thyroid fractions. Submitted for publication (1968a).

—, I. M. Roitt, D. Doniach, and D. J. El Kabir: Inhibition of LATS by membranous thyroid fractions. In preparation (1968b).

Benhamou-Glynn, N., D. J. El-Kabir, I. M. Roitt, and D. Doniach: Studies on the antigen reacting with the thyroid stimulating immunoglobulin in thyrotoxicosis. Immunology **16,** 187 (1969).

Berumen, F. O., I. L. Lobsenz, and R. D. Utiger: Neutralization of LATS by thyroid subcellular fractions. J. Lab. clin. Med. **70**, 640 (1967).

Bradbury, S., I. M. Roitt, and D. J. El Kabir: Induction of endocytosis in thyroid cells by LATS. In preparation (1968).

Brown, J., J. Ensor, and D. S. Munro: A comparison of the actions of TSH and LATS in an in vitro assay. Proc. roy. Soc. Med. **61**, 652 (1968).

Carneiro, L., K. J. Dorrington, and D. S. Munro: Recovery of LATS from serum of patients with thyrotoxicosis by concentrations of IgG. Clin. Sci. **31**, 215 (1966a).

— — — Relation between LATS and thyroid function in thyrotoxicosis. Lancet **1966 II** b 878.

Dorrington, K. J., L. Carneiro, and D. S. Munro: Absorption of LATS by human thyroid microsomes. J. Endocr. **34**, 133 (1966).

El Kabir, D. J., N. Benhamou-Glynn, D. Doniach, and I. M. Roitt: Absorption of thyroid-stimulating globulin from thyrotoxic sera by organ homogenates. Nature (Lond.) **210**, 319 (1966).

Greaves, M. F., and I. M. Roitt: The effect of phytohaemagglutinin and other lymphocyte mitogens on immunoglobulin synthesis by peripheral blood lymphocytes in vitro. Clin. exp. Immunol. **3**, 393 (1968).

Kriss, J. P., V. Pleshakov, and J. R. Chien: Isolation and identification of LATS and its relation to hyperthyroidism and circumscribed pretibial myxoedema. J. clin. Endocr. **24**, 1005 (1964).

McKenzie, J. M.: The bioassay of thyrotrophin in serum. Endocrinology **63**, 372 (1958).

— Humoral factors in the pathogenesis of Graves' disease. Physiol. Rev. **43**, 252 (1968).

Munro, D. S., J. Brown, K. J. Dorrington, B. R. Smith, and J. Ensor: Observations on the chemical structure of LATS and its influence on thyroid function in thyrotoxicosis. In: Thyrotoxicosis, p. 1. W. J. Irvine, Ed. Edinburgh: Livingstone 1967.

Sharad, A., and D. D. Adams: Inactivation of LATS by a heat-labile thyroid gland component. Proc. Univ. Otago med. Sch. **43**, 25 (1965).

Prof. Dr. I. M. Roitt
Department of Immunology,
Arthur Stanley House,
The Middlesex Hospital Medical School,
London, W. 1, England

Discussion

WALFORD (Los Angeles): Have you investigated different kinds of complements ? For example, we know that in human leucocyte typing with human anti-leucocyte serum, rabbit complement works very well. If you are doing complement fixation with human platelets and with human anti-human serum, human complement works very well but guinea pig complement does not work very well.

ROITT (London): The important point is that in vivo complement is not required.

OETTGEN (New York): Both TSH and LATS have a strong thyroid stimulating activity. Does LATS like TSH stimulate the lymphoid system ?

ROITT (London): This has not been studied. — There is good evidence that LATS and TSH stimulate the thyroid through the adenyl-cyclase system which produces cyclic AMP. This has been demonstrated for many different hormones and if you inject LATS plus theophylline, which is a phosphodiesterase-inhibitor, you prolong the life of cyclic AMP and you prolog the effect of LATS.

Bayer-Symposium I, 268—278 (1969)

Immunological Investigations in Myasthenia Gravis and Other Skeletal Muscle Disorders[1]

D. RICKEN

With 8 Figures

Since many years it has been looked for immune phenomena in skeletal muscle disorders. If positive findings were reported they referred to humoral antibodies or factors. Cellular immunity has not been investigated yet. However,

Table 1. *Immune phenomena in skeletal muscle disorders*

	Humoral antibodies against				Other immune-phenomena	Thymoma thymus-hyper-plasia	Muscle-fibre destruction
	Striated muscle	Smooth muscle	Epitheloid thymus cells	Nerve			
Myasthenia gravis	+	∅	+	(+)	ANF, LE RF, ATh	+	((+))
Muscular dystrophy	∅	∅	∅	∅	∅	∅	+++
Polymyo-sitis	∅	∅	∅	n.d.	RF	((+))	+++
Dermato-myositis	∅	∅	∅	n.d	RF, ANF LE	((+))	++
Other skeletal muscle disorders	∅	∅	∅	n.d.	∅	∅	∅

ATh = Antithyroglobulin.
n.d. = not done.

there is the occurence of thymoma or hyperplastic thymus particularly in myasthenia gravis which perhaps represents a condition of cellular immunity.

Objections are well taken for including myasthenia into the group of skeletal muscle diseases because a number of findings indicate that the neuromuscular transmission is inhibited (Struppler, Nastuk *et al.*, Osserman, Schwab). On the other hand the most striking immunological findings deal with proteins of the striated fibre itself.

In myasthenia, polymyositis and dermatomyositis clinical and pathological findings make it probable that autoimmune mechanism are participating in. But

[1] Supported by a grant of the Deutsche Forschungsgemeinschaft.

if one compares the true immunological data obtained in skeletal muscle diseases (Tab. 1), it is evident that myasthenia stands at the top concerning number and specificity of immune phenomena. The most important of them are autoantibodies against striated muscle (Strauss *et al.*, Beutner *et al.*, Ricken *et al.*) (Fig. 1) and against "epitheloid" cells of the thymus (v. d. Geld *et al.*, Strauss *et al.*, Osserman *et al.*.) Both autoantibodies occur in 40% of the patients and in almost 70% of myasthenics with thymoma (Beutner *et al.*, Strauss *et al.*). Adner *et al.* as well as Fischer *et al.* described antinuclear factors, autoantibodies against thyroglobulin and the rheumatoid factor in myasthenia. In some cases with low muscle autoantibodies serumfactors against medullar substance of the first and second neuron occur (Fig. 2) (Ricken).

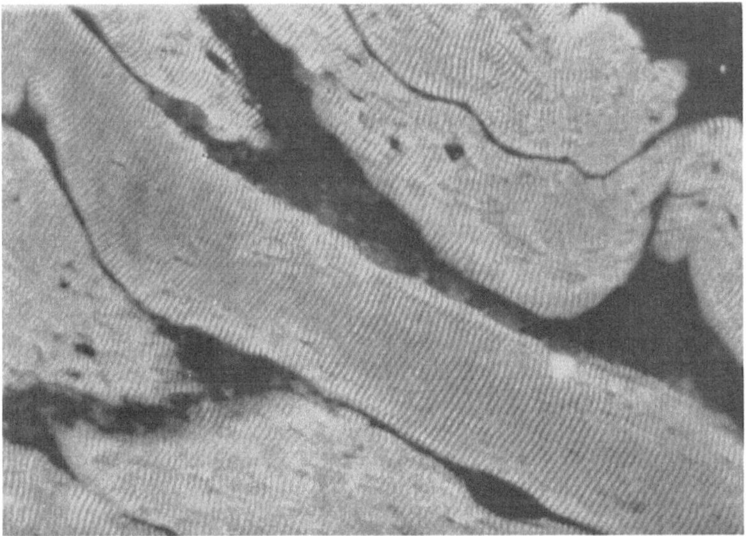

Fig. 1. Indirect immunofluorescence test. Myasthenia gravis serum 1:10; human skeletal muscle, acetone fixed

An intriguing finding, however, is the occurence of thymoma in 30% of the patients (Weigert, Erbslöh *et al.*, Schwab) or of thymus hyperplasia in an even higher percentage (Castleman *et al.*).

In contrast to that in muscular dystrophy immunological findings could not be reported until now (Strauss *et al.*, Beutner *et al.*, Ricken). In polymyositis and dermatomyositis antinuclear factors, the rheumatoid factor and the LE cell phenomenon has been seen sometimes in a low frequency. Even then it has to be taken into consideration, that in many cases myositis or dermatomyositis is an accompanying syndrome in primary chronical polyarthritis or in lupus erythematosus disseminatus (Pearson). Thus the immunological findings are belonging to the primary disease rather than to the attendant myositis or dermatomyositis. Muscle antibodies or antibodies against thymus "epitheloid" cells could not be observed. Sporadically thymoma is occuring (Klein *et al.*).

Comparing the occurence of immune phenomena with the intensity of skeletal muscle fibre destruction (Table 1) it becomes obvious that the skeletal muscle diseases with a high degree of fibre alteration or inflammatory infiltration are lacking antibodies; — particularly those against muscle fibres. In contrast to that they occur in an ample number in myasthenia which usually does not show any or only slight focal fibre destruction, sometimes together with small spots of mononuclear cell infiltration.

On this account it does not seem correct to assume that skeletal muscle destruction by itself is capable of inducing autoantibody formation. On the other hand extensive destruction can take place without antibody involvement.

In Myasthenia the thymus alterations and particularly the autoantibody against striated muscle have sponsored the suspicion of an autoimmune pathogenesis (Simpson, Osserman). This autoantibody is directed in vitro against the

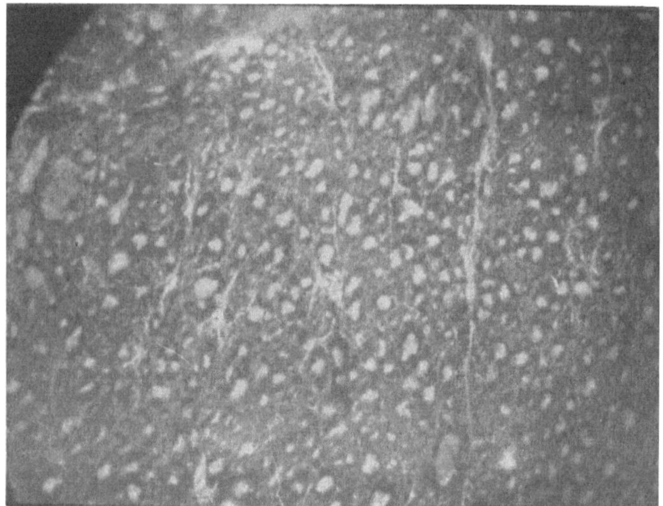

Fig. 2. Indirect immunofluorescence test. Myasthenia gravis serum Ol. 1:10; human spinal cord, acetone fixed

A-bands (Fig. 1) and does not react with other components of the striated muscle fibre and not with neuromuscular junction substrates, not to say with smooth muscle structures (Ricken, Beutner *et al.*). However, myasthenia gravis sera often react with heart muscle fibres in the same way as they do with skeletal muscle fibres (Beutner *et al.*).

The direct immunofluorescent method has been used in order to detect gamma globulin binding to the A-bands of myasthenia gravis patients intra vitam. So far only questionable results could be obtained concerning weak and scattered sub-sarcolemmal binding of anti-gamma globulin (Gordon *et al.*). Beutner *et al.* obtained some evidence of intra vitam bound gamma globulin by inhibition of passive hemagglutination.

In our laboratory investigations about the nature of the skeletal muscle antigen and about the autoantibody production against this antigen were performed. The methods of muscle protein fractionation as described by Mommaerts *et al.* or Groeschel-Stewart *et al.* were used. According to this methods skeletal muscle extracts in KCl-K-Phosphate-buffer (pH = 6.2; ionic strength = 0.55) were fractionated into actomyosin and myosin by stepwise dilution with destilled water. Actomyosin is precipitating at a ionic strength between 0.32 and 0.28, Myosin at a ionic strength lower than 0.28. Actomyosin and Myosin obtained by this method are fairly pure as it was demonstrated by immunization experiments (Fink, Furminger, Klatzo *et al.*). Both antigens were used in the agar gel double diffusion technique, in the complement fixation test and in the passive hemagglutination test. Smooth muscle fractions, thymus extracts (human and animal) and

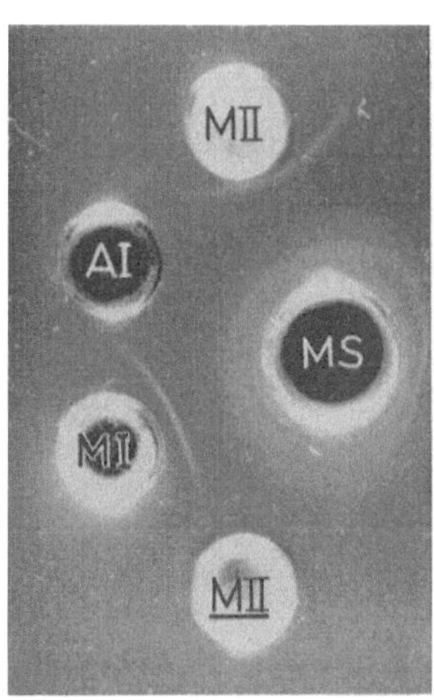

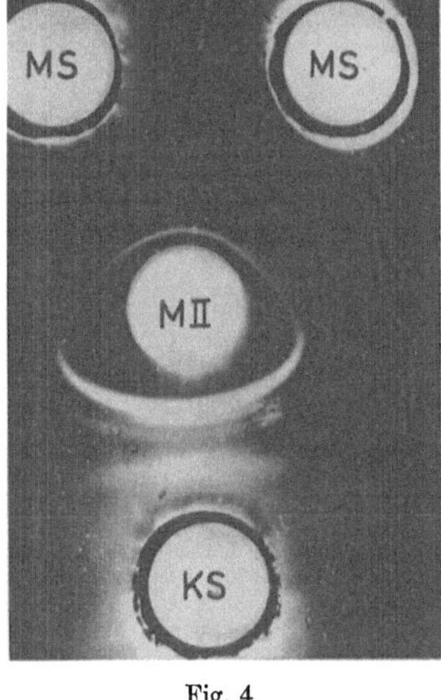

Fig. 3   Fig. 4

Fig. 3. Agar gel double diffusion test. MS = myasthenia gravis serum Schm., M I = human skeletal muscle myosin, A I = human skeletal muscle actomyosin, both obtained after 30 min extraction of muscle. M II = human skeletal muscle myosin after 24 h extraction, — in *M II* after storage at +4 °C for 8 days

Fig. 4. Agar gel double diffusion test. M II = human skeletal muscle myosin. MS_1 = myasthenia gravis serum Schm., MS_2 = myasthenia gravis serum Mi. KS = rabbit hyperimmune serum against human skeletal muscle myosin

human liver extracts were used as control antigens and for absorption experiments. In immunization experiments rabbits and rats were immunized either with crude skeletal muscle extracts or with sceletal muscle myosin of different origin together with equal amounts of Freund's adjuvant, in order to obtain antisera against muscle components.

Using the agar gel double diffusion technique usually one but sometimes also two lines can be observed with myasthenia gravis sera and human skeletal muscle myosin. There is no reaction with actomyosin (Fig. 3). Beside of these lines observed with myosin other precipitation lines could not be observed. Myasthenia gravis sera did not react with smooth muscle fractions, liver or thymus fractions

of human or animal (rat, rabbit) origin. The lines obtained with myosin could not
be eliminated by serum absorption with human actomyosin, smooth muscle-, liver- or
thymus fractions or with serum. They disappeared after absorption of the myasthenia sera with whole skeletal muscle extracts, skeletal muscle myosin or heart
muscle myosin of man and different animal species (rat, rabbit, mouse, cat, calf).

Our first assumption that the precipitation band obtained with myasthenia
gravis sera and myosin represent myosin altogether have not been confirmed
however by further investigations using hyperimmune sera of rabbits and rats
against skeletal muscle myosin.

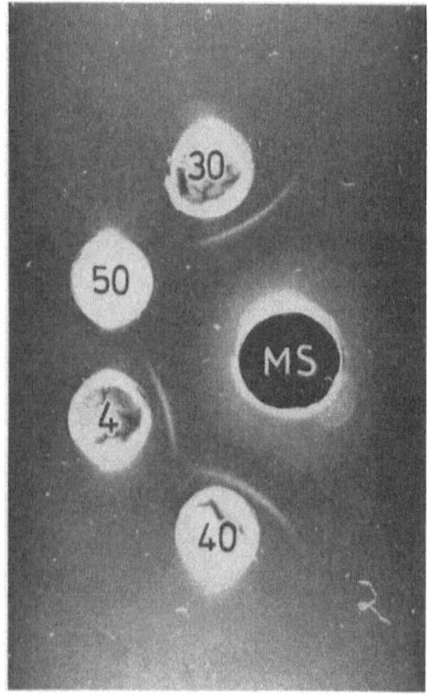

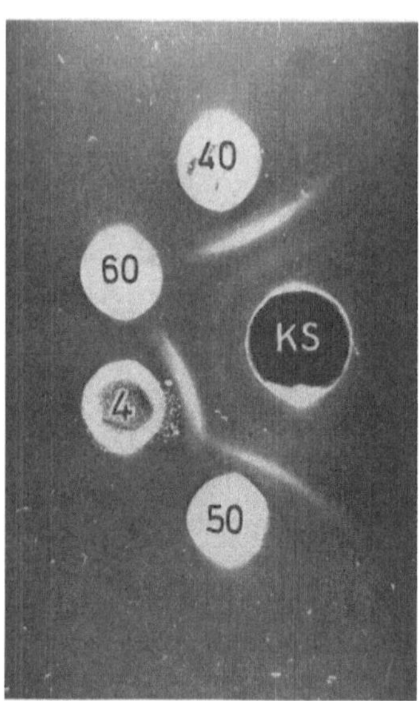

Fig. 5   Fig. 6

Fig. 5. Agar gel double diffusion test. MS = myasthenia gravis serum Schm. Human skeletal
muscle myosin, incubated 30 min at 4 °C (4), 30 °C (30), 40 °C (40) and 50 °C (50)

Fig. 6. Agar gel double diffusion test. KS = rabbit hyperimmune serum against human
skeletal muscle myosin, incubated at different temperatures for 30 min. For explanation see
Fig. 5! Note the loss of the precipitation line next to the antigen well after incubation at 50 °C,
and of the second line after incubation at 60 °C

Rabbits immunized with human skeletal muscle myosin or the whole extract
of human skeletal muscle together with Freund adjuvant produce antisera which
react with human myosin in the typical manner (Fig. 4), that is by forming two
lines near the antigen well. There are also bands more distant from the antigen
well and closer to the serum well (Fig. 4), but these precipitation bands can be
easily eliminated by serum absorption with human liver fractions and human
serum globulin. The absorption procedure does not affect the two lines near the
antigen well.

The comparison of these precipitation bands near the antigen well with that
formed by the myasthenic autoantibody shows that the band next to the antigen
well merges into the line obtained with the myasthenic autoantibody. The second

line of the rabbit hyperimmune serum does not have any counterpart (Fig. 4). These findings indicate that skeletal muscle myosin contains two immunologically active antigens one of them reacting with the myasthenic autoantibody and also with an antibody of the rabbit hyperimmune serum, the other one only reacting with the rabbit hyperimmune serum.

When human skeletal muscle myosin is incubated at different temperatures, the myosin component reacting with the myasthenic autoantibody denaturates at temperatures between 40° and 50 °C (Figs. 5 and 6). In contrast to that the second myosin component which is precipitated by the rabbit hyperimmunserum only

Table 2. *CFT with sera of rabbits immunized with autologous skeletal muscle myosin. The titers represent the antigen-dilution (dilution of autologous myosin), at which a 4+ or 3+ inhibition of hemolysis was present*

Rabbit sera	$\varnothing$	a	b	c	d	e
K 5 (1:10)	0	n.d.	1:10	1:20	—	—
K 6 (1:10)	0	n.d.	0	0	—	—
K 7/280 (1:10)	0	0	0	0	0	0
K 8/284 (1:10)	0	0	0	1:20	1:10	n.d.
K 9/299 (1:10)	0	0	0	1:10	1:10	1:5

$\varnothing$ = sera before immunization; a, b, c, ... = sera after first, second, third, ...immunization.

Table 3. *Passive hemagglutination test, using tanned human 0 red cells coated with autologous rabbit skeletal muscle myosin. Titers represent dilution of sera*

	$\varnothing$	a	b	c	d	e
K 5	0	n.d.	1:1280	1:640	—	—
K 6	0	n.d.	0	0	0	—
K 7 (280)	0	0	0	0	0	0
K 8 (284)	0	1:640	1:1280	1:320	1:160	n.d.
K 9 (299)	0	0	1:40	1:320	1:320	1:80

$\varnothing$ = sera before immunization; a, b, c, ... = sera after 1., 2., 3., ... immunization.

seems to be more heat stabile. It is destroyed by temperatures above 50 °C (Fig. 6). However, the "myasthenia"(auto-)antigen although it can be distinguished from the second myosin component by agar gel precipitation and by its minor heat stability probably is linked closely to the second component which is more heat stabile. When sedimented by preparative ultracentrifugation both antigens come down after 3 h at 50000 r.p.m. Thus far our results indicate that the antigen precipitated by the myasthenia autoantibody is localized in the myosin fraction of skeletal muscle.

In further experiments it was tried to produce autoantibodies in the experimental animal against this antigen. Groups of rabbits and rats were injected in weekly intervals with autologous myosin and equal amounts of Freund's adjuvant up to eight times. Thus far the results were not conclusive. Precipitating antibodies against muscle constituents could not be demonstrated either in the rabbit or in the rat sera. When tested in the complement fixation or in the passive hemagglutination test some of the rabbit sera but none of the rat sera had antibodies in low titer against autologous, isologous and heterologous myosin (Tabs. 2 and 3). Since these results did not seem very promising additional tests on these animal sera were not performed.

Quite different results were obtained with sera of rats, immunized with rabbit allogenic skeletal muscle myosin. It turned out that most of these sera possessed iso- and autoantibodies against isologous and autologous rat myosin, beside of antibodies against the rabbit myosin and against human skeletal muscle myosin (Tab. 4). The precipitation pattern in the agar gel double diffusion test was very similar to that described above already. In the system—rat serum against rabbit myosin—two precipitation lines were produced near the antigen well. With

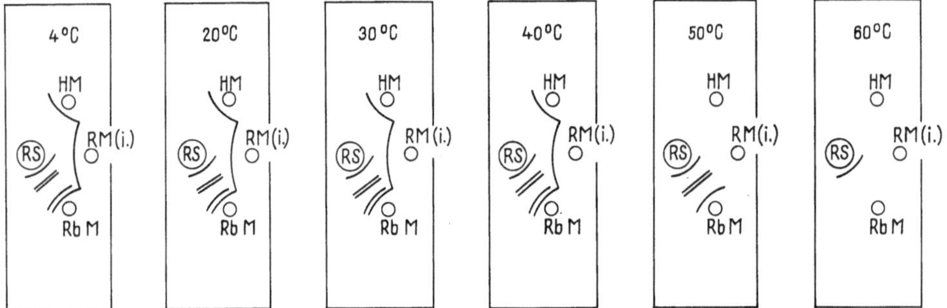

Fig. 7. Results of agar gel double diffusions tests carried out with skeletal muscle myosins of different species and rat hyperimmune serum against rabbit skeletal muscle myosin. The myosins were incubated for 30 min at different temperatures. Protein content of myosins about 18 mg/ml (Biuret-method). RS = rat serum. RbM = rabbit skeletal muscle myosin; RM(i) = isologous rat skeletal muscle myosin; HM = human skeletal muscle myosin

isologous and autologous rat myosin as well as with humau myosin the precipitation reaction became monospecific, because only one line could be observed near the antigen well (Figs. 7 and 8). This line did not appear when the myosin fraction was incubated for 30 min at 50 °C before testing, but it was not affected by temperatures of 40 °C or lower. In the heterologous system—rat serum against rabbit myosin—incubation at 50 °C only eliminated one of the precipitation lines near the antigen well, while the other one persisted and first disappeared after incubation at 60 °C first (Fig. 8). These results are comparable with the findings obtained with human autoantigen and myasthenia serum as well as with rabbit hyperimmune serum versus human skeletal muscle myosin. In this connection it has to be mentioned that the rat sera did not form precipitation lines with autologous or isologous smooth muscle antigens or liver antigens.

When a myasthenia gravis serum and a rat hyperimmune serum are tested against rat skeletal muscle myosins which are autologous and isologous to the rat serum identical lines are precipitated by both of the sera (Fig. 8). This finding supports the assumption that same myosin component is precipitated by the autoantibody of the myasthenia gravis patient and the immunized rat.

Table 4. *Agar gel double diffusion test. Sera of rats, immunized with rabbit skeletal muscle myosin and Freund adjuvant*

Rat-antiserum	Skeletal muscle myosin of			
	Autologous rat	Isologous	Rabbit	Man
R 30	+	+	(+)	+
R 36	+	+	+	+
R 37	+	+	+	+
R 44	(+)	+	+	+
R 46	(+)	+	+	+
R ∅	—	—	—	—

+ = precipitation line near the antigen well.

R ∅ serum of rat immunized with rabbit serum.

As far as agar gel technique permits the conclusion analogous results could be found with sera of rabbits immunized with human skeletal muscle myosin when tested against rabbit myosin of autologous and isologous origin.

It should be stressed that the rabbits or rats injected with their own skeletal muscle myosin and particularly the animals producing auto- or isoantibodies against "myosin" after allogenic immunization did not develop myasthenic symptoms. Although the animals were checked for several weeks during and after immunization muscle weakness was not observed. The histological examination of different muscles (levator palpebrae, muscles of the front and back limbs, of the abdominal wall, of the neck, of the diaphragma and intercostal muscles) did not demonstrate pathological changes. The thymusglands did not demonstrate any pathological findings. There were no inflammatory or degenerative changes in the heart muscle of the rats.

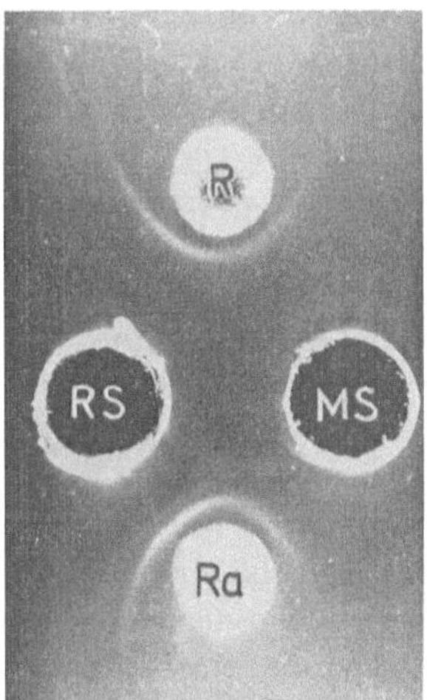

Fig. 8. Agar gel double diffusion test. MS = myasthenia gravis serum Schm. RS = serum of a rat immunized with rabbit skeletal muscle myosin and Freund adjuvant. Ra = autologous rat skeletal muscle myosin, R = isologous skeletal muscle myosin

Discussion

The detection of an organ-specific but non-species-specific autoantibody versus the A-bands of striated muscle in myasthenia gravis sera (Strauss *et al.*, Beutner *et al.*) has brought the skeletal muscle fibre into the discussion of the pathogenesis of this muscle disorder. Preliminary investigations about the intra vitam behavior of this autoantibody thus far failed to demonstrate couclusively its intra vitam binding to fibre structures, particularly to the A-bands (Gordon *et al.*, Beutner *et al.*). In our animal experiments we were able to produce autoantibodies

18*

against the same myosin component with which the myasthenic autoantibody reacts. However these animals did not develop myasthenic symptoms or muscle lesions. Goldstein *et al.* immunized groups of guinea pigs with xenogenic skeletal muscle and thymus. In both groups antibodies against striated muscle were produced and muscle weakness occurred in some of the animals when tested electromyographically. If these results are reproducible, they will show that it is possible to produce myasthenia-like symptoms in certain animals by immunization with skeletal muscle or even thymus. They do not mean necessarily that the humoral antibody against muscle constituents exerts this effect.

The skeletal muscle antigen reacting with the myasthenic autoantibody as well as with the autoantibody of the rat and the rabbit is strictly organ-specific but lacks species-specificity. It very probably is a component of myosin or at least is so closely connected with it that it cannot be separated from it by the methods applied in our investigations. The occurence of this autoantigen in the myosin fraction of sceletal muscle is in good accord with the binding of the autoantibody to the A-bands as observed by immunofluorescent methods. There is evidence however that myosin immunologically consists of two different organspecific components, one of them behaving as non-species-specific autoantigen, the other representing a species-specific antigen (Ricken *et al.*). Only the autoantigen obviously is capable of binding with the autoantibody of the same and other species. Until now the results obtained with myasthenia gravis sera and animal hyperimmune sera versus skeletal muscle myosin or skeletal muscle extracts seem to demonstrate that among the different antigens of the skeletal muscle fibre there is only one behaving as autoantigen. It is localized in the myosin fraction and can be destroyed by temperatures between 40° and 50 °C. By antisera it is precipitated characteristically in a close neighbourhood of the antigen well using the Ouchterlony method. The same antigen can be found in the myosin fraction of heart muscle.

Whether this antigen causes autoantibody production in myasthenia gravis remains unknown yet. In this event a trigger mechanism should be effective making it accessible to the antibody producing cell. The fact that other skeletal muscle diseases with high degree of fibre destruction do not have this or a similar autoantibody (Strauss *et al.*, Beutner *et al.*, Ricken) outlines that fibre destruction alone is not drastic enough to release autoantibody production. On the other hand a more generalized disorder of the immune system is might by the primary cause of the autoantibody production against a myosin constituent in myasthenia. For it has to be considered that beside of the muscle autoantibody antibodies against "epitheloid" thymus cells are produced too and sometimes antibodies against thyroglobulin, nerve substance, nuclear substances and altered IgM. Probably the thymus so often transformed to thymoma or hyperplasia plays a prominent role in this immune disorder. In this connection the intriguing observation should be emphasized, that in patients with thymoma but without myasthenia gravis autoantibodies against A-bands may occur (Strauss, Beutner *et al.*, Osserman *et al.*). Within a certain age range (25 to 40 years) thymectomy often has an improving effect on myasthenia (Schwab, Erbslöh *et al.*). There are several reports of myasthenia developing after thymectomy (Rowland *et al.*, Fershtand *et al.*, Madonick *et al.*, Roe *et al.*). Thus the central role of the thymus gland in myasthenia though somewhat ambiguous yet is obvious.

Particularly thymus hyperplasia often found in myasthenia and characterized by
the occurence of germinal centers might hold the key position in the pathogenesis
of this disease — either by producing or by inducing cellbound autoimmunity
(Good *et al.*).

The humoral autoantibody against myosin though probably being a secondary
phenomenon rather than an active participant in the course of myasthenia represents a valuable diagnostic mean because of its disease specificity. Myasthenia,
thymoma and sometimes myatrophic lateralsclerosis (Ricken, Fischer *et al.*) are the
only diseases thus far demonstrating this autoantibody. In our hands the agar gel
double diffusion technique proved to be a reliable and fast method to demonstrate
the autoantibody versus the heat labile myosin component in about 40% of the
cases, sometimes at the very beginning of the disease already.

References

Adner, M. M., J. D. Sherman, C. Isé, R. S. Schwab, and W. Dameshek: Immunologic study of
48 patients with myasthenia gravis. New Engl. J. Med. **271**, 1327 (1964).

Beutner, E. H., G. Fazekas, A. Scott, and E. Witebsky: Direct fluorescent antibody studies
of gamma globulin localization in muscle of patients with myasthenia gravis. Ann. N. Y.
Acad. Sci. 1965.

—, I. L. Leff, G. Fazekas, and E. Witebsky: Immunologic studies in fatal myasthenia gravis.
J. Amer. med. Ass. **191**, 461 (1965).

—, E. Witebsky, D. Ricken, and R. Adler: Studies on autoantibodies in myasthenia gravis.
J. Amer. med. Ass. **182**, 46 (1962).

Castleman, B., and E. H. Norris: The pathology of the thymus in myasthenia gravis, a study
of 35 cases. Medicine (Baltimore) **28**, 27 (1949).

Erbslöh, F., u. H. L. Allemand: Die Thymektomie im Therapieplan schwerer krisengefähr-
deter Myasthenien. Dtsch. med. Wschr. **90**, 800 (1965).

Fershtand, J. B., and R. R. Shaw: Malignant tumor of the thymus gland, myasthenia gravis
developing after removal. Ann. intern. Med. **34**, 1025 (1951).

Fink, H.: Immunochemical comparison of rabbit and chicken skeletal muscle myosin. Biochim.
biophys. Acta (Amst.) **111**, 239 (1965).

—, H. Holtzer, and J. M. Marshall: An immunochemical study of distribution of myosin in
glycerol extracted muscle. J. biophys. biochem. Cytol. **2**, 175 (1956).

Fischer, K., H. G. Mertens und K. Schimrigk: Ein Beitrag zur Immunpathologie bei Myasthenia gravis. Dtsch. med. Wschr. **90**, 1760 (1965).

Furminger, J. G. S.: The antigenic constituents of myosin preparations. Biochim. biophys.
Acta (Amst.) **90**, 521 (1964).

Goldstein, G., and S. Whittingham: Experimental autoimmune thymitis, an animal model of
human myasthenia gravis. Lancet **1966 II**. 315.

Good, R. A., R. D. A. Peterson, A. E. Gabrielsen: V. International Congress of Allergology,
Madrid 1964, 468. The thymus and autoimmunity.

Gröschel-Stewart, U., u. F. Turba: 14-C-Markierung und Peptidkarten der SH-Regionen von
Actomyosin, Myosin, Actin und H-Meromyosin. Biochem. Z. **337**, 104 (1963).

Klatzo, J., B. Horvath, and E. W. Emmart: Demonstration of myosin in human striated
muscle by fluorescent antibody. Proc. Soc. exp. Biol. (N. Y.) **97**, 135 (1958).

Klein, J. J., A. J. Gottlieb, R. J. Mones, St. H. Appel, and K. E. Osserman: Thymoma and
polymyositis. Arch. intern. Med. **113**, 142 (1964).

Madonick, M. J., M. Rubin, L. H. Levine, and W. Karliner: Myasthenia gravis developing
fifteen months after removal of thymoma. Arch. intern. Med. **99**, 151 (1957).

Mittelbach, F., u. G. Bodechtel: Zur Therapie der Muskelkrankheiten. Münch. med. Wschr.
110, 1988 (1968).

Mommaerts, W. H. M., and R. G. Parrish: Studies on myosin. I. Preparation and criteria of
purity. J. Biochem. **188**, 545 (1951).

Nastuk, W. L., K. E. Osserman, and O. J. Plescia: Search for a neuromuscular blocking agent in the blood of patients with myasthenia gravis. Amer. J. Med. **26**, 394 (1959).

Osserman, K. E.: Myasthenia gravis. New York: Grune and Stratton 1958.

— Myasthenia gravis, an autoimmune disease. Bull. Sch. Med. Maryland **47**, 12 (1962).

—, and L. B. Weiner: Studies in myasthenia gravis: Immunofluorescent tagging of muscle striations with antibody from serum of 256 myasthenic patients. Ann. N. Y. Acad. Sci. **124**, 730 (1965).

— — Studies in myasthenia gravis. New Engl. J. Med. **273**, 15 (1965).

Pearson,

Ricken, D.: Myasthenia gravis und humorale Antikörper gegen menschliche Skeletmuskelproteine (Vorl. Mittlg.). Klin. Wschr. **43**, 1717 (1965).

— Myasthenia gravis und humorale Antikörper gegen menschliche Skeletmuskelproteine. Dtsch. med. Wschr. **90**, 1717 (1965); Germ. med. Mth. **XI**, 134 (1966).

—, E. H. Beutner und E. Witebsky: Antikörper gegen Skelet- und Herzmuskelquerstreifen bei Myasthenia gravis. Verh. VII. Internat. Kongr. Inn. Med. **I**, 94 (1962).

—, u. I. Stroehmann: In: Heymer, A., X. Kongress dtsch. Ges. Allergie- u. Immunitätsforsch., Band II. Stuttgart: Schattauer 1968.

— — und H. Aulepp: Zur Immunpathogenese der Myasthenia gravis. Untersuchungen über Organspezifität und Antigenität von menschlichen und tierischen Skeletmuskelproteinen. Verh. dtsch. Ges. inn. Med. **74** (1968) (im Druck).

Roe, B. B.: Myasthenia gravis, secondary to thymic neoplasm. J. thorac. Surg. **33**, 770 (1957).

Rowland, L. P., H. Aranow, and P. F. A. Hoefer: Myasthenia gravis appearing after removal of thymus. Neurology (Minneap.) **7**, 584 (1957).

Schwab, R. S., and C. C. Leland: Sex and age in myasthenia gravis as critical factors in incidence and remission. J. Amer. med. Ass. **153**, 1270 (1953).

—, E. W. Wilkins, J. M. Head, and H. R. Viets: Thymectomy in myasthenia gravis. J. Amer. med. Ass. **187**, 850 (1964).

Simpson, J. A.: Myasthenia gravis: a new hypothesis. Scot. med. J. **5**, 419 (1960).

Strauss, A. J. L., B. C. Seegal, H. C. Hsu, P. M. Burkholder, W. L. Nastuk, and K. E. Osserman: Immunofluorescence demonstration of a muscle binding, complement fixing serum globulin fraction in myasthenia gravis. Proc. Soc. exp. Biol. (N. Y.) **105**, 184 (1960).

—, H. W. P. van der Geld, P. G. Kemp, E. D. Exum, and H. C. Goodman: Immunological concomitants of myasthenia gravis. Ann. N. Y. Acad. Sci. **124**, 744 (1965).

—, Ch. W. Smith, G. W. Cage, H. W. R. van der Geld, D. E. Mc. Farlin, and M. Barlow: Further studies on the specificity of presumed immune associations of myasthenia gravis and consideration of possible pathogenic implications. Ann. N. Y. Acad. Sci. **135**, 557 (1966).

Struppler, A.: Experimentelle Untersuchungen zur Pathogenese der Myasthenie. Z. ges. exp. Med. **125**, 244 (1955).

— Die Erkrankung der motorischen Endplatte einschließlich der Myasthenia gravis. Wien. klin. Wschr. **79**, 620 (1967).

Van der Geld, H. W. P., and H. J. G. H. Osterhuis: Muscle and thymus antibodies in myasthenia gravis. Vox Sang. (Basel) **8**, 196 (1963).

Weigert, C.: Pathologisch-anatomischer Beitrag zur Erb'schen Krankheit. Neurol. Centralblatt **20**, 594 (1901).

Priv.-Doz. Dr. D. Ricken
Medizinische Universitätsklinik
für Innere- und Nervenkrankheiten,
53 Bonn, Venusberg

Discussion

Bock (Tübingen): Has it been possible to exert with immuno-suppressive measures a definite influence on the course of myasthenia gravis ? As we are aware, the pattern of this disease changes quite considerably. I am just remembered of the preference of the face with the characteristic features of tiredness. With the administration of prostigmine or mestinon for example, the symptoms disappear relatively quickly. What happens to the antibodies during this space of time ?

RICKEN (Bonn): Balzereit (Symposium on Muscular Dystrophy, Myatony and Myasthenia. Berlin-Heidelberg-New York: Springer 1966) as well as Mertens [Europ. Neurology (1969) (in press)] administered Imuran in myasthenia. There were some patients who demonstrated some kind of improvement, but I do not know wether these results could be reproduced. Osserman (personal comm.) to my knowledge did not observe clear cut results. Clinical improvements have been achieved by thymectomy or administration of ACTH rather than with anything else. Humoral auto-antibodies probably do not play an essential role in this. There are cases in which the auto-antibodies persist after thymectomy. During remissions the auto-antibody does not alter significantly.

FISCHER (Hamburg): We examined some 60 cases of myasthenia and found by the fluorescence technique IgG antibodies against myosin in 40%. Certainly, in this disease there is a relatively high incidence of thymoma which contain IgG forming cell groups. The therapy of choice is early thymectomy. Immunosuppression — for instance with Imuran — may also have a favorable effect on this disease [Mertens, H. G., F. Balzereit, and M. Leipert: Europ. Neurology (in press)].

DE WECK (Berne): You have reported that in immunized rabbits it is not possible to produce muscular damage with myosin. I would like to refer to studies of Inderbitzin and his associates [Int. Arch. Allery 33, 576 (1968)] in pemphigus. Epithelial-specific antibodies may be induced in rabbits. These however become pathogenic only when the vascular permeability of the skin is increased. Then, histological changes resembling human pemphigus develop. In the studies with myosin the experimental production of similar changes of the vascular permeability may be worthwhile.

RICKEN (Bonn): Thank you for pointing out the possible role of vascular permeability. It certainly should be looked at this factor. In the context of the potential meaning of auto-antibodies in myasthenia the observations of Strauss should be mentioned. He found that thymoma carriers can have antibodies against skeletal musculature without being afflicted with myasthenia. No inflammatory changes were detectable even in muscle biopsies. Other additional mechanisms are certainly necessary for the outbreak of a case of the disease.

BOCK (Tübingen): Thus, the way from the formation of antibody to the development of the disease is far. Finding auto-antibodies does not justify speaking of disease.

RICKEN (Bonn): There are only few truly autoallergic diseases. In contrast to that the number of diseases in which the pathogenic role of the corresponding organ-specific auto-antibody cannot be proven is rather large. However even in these cases the intriguing question is impending what causes an organ-antigen to become autoantigenic or what causes the immuncompetent cells to produce auto-antibodies ?

Bayer-Symposium I, 280—288 (1969)

Comparative Studies of the Immunopathology of Inflammatory Cardiovascular Diseases

K. O. Vorlaender

Fundamental Statements

1. Pathogenic immunoreactions may be induced by environmental influences, usually by infections,—or they may correspond to the type of auto-immunoreaction that is commonly independent of environmental influences.

2. Both processes are based on the proliferation of cell systems that are immunologically active. The formation of circulating antibodies and soluble antigen-antibody complexes takes place chiefly in the plasma cells and corresponds to the immediate type of an immunological reaction.

Auto-immunoreactions are based on the proliferation of immunologically competent lymphocytes and correspond to the delayed type of immunopathological processes.

3. The following presentation contrasts immunopathological findings in rheumatic carditis with those in cardiovascular involvement in collagen diseases. I have tried of clarify the predominance of one of the two immunological reaction types in the development of certain clinical pictures.

Clinical Picture and Immunology of Rheumatic Carditis

Rheumatic carditis is the most common, clinically most important, and, under certain circumstance, the most severe organic manifestation of rheumatic fever. Its chief symptoms are: fever, persistent tachycardia, the development of disorders of rhythm or increasing ECG changes, alterations of the shape of the heart, and the occurrence of pathological murmurs. Pericarditis accompanies it in 10 to 20% of afflicted children; in adults pericarditis is found in only 3 to 5%. The fully developed picture of rheumatic pancarditis is thus found mainly in early youth.

Other rheumatic manifestations, e.g. acute polyarthritis or chorea minor, do not necessarily present together with these cardiological manifestations of rheumatic fever. This may explain why only 50% of patients with disorders of the mitral valves have a history of acute polyarthritis.

The complete picture of the disorder, as described above, is nowadays no longer so clear-cut. There is an impression that after World War II clinical pictures that are atypical and show few symptoms are in the foreground. So in the case of glomerulonephritis a primary-chronic clinical picture has developed with evanescent and minor initial symptoms, the true import of which is not being recognized for some time by the patient or his parents. In 50% of cases the typical, acute concomitant disorder of the joints is absent. The rheumatic character of the basic disorder is therefore often masked.

In this situation immunological investigations gain great clinical and pathogenetic importance as additional criteria. The immunopathological phenomena are multi-layered, and must be evaluated differently:

(a) The non-specific criteria of active rheumatic carditis are:

raised sedimentation rate;

strongly positive C-reactive protein, being a non-specific characteristic of inflammatory activity;

increased alpha-2-glucoproteids;

shift of the copper-iron ratio with increased copper and diminished iron in the blood;

increasing gamma-globulins.

Blood cultures remain bacteriologically negative; the disease process is thus not microbial.

(b) *Immunoelectrophoresis* shows:

a steady increase of 7-S-gamma-globulins, indicating an immunological struggle with the initial A-streptococcus infection, later also due to increasing auto-immunization (see below).

Quantitative studies have shown gamma-G-globulins and gamma-A-globulins to increase steadily;

gamma-macroglobulins, however, are increasing only slightly; this explains the obligatory lack of rheumatoid factor in rheumatic carditis;

in the acute state of the disorder immunoelectrophoresis reveals an increase of alpha-glucoproteids and a diminution of albumins.

Reduction of transferrin, the iron-binding fraction of serum, in blood is characteristic. The writer's investigations (Vorlaender *et al.*) have shown that transferrin is significantly increased in cardiac tissue altered by rheumatism. It was found, concordant with chemical analyses by Heilmeyer *et al.*, that at the site of inflammation iron was more plentiful and that it was obviously used for the purpose of defence against inflammation.

(c) The immunopathological struggle with the initial A-streptococci infection is indicated by:

(1) a rise of anti-O-streptolysin titers to 250 units and up to 1600 or more units. A late rise of these titers 4 weeks after the start of the disorder is characteristic, in contrast to uncomplicated streptococcal angina. In rheumatic fever increased antistreptolysin titers may be found persistently for years. In comparison, in streptococcal angina an immediate rise of the antistreptolysin titer and quick regression after 8 to 14 days are characteristic.

My own statistical investigations of the behaviour of the anti-O-streptolysin titer in rheumatic carditis when inflammatory activity is high, showed a positive yield of 77 to 97%.

Comparative investigations in cases without clinical activity, i.e. in valvular disorders of rheumatic origin, which are only of haemodynamic consequence, showed frequencies of 10 to 31%.

This difference is statistically highly significant. The X square of 53.282 was absolute proof of this.

Eckert *et al.* have carried out similar studies recently.

Their studies showed that a persistently increased antistreptolysin titer is five times more frequent when the clinical course is severe or when there is a tendency to recurrences than when the disorder is mild and when there are no inflammatory recurrences.

Further points in proof of the immunological struggle with the initial A-streptococcal infection are:

(b) The agglutination of whole bacteria corresponding to "living agglutination". Here, too, persistently high titers are obtained.

(c) A rise of anti-M-antibodies as the type-specific antibody for A-streptococci. Generally, the rise of anti-M-antibodies is slower than that of anti-O-streptolysin titers.

(d) A rise of anti-C-antibodies as the group-specific antibody of A-streptococci. Their rise runs more or less parallel with that of anti-O-streptolysin titers.

(e) The anti-enzyme-antibodies may be compared, i.e. the behaviour of

antistreptokinase;

antihyaluronidase;

antifibrinolysin,

which are altogether non-specific and inconstant and thus clinically of little value.

The behaviour of antistreptokinase may be of interest when streptokinase treatment is carried out on account of embolic processes after the formation of parietal thrombi in the enlarged left heart or in the left atrium: anaphylactic reactions are possible at high titers.

(4) Of great importance is the immunopathology of the chronic progression of rheumatic carditis or the immunopathology of cases in which new rheumatic inflammatory attacks constantly recur, which is bound to lead to a deterioration of valvular function:

(a) Formation of antibodies will now take place, the antigenic substrate of which must be situated within the heart. This immunological behaviour was first described in 1953 by me and has meanwhile been confirmed by Steffen, Vinogradow, and many others. The responsible antigen in the heart muscle has so far not been identified chemically, but there is no doubt that these antibodies are absorbed by extracts of human heart tissue and by A-streptococci, in the last case mainly by fractions which are rich in polysaccharides (Kaplan *et al.*). This twofold direction of action of the antibodies may be explained according to McCarthy as a cross reaction of a tissue-auto-antibody with a group-specific carbohdrase of the cell wall of A-streptococci.

Clinical observation shows, however, that this immune process is of long duration and may remain bound to tissue for years.

This makes more difficult the explanation of a simple cross reaction with a fraction rich in polysaccharides of A-streptococci, which would remain confined to the duration of the influence of the infection.

My own investigations have shown that there is a complex antigen effect, which remains localized in the heart and is composed of a bacterial component, namely, the streptococcal polysaccharides, and a tissue protein. This protein component determins the antigen. Cross reactions with healthy human heart tissue may be explained by the hapten nature of this tissue protein.

(b) Kushner and Kaplan have shown recently that there is a response of circulating antibodies to two further cardiac antigens: one is a muscular antigen, which may also occur in the peripheral musculature and which thus corresponds to myoglobin;

the other is a cardiac antigen, chemically not yet differentiated, which occurs in the kidney in low concentration. This would explain a possible, though weak cross-reaction of circulating antibodies against cardiac antigens with peripheral musculature or with kidney extracts.

This attachment of antibodies which has often been called a true auto-immuno-reaction and which belongs to those clinical forms that progress or have a tendency towards recurring inflammations, is localized, according to the fluorescence-serological investigations of Kaplan *et al.* and Hess *et al.*, in the subendocardial tissue, mainly Aschoff's nodules and the sarcolemma of the fibrils of the cardiac muscle. These are thus the sites, where the inflammatory process of rheumatic endomyocarditis is localized chiefly.

(c) These antibodies are attached to their antigenic substrate in the heart by complement fixation (Klein and Burkholder). At the same time, the complement level of serum, especially that of beta-1-C-globulin as essential representative of the third component of complement, is diminished, so that conclusions may be drawn clinically to the immunological activity of the process. As scar formation or calcification increase, in other words, with the regression of inflammatory activity, the consumption of complement in the heart ceases, and beta-1-C-globulin returns to normal.

(d) My own investigations have shown:

Circulating auto-antibodies against cardiac antigen in rheumatic carditis with signs of clinical activity in 44.5% of cases.

In rheumatic valvular disease with haemodynamic effects only, without signs of inflammatory activity, circulating antibodies were found in only 3.5% of all cases.

In comparison, positive immunofluorescence in cardiace tissue of the resected cardiac auricle or at post mortem in rheumatic carditis with signs of clinical activity were found in 63.4% of all cases.

In valvular lesions, haemodynamically active only without signs of inflammatory activity, in 16.4% of all cases.

These investigations were carried out by Hess, Ziff *et al.* on 624 cases, whilst my own evaluation was based on a total number of 128 cases of carditis with signs of clinical activity and 452 cases of valvular lesions with haemodynamic consequences without signs of inflammatory activity.

(e) The numerical differences are even more obvious in true rheumatic reactivation after mitral commissurotomy: again according to Hess and Ziff *et al.* in cases with active inflammation positive immunofluorescence was found in more than 70%;

in cases without inflammatory activity before or after operation it was present in only 16.4% of all cases.

Only little can be said about the numerical state of circulating auto-antibodies, because my own observations of true rheumatic reactivation after heart operations are too few to permit definite statements.

A number of case reports that verify these findings have been presented: (compare in Vorlaender in: Anschütz, F.: Die Endocarditis, pp. 166ff. Stuttgart: Thieme 1968.

Comparison of these immunological findings with the clinical picture shows that the tissue-bound immunophenomenon of rheumatic carditis in the vast majority of cases belongs to actively progressive or recurring inflammatory processes of the heart. This type of immunological reaction pertains only to rheumatic cardiac inflammations. It hardly occurs (maximally 3.8% of all cases) in non-rheumatic carditis and in valvular lesions without inflammatory activity.

It is therefore of differential diagnostic importance.

This proves that the active, though bacteriologically sterile inflammation of the heart in rheumatic carditis is closely related to an immunopathological process that initially is based on infection, and then shows all criteria of a proper auto-immune process. As this auto-immune process develops, the inflammatory process becomes independent and may well cause inflammation even without renewed environmental cause, i.e., without renewed contact with streptococcal antigens. This has been proved by the fact of postoperative rheumatic reactivation.

This auto-immunoprocess is *not* identical with immunological processes in the "post-myocardial-infarct syndrome": there, antigen effects arise, which are a consequence of the formation of necroses in the heart. The corresponding antibodies do not, however, show any cross reaction with alpha-streptococci.

The auto-immunoprocess present in rheumatic carditis is also *not* identical with the auto-immunoreactions in Libman-Sacks endocarditis, which always remains independent of infection. It is also not identical with immunological processes in coronary arteriitis, as found in the collagen diseases.

Clinical Picture and Immunology of the Involvement of the Heart in Collagen Disease

Both clinical manifestations and immunopathological processes differ characteristically from those of rheumatic carditis, in spite of a number of correspondences:

Clinical Picture

In Libman-Sacks endocarditis, which occurs mainly in visceral lupus erythematosus, varying cardiac murmurs, and (rarely) changes of shape, are the most impressive findings. Pathological changes of the ECG are caused by accompanying myocarditis, and only in a few cases by pericarditis. It is possible in the long term for isolated pericarditis to be present. Exudates in the pericardium or cardiac tamponade through haemorrhage are rare. In the overwhelming majority of cases fibrinous pericarditis is present. The endocardial changes characteristically never cause valvular disorders. On the whole the clinical signs of Libman-Sacks endocarditis are inconstant and highly variable.

In panarteriitis nodosa cardiac involvement occurs in 80%. It is diagnosed clinically, however, by no means as often as that. Anginal syndromes, persistent tachycardia, or disorders of rhythm with ECG changes of the type of deficiency of coronary blood flow are found. They occur the more frequently, the older the inflammatory process of the coronary artery is. The changes are very minor; blood-vessels may remain clinically silent for a long time. Again, valvular disorders do not develop, exceptionally parietal fibrosis of the endocardium may arise. This, too, may cause no clinical symptoms, but may lead to symptoms of muscular insufficiency of unknown origin.

(a) *Immunologically* the same non-specific criteria of inflammation are found, as mentioned under rheumatic carditis. In cardiac involvement of collagen disease or of coronary arteriitis the characteristic shift of the iron-copper ratio is not present, however. Copper does not increase in the clinical types mentioned.

The appearance of the rheumatoid factor in 30% of cases is a notable, though non-specific serological phenomenon. In rheumatoid carditis the rheumatoid factor never appears; equally, in cardiac involvement of collagen disorder the antistreptolysin titer is never raised, and there are no serological reactions that might indicate an immunological struggle with an A-streptococcal infection. Thus, none of the serological findings are present that have been referred to in (c) as characteristic signs in rheumatic carditis of a longterm immunological struggle with bacterial antigens of A-streptococci.

(b) *Immunoelectrophoretically* mainly 7-S-gamma-globulins, gamma-G- and gamma-A-fractions are increased. The gamma-macroglobulin fraction is also increased, so that the rheumatoid factor becomes positive, although frequently at low titer only. The rheumatoid factor represents a gamma-macroglobulin, which is able to react with 7-S-globulins. In the acute stages alpha-2-glucoproteids are increased, a non-specific symptom of inflammation that may be assessed by immunoelectrophoresis and also quantitatively. When there is a tendency to clinical progression, coeruloplasmin increases, indicating that it is mainly a symptom of chronic inflammation.

(c) The immunology of chronic progression differs characteristically from the immunological phenomena found in chronic rheumatic carditis:

In visceral lupus erythematosus and inflammatory cardiac involvement of the Libman-Sacks endocarditis type antinuclear auto-antibodies and therefore L.E. cells are frequently found. Antinuclear auto-antibodies are found in 80 to 95% of cases with suitable methods (antiglobulin consumption test, or better immunofluorescence on whole nuclei, also precipitation methods for the determination of antibodies against nucleoproteins or desoxyribonucleic acid, finally the latex test with nucleoproteins. The quick latex test, which is not very sensitive, is an exception. In my own investigations I obtained a response in only 40 to 50% of cases). L.E. cells, however, are commonly found in only 50 to 60% of cases, depending upon the stage of the disease (compare Gonzales, in: Rothfield).

Characteristically, antinuclear factors have not been demonstrated in panarteriitis nodosa and generally in inflammatory vascular processes of the coronary arteries, in so far as these processes belong to the group of collagen diseases.

Highly important nowadays is the proof of the presence of cytoplasmatic auto-antibodies, which react within the cell body, are not cell-specific and not organ-specific, but are attached to the fraction of mitochondria and lysosomes in the cytoplasm.

My own investigations (also compare Halberg, who had similar percentages) have shown that cytoplasmatic auto-antibodies without organ-specificity occur:

In visceral lupus erythematosus with cardiac involvement in up to 80% of cases;

in panarteriitis nodosa and related vascular processes, mainly of the heart, in about 50% of cases.

Cytoplasmatic auto-antibodies, in spite of their lack of organ-specificity, usually accumulate in organs with clinically high inflammatory activity, so that an impression of organspecificity may arise, which, however, is disproved by absorption tests.

Paronetto and Koffler were able to show by means of immunofluorescence that in inflammatory vascular processes of collagen disease all three gamma-globulin fractions are deposited in the arteries of the spleen, of the heart, the liver, and, preferentially, of the kidney. Fibrinogen is increasingly deposited in the inflamed vascular walls. The immune complexes bind complement, which may be measured by the amount of beta-1-C-globulin as the representative component of C-III. According to McClusky, the increase in deposition of fibrinogen into the cell wall is the consequence of a primary immunopathological process and is supposed to play a decisive role in the development of the proliferative stage of vascular changes up to secondary sclerosis.

Generally speaking, the immunoglobulins deposited in vascular walls are components of antigen-antibody complexes, which are found in inflamed vascular walls.

By themselves, anticytoplasmatic auto-antibodies are not able primarily to penetrate intact cell membranes, e.g. the intima cells of blood-vessels. They cannot therefore be primary causes of disease. Necrobiotic processes, in other words, destruction of cells, are preconditions for the effectiveness of these anticytoplasmatic factors. As consequence of such cell destructions, large quantities of cytoplasmatic antigens are liberated and then unite with the corresponding auto-antibodies to immunocomplexes. By complement fixation these immunocomplexes are then deposited in arteries and sustain the arteriitis, the inflammatory process. The cause of the primary triggering off of these immunopathological processes is not properly understood as yet.

The rheumatoid factor may also play a part in the pathogenesis of these vascular changes: Baum, Staestny, and Ziff have shown that the injection of antigen-antibody complexes together with rheumatoid factor under experimental conditions may lead not only to arteriitis, i.e. to inflammatory changes in the intima of small arteries, but to the production of thrombotic occlusions, as found so often in hospital. The authors believe therefore that the rheumatoid factor is indirectly involved in the pathogenesis of these vascular changes.

Compared with the immunology of chronic progressive or acute rheumatic carditis the immunopathological processes concerned with the cardiovascular involvement in the collagen disease are fundamentally different:

Primary infection plays no part, so that prophylaxis with penicillin is not applicable. Primary sensitization by bacteria therefore plays no part in the auto-immunophenomena, although sensitization by drugs or other chemical substances may be a factor. These are, however, usually true auto-immunoreactions, usually on the basis of a genetic, and very rarely of an acquired, abnormality of immuno-cytes.

These pathogenetic relationships are accepted nowadays in the case of visceral lupus erythematosus with cardiac involvement. They may also be concerned in other inflammatory vascular processes of collagen disease. Therefore, immuno-histological methods usually demonstrate lymphocytic perivascular infiltrates found around inflamed small arteries.

Out of all this, important differential diagnostic criteria arise so far as endangiitis obliterans and vascular sclerosis are concerned. These are never accompanied by similar auto-immunophenomena. Necrosis is of decisive importance; with the occurrence of necrosis the liberation of cytoplasmatic auto-antigens becomes the cause of the auto-immunoreactions, which are stimulated over and over again, a process that leads to the deposition of pathogenic immunocomplexes in the arteries.

Discussion and Summary

When these immunopathological findings in cardiovascular inflammatory disorders are compared, two fundamentally different principles are discovered, from which nevertheless arises a common, higher principle of cellular fundamentals:

(a) The development of immunopathological processes in rheumatic carditis is the consequence of an environmental, or *exogenous*, stimulus by a primary A-streptococcal infection of the cell systems that produce antibodies: It is followed by a proliferation chiefly of *plasmacellular* elements, which typically and chiefly produce circulating antibodies and antigen-antibody complexes that initially are soluble. This explains the production of antibodies against the various antigens of A-streptococci, which may go on for a long time.

It also explains the formation of soluble antigen-antibody complexes and their deposition into the endomyocardium. According to model experiments this may be the cause of active rheumatic inflammation and its acute recurrences. The second immunological process, largely linked with immunologically competent lymphocytes, commences only when the progress of this inflammatory process becomes chronic. It may well smoulder for years before it is diagnosed as valvular disorder with haemodynamic action. The process itself has many traits of a true auto-immunization: the immunoreactions, the antigenic substrate of which is situated within the heart, occur only at this stage.

The first phase of these immunopathological processes will obviously respond to treatment or prophylaxis with penicillin and treatment with anti-inflammatory agents, whilst the second phase is often refractory to therapeutic attack.

(b) In contrast, the immunopathological processes in collagen disorders and in the inflammatory cardiovascular involvement are linked with the proliferation of immunologically competent *lymphocytes*, for which a genetic predisposition to produce anomalous immunocytes is largely responsible. These relationships have been confirmed by family investigations, particularly for visceral lupus erythematosus. Environmental influences may additionally stimulate this proliferation of lymphocytes which are changed or the reactions of which are changed. In practice, drug stimulation is of far greater importance than infection. Plasmacellular proliferation loses its importance, and the immunohistological picture of peri-vascular infiltrations is dominated by lymphocytes that are ready for reaction immunologically.

Consequently, prophylaxis with antibiotics cannot be used in this group of disorders. *Immunosuppressive treatment* has its proper domain here, together with cortisone, the indication for which, however, is limited to fresh inflammatory attacks.

The tendency to chronic imflammatory progression in the cardiovascular system without any ascertainable environmental cause is due to these various auto-immunoprocesses. The reason for the progressive development of the disorder is the parmanent infiltration by cells that are ready for immunological reaction, the occurrence of new necrotic processes, and the liberation of cytoplasmatic auto-antigens with the formation of antigen-antibody complexes, the renewed deposition of which in healthy vascular regions causes the progression of the pathological process.

It must be admitted that exclusive and one-sided proliferation of only one of the two cell systems is rare: it is important for clinical purposes, however, to know which of the immunological systems has gained ascendency. I hope that this has been made clear by comparing the immunopathological findings of the different diseases. The particular system that is preponderant will determine the clinical picture of the fundamental disease process: plasmacellular proliferation with its immunological consequences requires recurrent exogenous stimulation. Clinically, therefore, fresh episodes and acute recurrences will be dominant, although these immunopathological processes may be self-limiting.

Lymphocytic proliferation, being a symptom of genetic misdirection of the immunosystem, will continue without exogenous stimulation. It may never quite burn out, and it is not selflimiting. It is the cause of chronic, autonomously proceeding disease processes.

Comparison of clinical and immunological pictures will help to elucidate the extent to which the development of disease depends on the kind of immunological reaction and its cellular basis.

References

Anschütz, F.: Endocarditis. Stuttgart: Thieme 1968.
Baum, J., P. Stastny, and M. Ziff: J. Immunol. **93**, 985 (1964).
Eckert, W., F. Harter und W. Kuhn: Med. Welt **1965**, 2525.
Gonzales, E. N., and N. F. Rothfield: New Engl. J. Med. **274**, 1333 (1966).
Hess, E. V., C. W. Fink, A. Taranta, and M. Ziff: J. clin. Invest. **43**, 886 (1964).
Kaplan, M. H., R. Bolande, L. Rakita, and J. Blair: New Engl. J. Med. **171**, 637 (1964).
Klein, P., u. P. Burkholder: Dtsch. med. Wschr. **84**, 2001 (1959).
McCarthy, M.: Circulation **29**, 488 (1964).
McCluskey, R., and B. Benacerraf: Amer. J. Path. **35**, 275 (1959).
— —, J. Potter, and F. Müller: J. exp. Med. **111**, 1881 (1960).
Paronetto, F., L. Deppisch, and L. R. Tuchmann: Amer. J. Med. **36**, 984 (1964).
—, and D. Koffler: J. clin. Invest. **10**, 1657 (1965).
Steffen, C.: Wien. klin. Wschr. **68**, 865 (1956); **75**, 894 (1963).
Vorlaender, K. O.: In: F. Anschütz, Endocarditis, S. 138ff. Stuttgart: Thieme 1968.
Vinogradow, W. J.: Therap. Inn. Moskva **34**, 41 (1962).

Prof. Dr. K. O. Vorlaender
Innere Abteilung des Luisenhospitals,
51 Aachen, Boxgraben 99

Discussion

FISCHER (Hamburg): What proportion of lupus erythematosus cases are drug induced? We have seen two cases: one had been caused by hydantoin in a child who at the same time had haemolytic anaemia which disappeared with the cessation of the drug. The second case occurred after INH medication.

BOCK (Tübingen): In the individual case it is often very difficult to find the immediate connection between erythematodes and a drug. To state the actual percentage is probably impossible.

VORLAENDER (Aachen): In addition to the nucleoproteids, cytoplasmatic antigens are released which can also be important in erythematosus. Anti-nucleic antibodies are also found in the healthy subject. It should be emphasized that in lupus erythematosus the pathogenic immune complexes are chiefly found in the kidneys.

FISCHER (Hamburg): Have animal experiments been carried out in which an exogenous agent started a morbid process that after withdrawal of the agent became an autonomous auto-immune disease.

VORLAENDER (Aachen): Paronetto and his team experimentally sensitised against vascular extracts and produced an arteriitis which then became autonomous. Application of the rheumatoid factor led to thrombotic vascular occlusions. Here we are concerned with an induction by sensitisation.

Bayer-Symposium I, 290—293 (1969)

Possible Bithermic Pathomechanism
in Cryoglobulinemic Vasculitis

K. ROTHER, H.-D. FLAD[1], U. ROTHER, and P. A. MIESCHER[2]

With 2 Figures

Recent observations (Miescher *et al.*) of the vascular lesions in cryoglobulinemic patients (mixed type of cryoglobuline) have suggested that immune processes are involved in the pathogenesis. The present study on the serum of a patient with IgM-IgG-type of cryoglobulinemia may contribute to the understanding of the mechanism that is operative in the pathogenesis of the vasculitis.

Clinically, the disease is characterized by acrocyanosis upon exposure to low temperatures, accompanied by Raynaud-type episodes. A purpura is often found with a slight tenderness on pressure of the affected tissue. The histology of the skin reveals a vasculitis with infiltration by PMN's, lymphocytes and plasma cells. By means of the immunofluorescence technic, deposition can be shown (Miescher *et al.*) in the involved vessels of autologous γ-globulin, C and fibrinogen. A similar pattern is seen in the vasculitis of the Arthus reaction. However, in contrast to the Arthus reaction, the mechanism causing the activation of the C system and its vascular deposition is not known in these patients. Neither is the pathogenic relevance of the γ-globulin and the C localization understood. The sera of the patients contain proteins that precipitate at low temperature. According to the nature of the precipitates, the disease has been subdivided. One group comprises the sera with homologous precipitates of either 19S or 7S γ-globulins, most of them myeloma or macroglobulin proteins. Another group has been described in detail by LoSpalluto and is characterized by the mixed composition of the precipitate of 19S and 7S globulins. The cryoprecipitate of our patient was of the mixed type. It has previously been analyzed in a publication by Meltzer and Franklin.

In the 40 year old female patient the serum C titer varied between normal levels (200 CH_{50} units) and zero. A blood sample was drawn at a time when the C titer was high. Incubation of the serum at 37 °C resulted in only an insignificant loss of C activity, comparable to that of a normal serum control. Cooling of the serum to 1 °C caused a massive precipitation of cryoglobulin, but again did not influence the C titer.

For the following study the cryoprecipitation reaction was separated from the C reaction. The patient serum was incubated at 2 °C for 200 min, resulting in the precipitation of 3.2 mg protein per ml. The precipitate was washed and standard-

---

[1] Present address: Department of Clinical Physiology, University of Ulm, 10/11 Parkstr., 7900 Ulm, Germany.

[2] Present address: Hopitâl Cantonal, Université de Genève, Division of Hematology, Geneva, Switzerland.

ized to 0.5 mg/ml. Aliquots were distributed to tubes and stored at —70 °C. Sera of healthy human donors were used as a source of C.

The addition of cryoprecipitate to normal sera equilibrated at 37 °C caused a significant inactivation of C. Fig. 1 depicts the inactivating effect of various amounts of cryoprecipitate on constant amounts of C upon incubation of the mixtures for 10 min at 0 °C and then for 20 min at 37 °C. The more cryoprecipitate was added, the more inactivation of C was observed.

Analyses of the C subcomponents involved in the reaction seemed especially important in view of the findings of Hanauer and Christian in cryoprecipitating sera from patients with Lupus erythematosus. The authors found a participation of 11S serum protein in the flocculation reaction. Since 11S protein (= C1q) is also a part of the first component of C (C1), it had to be ruled out that the loss of C

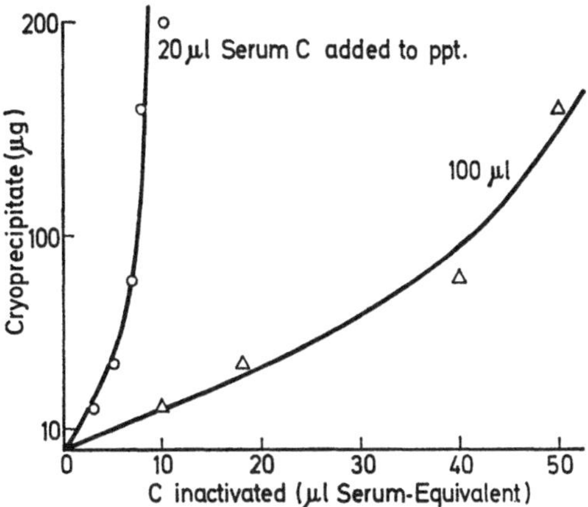

Fig. 1. Dose response curve of the inactivation of constant amounts of C by varying amounts of preformed cryoprecipitate. △ = 100 μl serum were incubated with varying amounts of precipitate; ○ = 20 μl were similarly incubated

activity was merely caused by an exhaustion of 11S due to its incorporation into the precipitates.

The C reactivity remaining after incubation with cryoprecipitate was titrated by the use of (a) sensitized erythrocytes (EA) and (b) of erythrocytes that, in addition to the antibody, also carried C1 (EAC1). If the cryoglobulin had reduced only the 11S concentration of the serum, one would have expected a low C titer when EA were used for substrate, as contrasted with an higher titer upon incubation with EAC1. However, the loss of C activity was similar with the two substrates. Exhaustion of 11S by incorporation into the precipitates could thus be ruled out. The diminished C titer was caused by the limiting effect of factors other than C1.

One of them may be C2. When the same reaction product was assayed for C2, a significant inactivation of this component was found. The participation of the third component of C (C3) entailed its attachment to the cryoglobulin complexes. Cryoglobulins were incubated with serum, centrifuged and resuspended following a washing cycle. They were found positive in the immuneadherence test (Nishioka and Linscott), indicating the presence of C3. Cryoprecipitates not

19*

incubated with serum or cryoglobulins incubated with serum in the presence of EDTA did not show this activity. Concomitant with the binding of C3 to the complexes, a loss was observed in the C3 titer (immuneadherence) of the supernatant. The C3 molecule could be dissociated from the complexes. Immuneadherence positive cryoglobulin complexes were solubilized by incubation at 37 °C and the solution analyzed in the Ouchterlony test. A precipitation line identical with a β_{1A} control was observed following incubation with an anti-β_{1A}-serum.

Of the remaining C factors, the overall activity of the post-C2 factors (C_{EDTA}) and C6 were tested for inactivation by cryoglobulin. No significant influence was seen, indicating that none of these factors was responsible for the decreased activity.

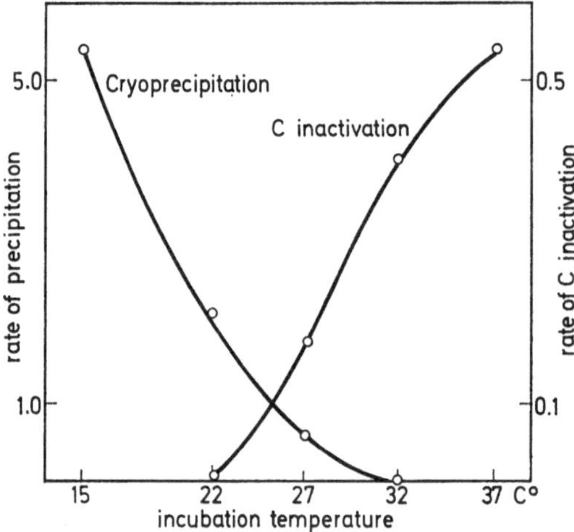

Fig. 2. Influence of temperature on the cryoprecipitation and on the C inactivation by preformed cryoprecipitates. Significant cryoprecipitation occured only at temperatures below 27 °C. In contrast, C reaction was discernible only at temperatures of and above 27 °C

Summarizing the results, it was concluded that the cryoglobulin of our patient was reactive with the C system including the most critical of the C factors from a pathogenetic point of view, i.e. C3.

It was puzzling to note in the circulation of our patient a normal (200 CH_{50} units) C titer although she had a serum concentration of 3.2 mg/ml of potentially highly C reactive cryoglobulin. In the following experiments it was tested whether temperature factors may account for the apparent contradiction.

The cryoprecipitation reaction was analyzed kinetically at various temperatures. The speed of the reaction was calculated graphically from the kinetic curves. It is expressed in terms of "rate of reaction" in Fig. 2. While a rapid flocculation was seen at 15 °C, the reaction was barely discernible at 27 °C and did not occur at all at 32 °C. The opposite was observed when the interaction of preformed cryoglobulin and C was analyzed by kinetic technics. No C inactivation took place at 22 °C. The reaction was slow at 27 °C and fast at 37 °C (Fig. 2). A differentiation by temperature factors could thus be achieved of the cryoprecipitation and the interaction of cryoprecipitates and C.

The separation of the cryoprecipitation reaction and the C inactivation was abandoned at this stage and the findings used in a retest of the patient serum. It was incubated first for 200 min at 4 °C, followed by 20 min at 37 °C. The result was a 30% loss of C activity. No loss occured when the serum was incubated first for 20 min at 37° and then for 200 min at 4 °C.

In conclusion, bithermic conditions were required for the activation of the C system in the serum of this cryoglobulinemic patient. A phase of exposure to low temperature caused the cryoprecipitation. It had to be followed by a phase of elevated temperature to allow for the interaction of the cryoprecipitates and C. The bithermic activation of the serum C system may, by the various biological activities associated with the intermediate steps of the reaction sequence, be relevant in the pathogenesis of the vascular lesions in cryoglobulinemic patients.

When referring to the Donath-Landsteiner hemolytic antibody, Dr. Schubothe yesterday pointed out their peculiar characteristics (page 167). The unusual bithermic conditions required for their hemolytic function made them appear an exception in the field of immunology and without a parallel. The present findings seem to indicate that such requirements may not be that rare. We believe we have presented to you a similar bithermic mechanism that is operative in another condition, cryoglobulinemia.

References

Hanauer, L. B., and Ch. L. Christian: Studies of cryoproteins in systemic lupus erythematosus. J. clin. Invest. **46**, 400 (1967).

LoSpalluto, J., and B. Dorward: Cryoglobulinemia based on interaction between a gamma macroglobulin and 7S gamma globulin. Amer. J. Med. **32**, 142 (1962).

Meltzer, M., and E. C. Franklin: Cryoglobulinemia. A study of twenty-nine patients. Amer. J. Med. **40**, 828 (1966).

Miescher, P. A., F. Paronetto, and D. Koffler: Immunofluorescent studies in human vasculitis. In: Immunopathology, IVth Internat. Symposion. Basel-Stuttgart: Schwabe & Co. 1966.

Nishioka, K., and W. D. Linscott: Components of guinea pig complement. I. Separation of a serum fraction essential for immune hemolysis and immune adherence. J. exp. Med. **118**, 767 (1963).

Prof. Dr. K. O. Rother
Max-Planck-Institut für Immunbiologie,
78 Freiburg-Zähringen, Stübeweg 51

Discussion

RIETHMÜLLER (Tübingen): As we have published, without employing bithermic activation we found in 8 cryo-globulinaemia patients a diminution of C2 and sometimes also a diminution of the total complement [Clin. Exp. Immunol. **1**, 337 (1966)].

ROTHER (Freiburg): I agree. When a reduced complement titer was found in our patients, the limiting factor always turned out to be C2.

SPRINGER (Evanston): Do all cryo-globulin types behave the same ?

ROTHER (Freiburg): We intend to examine sera of other cryoglobulinic patients. This is on our programme.

DE WECK (Berne): Does a similar mechanism operate in cold allergy ? I think of the clinical picture of urticarial skin changes only occurring under the action of cold. This allergy can be transferred to a normal person with the serum of the patients.

ROTHER (Freiburg): This has not yet been studied although it would be feasible. It would be interesting to see whether or not in such skin lesions β_{1A} globulin is deposited on te vessel walls.

Bayer-Symposium I, 295—301 (1969)

Amyloid Involvement and Monoclonal Immunoglobulins

F. W. ALY, H. J. BRAUN, and H. P. MISSMAHL

With 4 Figures

At a relatively early date the coincidence of serum protein changes and amyloid tissue deposits invited speculation as to whether there might be an underlying intimate correlation or even a causual relationship (Magnus-Levy, Letterer). No

Table 1. *Classification of amyloidoses*

	Peri-reticulin amyloidosis	Peri-collagen amyloidosis
Hereditary	Hereditary amyloidosis with nephropathy (e.g. familial mediterranean fever)	Hereditary amyloidosis with neuropathy or cardiomegaly
Idiopathic "primary"	Amyloidosis with nephropathy without underlying disease	a) Amyloidosis with neuropathy, cardiopathy or malabsorption without underlying disease b) Localized amyloidosis (e.g. tumorlike amyloidosis, lichen amyloidosis, amyloidosis in old age)
Acquired "secondary"	Amyloidosis associated with infection (e.g. tuberculosis, osteomyelitis) rheumatic disease, malignant neoplasm etc. Amyloidosis in systemic lupus erythematodes	Amyloidosis associated with multiple myeloma of macroglobulinemia a) generalized b) localized

definite statement could be presented so far as to the extent of characteristic changes arising in the serum protein pattern in generalized amyloidosis in humans; the observations which are available on the employment of modern chemical methods of protein estimation are as yet too insufficient to warrant any explanations. More exhaustive investigations on this problem have been conducted by the group of Ossermann who on the strength of his findings postulates that abnormal gamma globulins or gamma globulin particles, which may be detected in serum or urine, actively participate in amyloid formation.

In the light of this, the question as to whether specific protein changes may be demonstrated in serum or urine in generalized amyloidosis was restudied in a large group of patients all of whom were subjected to uniform examination methods. Amyloidoses were graded according to the criteria discussed in a previous paper (Missmahl, 1965, 1967) (reference is made to Tab. 1).

Method

Diagnosis of amyloidosis: Amyloidosis was diagnosed in the 57 patients under study by demonstrating amyloid presence at rectal biopsies (Missmahl, 1965, 1967). In histological sections stained with Congo red amyloid degenerations may be detected in the polarizing microscope by their characteristic green coloration. The amyloid deposits may be demonstrated in the perireticulin (prA) or pericollagen (pkA) form, or the combined perireticulin/pericollagen mixed form. A sharp distinction should be drawn between these amyloid forms and amyloid caused by old age (Gafni, Sohar and Missmahl, 1967).

Qualitative and Quantitative Methods for Demonstrating Polyclonal and Monoclonal Gamma Globulins

1. Paper electrophoresis by the method of Durrum using a Veronal buffer, pH 8.6, μ 0.1.

Urine electrophoresis: (a) separation of 30 µl native urine, (b) reduction of protein-containing urine to serum concentration; quantity applied: 10 µl, (c) concentration of protein-poor urines at a ratio of 250:1; quantity applied: 10 µl. Determination of protein concentrations with the Biuret reagent.

2. Starch gel electrophoresis in vertical chamber by the method of Smithies in sodium hydroxide-borate buffer, pH 8.6, staining with Amido Black 10B.

3. Immunoelectrophoresis on slides by the modified method of Scheidegger, using 2 to 3 dilutions, pH 8.6, ionic strength 0.06 in 2% pure agar (Behring-Werke, Marburg).

Immunoprecipitation with

(a) horse antihuman sera (Institut Pasteur);

(b) antiserum to isolated rabbit serum proteins (anti-IgG, anti-GgA, anti-IgM) supplied by Behring-Werke, Marburg;

(c) antiserum to light chains (type K, type L), supplied by Travenol/Munich and Chemapol/Pragune respectively.

4. Quantitative determination of immunoglobulins by radial immunodiffusion by the method of Mancini *et al.* on Partigen slides, kindly supplied by Behringwerke, Marburg.

For details of method and normal values of the three immunoglobulin fractions, reference is made to Braun and co-workers.

Results

1. Among 57 patients with generalized amyloid involvement perireticulin amyloid deposits were found in 26 cases; pericollagen amyloid deposits were shown to exist in 24 and amyloid deposits of the mixed type in 7 cases (Table 2).

2. In 26 patients with perireticulin amyloidosis (most of whom had to be clinically assigned to the secondary amyloidosis category) an M-component was detectable in no case. By contrast, an M-component was shown to exist in 10 out of 24 patients with pericollagen amyloidosis, and in 3 out of 7 patients with mixed type amyloid deposits; an M-component was thus obtained in 23% of the cases studied.

Table 2. *Type of amyloid deposits in 57 patients with respect to immunoglobulins*

Type of amyloid deposits	n	M-component	Ig-class
Peri-reticulin	26	—	—
Peri-collagen	24	10	4 IgG 3 IgA 2 IgM 1 BJ
Peri-collagen and peri-reticulin	7	3	2 IgG 1 IgM

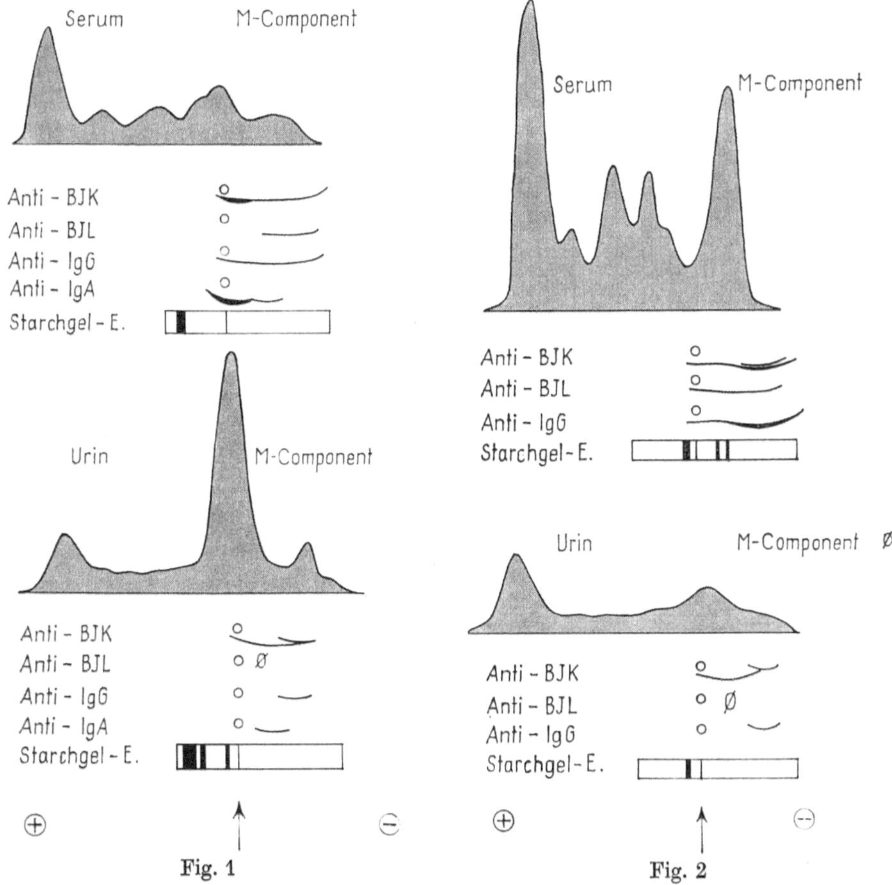

Fig. 1. *Za., E.*, male, age 48, serum 18.9.67; Diagnosis: Amyloidosis of peri-collagen type and multiple myeloma (IgA type K — myeloma protein). Schematic representation of paperelectrophoretic-, immunelectrophoretic- and starchgelelectrophoretic patterns of serumproteins and the proteins of concentrated urine. Antisera: RAHu BJK 01-0767, RAHu BJL 01-0767, Chemapol Prague; RAHu IgG — RCM 04, RAHu IgA — RCL 04 Behring-Werke Marburg/L. For further details s. text

Fig. 2. *Epp. Al*, male, age 58, serum 28.11.66; Diagnosis: Amyloidosis of peri-collagen type and multiple myeloma (IgG type K-myeloma protein). For further details see above

3. In 25 patients showing amyloid involvement it was possible to investigate serum and urine proteins electrophoretically (starch gel and immunoelectrophoresis), specific emphasis being given to the occurrence of monoclonal proteins. Figs. 1 to 3 schematically illustrate typical experimental results for different types of constellations. In Fig. 1 (patient Za., pkA and IgAK plasmocytoma) an M-component is obtained on paper and starch gel electrophoresis both in serum and urine. Immunologically the protein is of the IgAK type, and of the Bence-Jones type K in urine. In addition small amounts of IgA and IgG are detectable. As to Fig. 2 (patient Ep., pkA and IgGK plasmocytoma) paper electrophoresis yields an M-component only in serum, but not in urine. Bence-Jones protein, type K, is detected by immunoelectrophoresis in concentrated urine, apart from small amounts of IgG, involving most likely a monoclonal IgGK. In view of the low concentration, a corresponding fraction is not located by starch gel electrophoresis. Fig. 3 shows the results obtained on analysis of serum and urine proteins in a patient with secondary perireticulin amyloidosis. It is not possible to demonstrate the presence of an M-component in serum, nor of a Bence-Jones protein in serum or urine.

When applying these methods in 10 patients with amyloidosis showing an M-component in serum or urine, the presence of even small traces of monoclonal light chains in concentrated urine could not be proven in 5 cases. It was not possible to demonstrate monoclonal light chains in serum or urine in 10 cases of acquired perireticulin amyloidosis, 3 cases of idiopathic pericollagen amyloidosis and 2 cases of the acquired mixed type without an M-component in serum (Plassmann).

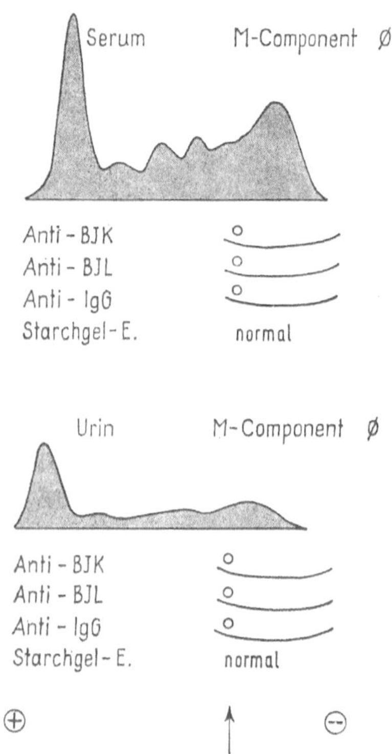

Fig. 3. *Schü. Kath.*, female, age 58, serum 6. 4. 67; Diagnosis: Amyloidosis of perireticulin type and morbus Felty. No monoclonal protein detectable. Further details see above

4. The quantitative determination of immunoglobulins does not permit the establishment of a systematic correlation to amyloidosis. As has already been shown by the estimation of the serum protein pattern (Aly *et al.*), the prevalence of the underlying disease seems to be the decisive factor. The isolated increase of immunoglobulin A described by Ossermann in several of his patients can be demonstrated in not more than 3 cases of perireticulin amyloidosis out of 15 (Table 3).

Table 3. *Behavior of immunoglobulins in amyloidosis*

	M-components and amyloidoses (12 cases)	Pericollagen amyloidoses (idiopath. and familial form) (8 cases)	perireticulin amyloidoses (15 cases)	periret. and pericollagen amyloidoses (mixed forms) (4 cases)
normal Ig-values	0	5	4	0
increase in IgG	5[a]	1	2	2
increase in IgA	1[a]	0	5	2
increase in IgM	3[a]	1	4	1
decrease in IgG	7	1	4	1
decrease in IgA	9	0	1	0
decrease in IgM	8	0	1	0

[a] M-component.

Discussion of Results

In the light of the above experimental results, it should be pointed out that in our patients the coincidence of pericollagen amyloid deposits and monoclonal proteins is strikingly high, while on the other hand monoclonal light chains do not seem to be detectable in all patients with amyloidosis. Our studies have shown unequivocally that amyloid deposits may occur without any evidence of monoclonal proteins. Similar results have also been obtained by Haellen and Rudin, and by Senn *et al.* In the course of more recent investigations Ossermann *et al.* have equally encountered cases not evidencing any monoclonal proteins.

When weighing the significance of the above findings with regard to our current concepts on amyloid formation, it should be emphasized again that on the strength of our studies the formation of amyloid deposits cannot reasonably be associated with the existence of light chains. The hypothesis that light chains, which may have formed, have been retained on fibril formation of the amyloid and are thus not detectable deserves further discussion. On the basis of studies carried out by the group of Cohen this seems very unlikely, as there is no evidence of any antigenic relationship existing between the purified amyloid fibrils on the one hand and gamma globulins as well as gamma globulin particles on the other hand. On isolation of amyloid fibrils by the method of Bestatti, IgG molecules may be demonstrated on their surface, but this is not true in the case of isolated light chains (Schultz *et al.*). This finding has recently been confirmed by Sellin and Haferkamp who employed immunofluorescence to analyze histologic sections of amyloid tissues.

Our findings readily fit in with the pattern shown in Fig. 4 which illustrates the pathogenesis of amyloidosis (Missmahl, 1967). This pattern reveals that amyloid deposits have to be considered a cellular product of the R.E.S. and of fibroblasts respectively (Sohar *et al.*). It may further be gathered from this pattern that both amyloid producing cells and plasma cells are part of the mesenchyma. The factors releasing amyloid formation, such as mutation in familial amyloidosis, stimulation in acquired and unknown factors in idiopathic amyloidosis may lead to simultaneous stimulation of the plasma cells forming the gamma globulins and of the amyloid-producing mesenchymal cells resulting in an amyloidosis which is associated either with gamma dysproteinemia or, in specific cases, with formation of monoclonal proteins. If stimulation affects only the amyloid-producing cells, amyloidosis without evidence of monoclonal proteins will occur. On the other hand, monoclonal proteins without amyloid involvement may be encountered just as well.

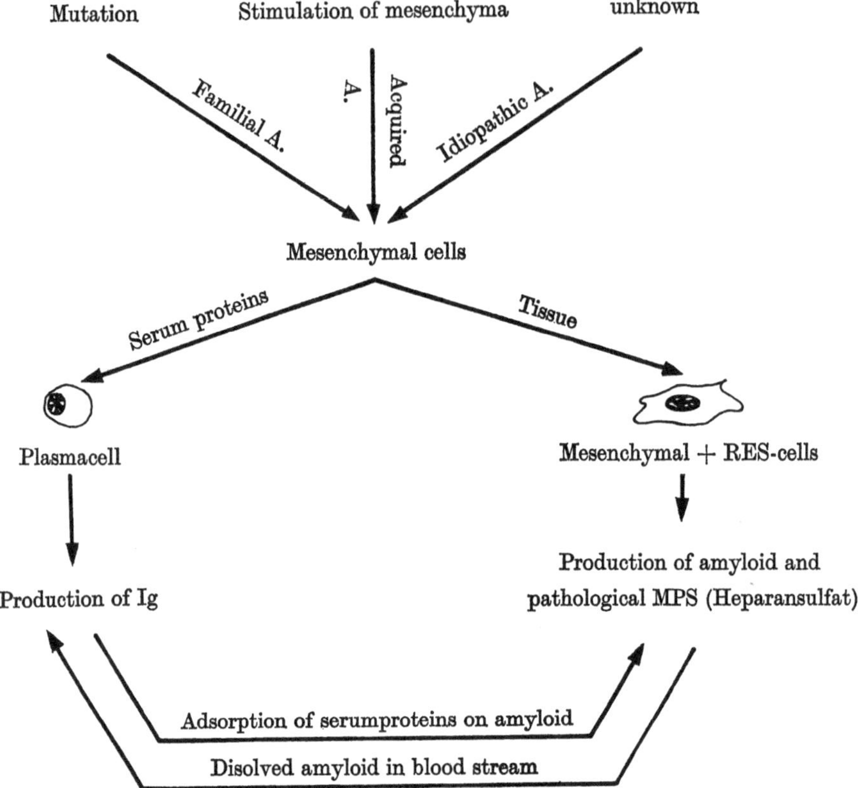

Fig. 4. Pathogenesis of amyloidoses with respect to monoclonal gamma-globulins

The question why particularly pericollagen amyloidosis frequently occur in combination with monoclonal proteins—while this happens never or only very rarely with perireticulin amyloidosis—cannot be decided at present.

References

Aly, F. W., H. J. Braun und H. P. Missmahl: Dys- und Paraproteinämien bei Amyloidbefall. Klin. Wschr. 46, 762 (1968).

Braun, H. J., F. W. Aly und H. P. Missmahl: Die Immunglobuline bei Amyloidbefall. Verh. dtsch. Ges. inn. Med. 74 (1968).

Cathcart, E. S., F. A. Wollheim, and A. S. Cohen: Plasma protein constituents of amyloid fibrils. J. Immunol. 99, 376 (1967).

Gafni, l., E. Sohar, and H. P. Missmahl: Incidence and origin of nonsystemic microdeposits of amyloid. J. clin. Path. 20, 15 (1967).

Haellen, J., and R. Rudin: Peri-collagenons amyloidosis. A study of 51 cases. Acta med. scand. 179, 483 (1966).

Letterer, E.: Neue Untersuchungen über die Entstehung des Amyloids. Virchows Arch. path. Anat. 34, 293 (1934).

Magnus-Levy, A.: Bence-Jones-Eiweiß und Amyloid. Z. klin. Med. **116**, 510 (1931).
Missmahl, H. P.: Diagnose der generalisierten Amyloidosen. Dtsch. med. Wschr. **90**, 394 (1965).
— Amyloidose, Klinik, Therapie und Prognose. Fortschr. Med. **85**, 621 (1967).
Ossermann, E. F.: Amyloidosis and plasma cell dyserasia. Immunopathology. IVth Internat. Symp., 283—293, Monte Carlo 1965. Basel/Stuttgart: Schwabe u. Co. Publ. 1966.
—, K. Takatsuki, and N. Talal: The pathogenesis of amyloidosis. Semin. Haematology **3**—86 (1964).
Plassmann, H. W.: Dissertation Tübingen (In Vorbereitung).
Schultz, R. T., E. Calkins, F. Milgroma, and E. Witebsky: Association of gamma-globulin with amyloid. Amer. J. Path. **48**, 1—17 (1966).
Sellin, D., u. O. Haferkamp: Bence-Jones-Protein und Amyloid. Z. ges. exp. Med. **147**, 173 (1968).
Sohar, E. H., J. Merker, H. P. Missmahl, J. Gafni. and H. Heller: Electron-microscope observations on peri-reticulin and peri-collagen amyloidosis in rectal biopsies. J. Path. Bact. **94**, 89 (1967).

Priv.-Doz. Dr. F.-W. Aly
Medizinische Universitätsklinik,
74 Tübingen, Olfried-Müller-Straße

Discussion

Grundmann (Wuppertal): Have any qualitative and quantitative amyloid studies been carried out on bioptic material from rectum, kidney, spleen, liver, etc. ?

Aly (Tübingen): If we find amyloid in the rectum the amyloidosis is always generalised, the biopsy offers the special advantages of the different forms of amyloid deposits being easily distinguishable [Missmahl, H. P.: Münch. med. Wschr. **107**, 846—848 (1965)].

Springer (Evanston): What is known about the chemistry of the amyloids and how are they related with the amyloid of old age ?

Aly (Tübingen): The method of Cohen and Calkins enables pure amyloid to be obtained from the organs [Cohen, A. S., and E. Calkins: J. Clin. Invest. **41**, 1350 (1962)]. The amino acids of different kinds of amyloid have been determined and no differences have been found. It was noted that the amyloid contain neither proline nor hydroxyproline. Amyloid deposits in old age are morphologically distinguistable from those in secondary amyloidosis. Amyloid in old age accumulates in the peri-collagen form, whereas in rheumatism for example amyloid is present in the peri-reticulin form. All amyloids are identical as to their fibrils.

Westphal (Freiburg): To what extent and in what form does amyloid occur in species other than man ?

Aly (Tübingen): Peri-reticulin amyloid has been found in horses, cows, dogs, rabbits, mice, guinea-pigs, rats, hamsters, baboons, moreover in birds e.g. ducks, even in reptiles as in turtles.

Bock (Tübingen): Can Dr. Schwick in this connection tell us something about the serum horses of Behring-Werke.

Schwick (Marburg): Amyloid only occurred in horses when the animals had been immunised with diphtheria or tetanus toxoid for more than 2 years. With today's immunisation method of 4 to 6 months duration it does not appear.

Bayer-Symposium I, 302—308 (1969)

Research in Drug Allergy: A Search for Impurities?[1]

A. L. DE WECK

Most drugs being low molecular weight chemicals eventually functioning as haptens, sensitization and allergic reactions to drugs should (according to the Landsteiner's theory) only occur if the drug or one of its reactive metabolites is able to form suitable conjugates with autologous proteins in vivo. Accordingly, research on the immunochemical mechanisms of drug allergy has been mostly oriented towards study of the reactivity of the drug itself and towards a search for reactive derivatives, eventually able to form immunogenic conjugates.

In the case of sensitization to penicillins, attention had been therefore directed on one hand to the direct reactivity of penicillin with amino and hydroxyl groups [1] yielding immunogenic conjugates of penicilloyl (BPO) specificity and on the other hand to the occurrence of reactive derivatives, such as penicillenic acid [2]. However, a series of papers published about a year ago [3—5] by the Beecham group raised the possibility that protein impurities, in particular residual proteins extracted from the fermentation medium, could represent a major cause of sensitization to the natural penicillins (benzylpenicillin, penicillin V). Theoretically at least, protein impurities could also be involved in sensitization to semi-synthetic penicillins prepared from 6-amino penicillanic acid (6-APA). As 6-amino penicillanic acid is nowadays mostly prepared by enzymatic degradation of benzylpenicillin (splitting off of the side chain by microbial penicillin acylase), it was shown that penicilloylated enzyme impurities may be present in commercial 6-APA preparations [3]. If, as suggested by the Beecham group, protein impurities were playing an important role in sensitization to penicillins, relatively simple purification procedures could be visualized by which the incidence of allergic reactions to penicillin could be substantially reduced.

However, numerous experiments carried out by our group and by some other workers in the field have demonstrated that such optimism is not justified. In fact, we have reached the conclusion that under present conditions of therapy protein impurities play no or only a very minor role in penicillin allergy. Experiments and arguments on which this statement is based have been discussed elsewhere [6]. I will therefore only briefly summarize our main findings in this respect.

First, we could show that "purified" benzylpenicillin preparations, in which eventual protein impurities have been eliminated by different procedures (e.g. dialysis, Sephadex chromatography, ultrafiltration), still possess immunogenicity and induce the formation of anti-BPO antibodies. On the other hand, "crude" commercial penicillin preparations still containing eventual protein contaminants

---

[1] This work has been supported in part by the Swiss National Foundation for Scientific Research (Grant No. 4182) and by the Emil Barell Foundation of F. Hoffmann-La Roche, Inc., Basle.

but where the β-lactam ring has been hydrolyzed under mild conditions no longer cause the formation of anti-BPO antibodies in rabbits [6, 7]. This demonstrates that the intact reactivity of the β-lactam ring of penicillin is responsible for the bulk of the immunogenicity of BPO specificity and not eventual penicilloylated protein contaminants. Furthermore, we have observed that animals and patients sensitized to penicillins very frequently fail to react to the residual proteins from the fermentation medium or from the penicillin mycelium [6, 7]. It appears evident therefore that the bulk of immunological activity is exerted by the penicillin molecule itself.

This conclusion was reinforced by experiments based on the performance of skin tests in hypersensitive patients with various fractions of penicillin solutions

Table 1. *Skin reactions to various fractions and/or components of benzyl-penicillin solutions in patients allergic to penicillin and normal controls*

Test with	Skin test positive/number of patients tested	
	Allergic	Non allergic
1. Commercial penicillin 200,000 U/ml scratch	7/15	0/10
2. Penicilloyl-polylysine 0.6 U.equiv. id	14/15	0/10
3. Penicillin kept 4° 24 h in buffer pH 7.4	7/15	0/10
4. Penicillin kept 4° 24 h in H_2O pH 5	7/15	0/10
5. Penicillin freshly dissolved	7/15	0/10
6. Penicillin freshly chromatographed G-10	8/15	0/10
7. Penicillin fresh dialyzate	4/4[a]	0/10
8. Penicilloic acid, crystalline	7/15	0/10
9. Penicilloic acid peak from counter current distribution	5/15	0/10
10. Penicilloic acid peak from G-10 chromatography	6/15	0/10
11. Spent broth, various chromatographic fractions	9/15	5/10
12. Mycelium, various chromatographic fractions	5/15	3/10
13. CM-cellulose	0/15	0/10

[a] All positive to freshly dissolved penicillin.

obtained by separation procedures such as column chromatography on Sephadex, ultrafiltration, rapid dialysis or countercurrent distribution. Some of these experiments have been published elsewhere [6], others are presented in Table 1. Summarizing our results, it may be stated that numerous penicillin derivatives and penicillin itself, certainly devoid of any protein contaminants, are susceptible to elicit reactions in hypersensitive individuals. It does not seem that any of the purification procedures used may significantly reduce the allergenicity of penicillin for sensitized individuals. The differences reported by Knudsen *et al.* [5] in the capacity of crude or Sephadex-purified penicillin to elicit skin reactions in sensitized patients have been confirmed neither by us nor by several other investigators [8, 9]. At the present time it also appears that most commercial penicillin preparations contain, if any, so small amounts of residual proteins [10] that such contaminants may not be expected to play an important immunological role.

The main antigenic determinant in penicillin allergy is the penicilloyl (BPO) group. Sensitization to the penicilloyl group occurs essentially due to the formation of penicilloyl conjugates in vivo either from penicillin directly or through the penicillenic acid intermediate. Several other antigenic determinants may arise from the penicilloyl group and from penicillin derivatives such as penicilloic acid [11]. Some allergic patients have a sensitivity restricted to the penicilloyl determinant, others appear to be sensitive to many different determinants. Anaphylactic reactions are most likely to occur in the patients sensitive to a large number of determinants (and therefore yielding positive skin reactions not only to penicilloyl-polylysine but also to penicillin solutions).

Aside from protein impurities, another factor recently discussed has been the formation of dimers and small polymers by polycondensation of the penicillin molecule. These compounds might also be considered as "impurities" arising from penicillin. Their removal appears to be peculiarly desirable, as they are capable of eliciting anaphylactic reactions without prior conjugation to autologous proteins in vivo [6, 7]. Experience up to now is not encouraging, as far as the practical possibility is concerned.

If in the case of penicillin allergy in humans eventual impurities do not appear to play a major role, allergy to penicillin in the cow is another matter. Coming from Switzerland, you will certainly not be astonished if my report shall deal with some studies on allergic reactions to penicillin in cows. Our interest in this field was awakened in 1967 by numerous reports from veterinary surgeons concerning anaphylactic shock or generalized urticaria occurring in cows a few minutes after the injection of various drugs but mostly of penicillin preparations. Although such reactions had occasionally been encountered in Switzerland before, the incidence of acute allergic reactions appeared to increase markedly in the months following a compaign of generalized vaccination against foot-and-mouth disease during the winter 1966/1967. Although precise indications on the composition of the foot-and-mouth disease vaccines used during that campaign could not be obtained from the manufacturers, it was ascertained in some cases at least that relatively high concentrations of antibiotics (especially penicillin) had been associated at some stage of the preparation of the vaccine. Accordingly, it appeared possible that penicilloyl-protein conjugates formed during fabrication could have been contaminating the final product and be responsible for sensitization of cows to penicillin. This logical hypothesis, however, could not be confirmed by experimental studies. No anti-penicillin antibodies were detected in the sera of allergic cows by various procedures [12]. The foot-and-mouth disease vaccine did not appear to contain penicilloyl-protein impurities and did not induce penicilloyl-specific hypersensitivity in guinea pigs. Upon skin testing allergic cows with pure benzylpenicillin, with various chromatographic fractions of penicillin and with penicilloyl-polylysine only negative results were obtained. On the other hand, and very much to our surprise, skin tests performed with commercial penicillin preparations yielded strongly positive urticarial reactions and in some instances anaphylactic shock in allergic cows.

An inquiry by penicillin manufacturers revealed that carboxymethyl cellulose (CMC) is frequently added to commercial penicillin preparations in order to stabilize suspensions or to facilitate dissolution of cristalline penicillin. Intradermal skin tests with CMC of various origins in allergic cows elicited strong local urticarial reactions at doses as low as 1 μg. No reactions to CMC were observed in non allergic cows or in non vaccinated calves. The allergic nature of the hypersensitivity to CMC was confirmed by the sometimes fatal systemic anaphylactic reactions which were elicited in some vaccinated cows by the intravenous injection of as little as 10 mg CMC.

The finding that CMC may be the cause of anaphylactic reactions in an animal species may appear particularly disquieting. CMC is used nowadays in an enormous variety of materials (e.g. paints, industrial products, foods) and especially in a large number of drug formulations. However, CMC has always been considered as very well tolerated and ours appears to be the first report of clinical allergic reactions due to CMC. We investigated the immunogenicity of various samples of CMC from different origins in guinea pigs. A few guinea pigs appeared indeed to develop skin hypersensitivity and circulating antibodies to CMC but as a whole CMC appeared to be a much poorer immunogen in guinea pigs than in cows. From various types of experimental evidence [12], the sensitivity appeared to be directed against CMC itself and not toward some protein impurities. Up to now we have found no evidence of hypersensitivity to CMC in patients allergic to penicillin. The apparently strong immunogenicity of CMC for cattle could eventually be related to species differences in the capacity to metabolize CMC. As shown by studies on immunogenic synthetic polypeptides, there seems to exist a striking relationship between the ability of compound to be metabolized and its capacity to induce an immune response. In any case our findings suggests that CMC should no longer be used in veterinary drug formulations.

The last part of my talk will not be devoted to a drug allergy, but to the disquieting experience which we recently made, in collaboration with the group of Dr. Frey, when studying the immunogenicity of hapten-amino acids, in particular of dinitrophenyl (DNP) amino acids in guinea pigs. We were interested in such compounds after having observed that some DNP-amino acids are indeed immunogenic for guinea pigs, inducing contact sensitization to dinitrochlorobenzene (DNCB) and the formation of anti-DNP antibodies. As it could not be considered a priori that DNP-amino acids possess a reactive chemical group enabling them to form conjugates with protein in vivo, the possibility was open that such compounds function as immunogens as such and represent thereby the smallest molecules described as possessing immunogenicity [13, 14]. Some other groups have reported similar observations e.g. with para-azobenzenearsonate tyrosine [15, 16]. It must be remembered, however, that the bulk of experimental evidence up to recent years indicates that low molecular weight substances may only sensitize when possessing a reactive group and being able to form hapten-protein conjugates in vivo.

Among 32 DNP-amino acids or oligopeptides we have studied up to now, 17 induced both immediate and delayed hypersensitivity of DNP specificity, 6 only delayed hypersensitivity and 9 were found to be non immunogenic. Overall results are summarized in Table 2; techniques and experimental details will be published elsewhere [14]. From an operational point of view, there is no doubt that many DNP-amino acids may induce contact and delayed hypersensitivity to DNCB as well as the formation of anti-DNP antibodies. DNP-amino acids could be classified into those which were never immunogenic, those which were irregularly immuno-

A. L. de Weck

Table 2. *Immune response of guinea pigs to DNP-amino acids*

Expt. No.	Compound	Lot	PCA	S.A.	C.S.	D.S.
1	DNP-beta-alanine		—	—	+	—
2	DNP-L-alanine	a	—	—	(+)	—
		b	+	+	+	+
3	DNP-epsilon-amino caproid acid		+	+	+	+
4	DNP-L-asparagine	a	—		—	—
		b	+		+	—
5	DNP-L-aspartic acid	a	—		(+)	—
		b	+		+	+
6	DNP-DL-aspartic acid		—	—	+	—
7	di-S,N-DNP-L-cysteine		+		+	+
8	DNP-mono-S-L-cysteine		+	+	+	+
9	di-DNP-L-cystine		+		+	+
10	DNP-DL-glutamine acid	a, c	—	—	+	(+)
		b	+		+	+
		d	—		—	—
11	DNP-L-glutamic acid		—		—	—
12	DNP-L-glutamine	a	—		+	+
		b	—		(+)	—
13	DNP-glycylglycine		—	—	—	—
14	DNP-glycine		—	—	—	—
15	di-DNP-L-histidine	a, b, c	+	+	+	+
16	DNP-D-allo-isoleucine		+		+	+
17	DNP-L-isoleucine		—		—	—
18	DNP-L-leucine		+		+	+
19	bis-DNP-L-lysine		+		+	+
20	DNP-epsilon-L-lysine		(+)	—	+	—
21	DNP-DL-methionine		—	—	—	—
22	DNP-L-methionine sulfoxide		—	—	+	—
23	DNP-DL-methionine sulfoxide		(+)	+	+	+
24	DNP-L-proline		—	—	—	—
25	DNP-L-hydroxyproline		—		—	—
26	DNP-L-serine		—	—	—	—
27	di-O,N-DNP-L-tyrosine		+		+	+
28	mono-O-DNP-L-tyrosine		+	+	+	+
29	DNP-L-valine	a, b	—	—	—	—
30	DNPS-glycine		—	—	+	—
31	S-DNP-glutathione		+	+	+	+
32	DNP-1-piperidine-carbodithioate		+	—		+
33	Dinitrophenol		—		—	—
34	Dinitroaniline		—		—	—

PCA: passive cutaneous anaphylaxis.

S.A.: systemic anaphylaxis.

C.S.: contact sensitivity to DNCB.

D.S.: delayed hypersensitivity to the immunizing DNP-amino acid.

+: > 50% of the guinea pigs positive.

(+): < 50% of the guinea pigs positive.

—: no animal positive.

a, b, c, d: various lots of the same compound.

genic (according to the lot used) and those which were always immunogenic despite extensive recristallisation and purification procedures.

In the case of irregular immunogenicity and of differences observed among various lots of the same DNP-amino acid, the easiest explanation for our data would be the presence of small amounts of unreacted DNFB able to form DNP-conjugates in vivo. This would be compatible with a number of observations, such as the extensive cross-reactivity among immunogenic DNP-amino acids and DNCB, the requirement for relatively high doses of DNP-amino acids (0.5 to 1 mg) in comparison to DNFB (0.05 to 0.02 mg) and the fact that in a few instances a non immunogenic lot at the dose of 5 mg could be shown to be immunogenic when injected in higher amounts. On the other hand, analytical and chromatographic data were incompatible with the assumption that the impurity responsible for sensitization of DNP specificity could be DNFB. Most careful analytical procedures were performed, but in several instances we were left with the hypothesis of a highly immunogenic impurity of DNP specificity which was not DNFB and which was not to be detected even by very thorough chromatographic analysis. Nevertheless, the results obtained especially with some of the immunogenic α-DNP-amino acids could not be explained otherwise than by a highly immunogenic contaminating impurity responsible for variable results from lot to lot. The fact that often immunogenic and non immunogenic lots of the same DNP-amino acid could not be distinguished analytically and appeared chromatographically homogeneous and identical, even under analytical conditions especially devised to pick up possible differences, demonstrates that the criteria of purity usually accepted by organic chemists are insufficient for immunological work. It was evident that our guinea pigs were more discriminating than our analytical procedures.

In other instances where the immunogenicity was constant from lot to lot and was not impaired by repeated recristallisation or extensive purification procedures such as countercurrent distribution, we are dealing with another phenomenon and it appears likely that the DNP-amino acid itself is responsible for sensitization.

After eliminating several other possibilities, we had to come to the conclusion that a "transconjugation" is occurring in vivo by which the DNP-group jumps off its amino acid carrier and attaches covalently to an autologous protein carrier in the same way that DNFB forms immunogenic conjugates with autologous proteins. Although the covalent bond between the DNP-group and various amino acids is classically considered as quite stable, as testifies the wide use of dinitrophenylation for structural analysis of proteins, "transconjugation" of the DNP-group may be confirmed by experiments involving the incubation of DNP-amino acids with proteins in vitro. Upon incubation of di-DNP-L-histidine with bovine gamma globulin (BGG), immunogenic DNP-conjugates were formed. The amounts of DNP-groups bound to BGG in this way was too low to be detected analytically but was sufficient to induce in guinea pigs antibodies of DNP specificity [14]. The formation of a new covalent bond between the DNP group splitting off from its amino acid carrier and the protein was suggested from the incubation conditions required to yield immunogenic DNP-protein conjugates. Mere short mixing of the DNP-amino acid and BGG prior to chromatographic separation was insufficient to yield conjugates inducing anti-DNP antibodies.

20*

Our experience with DNP-amino acids constitutes a warning to immunochemists and points to the fact that usual criteria of chemical purity may be insufficient for immunological work. Small amounts of reactive immunogenic impurities could also be responsible for some of the drug allergies instead of the reactive metabolites which are usually postulated.

References

1. Schneider, C. H., and A. L. de Weck: Studies on the direct neutral penicilloylation of functional groups occurring on proteins. Biochim. biophys. Acta (Amst.) 168, 27 (1968).
2. de Weck. A. L., and H. N. Eisen: Some immunochemical properties of penicillenic acid, an antigenic determinant derived from penicillin. J. exp. Med. 112, 1227 (1968).
3. Batchelor, F. R., J. M. Dewdney, J. G. Feinberg, and R. D. Weston: A penicilloylated protein impurity as a source of allergy to benzylpenicillin and 6-amino-penicillanic acid. Lancet 1967 I, 1175.
4. Stewart. G. T.: Allergenic residues in penicillins. Lancet 1967 I, 1177.
5. Knudsen, E. T., O. P. W. Robinson, E. A. P. Croydon, and E. C. Tees: Cutaneous sensitivity to purified benzylpenicillin. Lancet 1967 I, 1184.
6. de Weck. A. L., C. H. Schneider, and J. Gutersohn: The role of penicilloylated protein impurities, penicillin polymers and dimers in penicillin allergy. Int. Arch. Allergy 33, 535 (1968).
7. de Weck, A. L., and C. H. Schneider: Unpublished results.
8. Schultz. K. H.: Personal communication.
9. Girard. J.-P.: Personal communication.
10. Dürsch, F.: Search for protein contaminants in benzylpenicillin. Lancet 1968 I, 1005.
11. Idsøe, O., T. Guthe, R. R. Willcox, and A. L. de Weck: Nature and extent of penicillin side-reactions, with particular reference to fatalities from anaphylactic shock. Bull. Wld Hlth Org. 38, 159 (1968).
12. Leemann, W., A. L. de Weck, and C. H. Schneider: Hypersensitivity to carboxymethyl cellulose as a cause of anaphylactic reactions to drugs in cattle. Nature (Lond.) (in press).
13. de Weck, A. L., K. Vogler, J. R. Frey, and H. Geleick: The induction of contact hypersensitity to dinitrochlorobenzene (DNCB) in guinea pigs by dinitrophenyl-amino acids. Int. Arch. Allergy 29, 174 (1966).
14. Frey, J. R., A. L. de Weck, H. Geleick, and W. Lergier: The immunogenicity of dinitrophenyl-amino acids J. Exp. Med. (in press).
15. Borek, F., Y. Stupp, and M. Sela: Immunogenicity and role of size: response of guinea pigs to oligotyrosine and tyrosine derivatives. Science 150, 1177 (1965).
16. Leskowitz, S., V. E. Jones, and S. J. Zak: Immunochemical study of antigenic specificity in delayed hypersensitivity. V. Immunization with monovalent low molecular weight conjugates. J. exp. Med. 123, 229 (1966).

Priv.-Doz. Dr. A. L. de Weck
Dermatologische Universitäts-Klinik,
Abteilung für Allergie
und klinische Immunologie,
CH 3008 Bern, Inselspital

Discussion

HILSCHMANN (Göttingen): Is it definite that a conjugate with DNP occurs if protein is treated with DNP histidine. Is it not possible that only an absorption is involved?

DE WECK (Berne): Absorptive phenomena proceed as a rule relatively quickly and do not require prolonged incubation. I am reminded of the absorption of penicillin to serum as an example.

LAUENSTEIN (Wuppertal): Had the cows you used in studying your reactions been previously treated with culture vaccine? If so, may the baby-hamster kidney protein play a role?

DE WECK (Berne): You are right, as yet the studies are not quite completed. For example I do not yet understand the relationship between the vaccination and the sensitisation to carboxy-methyl-cellulose. It is certain that the response to our carboxy-methyl-cellulose preparations was not caused by protein contamination. I do not see how hamster-kidney proteins could be present in the eliciting penicillin preparations. The clinical manifestations did not only appear after the administration of vaccine, but also after some drugs, such as progesterone or penicillin or streptomycin.

Bayer-Symposium I, 310—322 (1969)

Immunogenicity of Semisynthetic Penicillins

HANS-J. WELLENSIEK

Allergic reactions following drug therapy with penicillin are a well known, unpleasant, rather frequent and occasionally dangerous phenomenon. The immunological processes leading to sensitization against Penicillin G (PG) and the factors operative in the elicitation of hypersensitivity reactions against the drug have mainly been elucidated by the extensive work of Eisen, Parker [25—27], DeWeck [41—45] and B. Levine [16—23]. Antibodies with penicilloyl specificity have been demonstrated in the serum of animals experimentally immunized with PG and more important in the majority of human beings suffering from allergy against penicillin. In vivo allergic reactions could be elicited with penicilloyl-conjugates both in man and animals sensitized with PG. The penicilloyl group has now been unequivocally established as the major antigenic determinant in penicillin allergy.

There is no doubt that semisynthetic penicillins can also evoke allergic reactions, ampicillin being an frequent offender. However the problem has not been studied systematically whether immunogenicity is a property common to all biologically and semisynthetically produced penicillins [3, 5, 6, 11, 13, 39, 42] or whether some penicillins exist without these unwanted allergenic qualities. Little is also known about the specificity of antibodies arising after immunization with semisynthetic penicillins.

Semisynthetic penicillins differ from PG by the chemical structure of their sidechains. Coupling of different sidechains to 6-Amino-Penicillinanic acid (6-APA), the molecular nucleus of PG without sidechain, lead to semisynthetic penicillins differing from the parent molecule in many important respects. So penicillins were discovered which were acid stable, penicillinase resistant or showed a wider range of antibiotic activity compared to PG. Ampicillin for example kills gram negative pathogenic bacteria while PG has almost no effect on these organisms. Since so many essential biological properties of penicillins are obviously determined by their sidechain structure, the question arose, whether some semisynthetic penicillins for chemical reasons might lack the immunogenic qualities of the parent molecule penicillin G.

1. Immunization of Rabbits with Semisynthetic Penicillins

In order to determine the immunogenic qualities of semisynthetic penicillins adult healthy rabbits of 2.5 to 3.5 kg body weight were injected with 50 mg/kg Penicillin G or the respective molar equivalents of semisynthetic penicillins as listed in Table 1. PG or penicillin derivatives were emulsified at neutral pH in complete Freund's adjuvant. Six weeks after the first injection with penicillins the rabbits were challenged with a second dose of 50 mg/kg of the same penicillin in neutral saline solution. Five days after the booster injection the rabbits were bled and the antibody content of the sera determined using a passive hemagglutination technique modified for the demonstration of penicillin specific antibodies.

It has been reported by DeWeck *et al.* [44] that erythrocytes are more efficiently coated with penicilloyl determinants at alkaline pH. We have made the same experience. Our standard conditions for direct coating of erythrocytes with penicillins are the following: 100 mg of the respective penicillin are dissolved in 10 ml of neutral isotonic phosphate buffer. The sediment of 10×10^9 sheep, rabbit or human erythrocytes is suspended in the penicillin solution. The mixture is adjusted to pH 9.0 with 1 n NaOH and incubated at 37° in a waterbath for 4 h. The cells are kept in even suspension and every 30 min the pH is readjusted to pH 9.0 with 1 n or 0.15 n NaOH respectively. After the first 4 h of incubation the cells are stored in the same penicillin solution at pH 9.0 in the refrigarator over night. The next morning the cells are washed three times with isotonic neutral phosphate buffer and resuspended in this medium at a cell density of 5×10^8 erythrocytes/ml. Serial dilutions of antisera are prepared in microtiter plates [28, 31] using isotonic phosphate buffer as diluent. One drop of the penicillin coated erythrocyte suspension is added to 1 drop of antiserum dilution. The plates are incubated for 30 min at 37° and another 30 min at room temperature and then read. The pattern of sedimented cells on the bottom of the holes in the plates gives a clear-cut end point of agglutination.

Direct coating of erythrocytes with ampicillin, dicloxacillin and many other semisynthetic penicillins is not feasable with the above described method because hemolysis is easily induced by these penicillins. Therefore rabbit serumproteins were first incubated with penicillins and in a second step attached to erythrocytes treated with dilute tannic acid according to the method of Boyden as modified by Stavitsky [32]. 100 mg of PG or molar equivalent of penicillin derivatives are dissolved in 10 ml undiluted rabbit serum. The serum mixture is incubated at pH 9.0 for 4 h at 37° and 18 h at 4° keeping the pH constant during this time. After the incubation period the pH is adjusted to pH 7.2 and the serumproteins are then ready for coating of tanned erythrocytes. Earlier, low molecular weight substances were separated from Penicillin treated serum proteins by filtration through columns of Sephadex G 25. This proved later to be unnecessary. Highly purified serum proteins can of course be coupled with penicillin by the same method. 20 ml of penicillin treated serum diluted 1:200 with isotonic phosphate buffer pH 6.6 are mixed with 5 ml tanned erythrocytes (1×10^9/ml) and incubated for 30 min at 37°. The cells are washed twice in isotonic phosphate buffer pH 7.2 and finally suspended in the same buffer containing 1% normal rabbit serum. 1% normal rabbit serum in isotonic phosphate buffer pH 7.2 is also used as diluent for preparing the antisera dilutions in microtiterplates as described above. Controls included cells coated with normal rabbit serum proteins, uncoated tanned cells and serum controls with normal rabbit serum instead of immune sera.

Table 1 shows the results obtained after immunization of rabbits with various natural and semisynthetic penicillins. The majority of animals reacted with the production of significant amounts of humoral antibodies against the respective penicillins. All rabbit antisera with titers higher than 1:10 are listed and usually titers were much higher. The number of animals in each group is not sufficient to

determine the relative immunogenicity of these penicillins, however the results
show clearly, that each one of the listed penicillins has to be regarded as a potential immunogen. Four penicillins are listed in Table 1 by their code numbers[1].
These were chosen for their minimal or absent tendency in vitro to form penicillenic
acid (PNCE) derivatives. In addition the semisynthetic penicillins OB 1716 and
OB 15087 were selected because they are structural analogues of penicillin 0, a
penicillin which was supposed to be less allergenic than PG. This impression failed
to become substantiated by later observations [37].

It seems worth mentioning, that a number of semisynthetic penicillins listed
in Table 1 like 6-APA, Penicillin V, Oralopen, Propicillin, Sz 1001, MeB 184,

Table 1. *Antibody production by rabbits after immunization with various semisynthetic penicillins*

Penicillins	Number of rabbits with circulating antibodies / Number of rabbits immunized
6-APA	10/12
Penicillin G	10/11
Penicillin V	6/6
Penicillin O (Allyl-thio-P.)	6/6
Ampicillin	4/5
Oralopen (Phenoxyethyl-P.)	5/6
Propicillin	9/11
Methicillin	2/2
Oxacillin	4/4
Dicloxacillin	3/3
Sz 1001	3/5
MeB 184	3/5
OB 1716	4/5
OB 15087	4/5

OB 1716, OB 15087, with low or absent capacity for rearrangement to PNCE
analogues are nevertheless potent immunogens. PNCE has been discussed as an
intermediate in the formation of the complete antigen in penicillin allergy [17, 20,
25, 26, 41]. However as already noted by DeWeck [42, 43] and others [5] low or
lacking tendency for in vitro formation of PNCE is not correlated with low or
absent immunogenicity. 6-APA which because of lacking sidechain cannot
rearrange to PNCE and similarly propicillin, penicillin V and the four experimental
penicillins used in these studies readily induced antibody formation. Rearrangement to PNCE therefore can not be an obligatory step in the formation of an
complete penicillin antigen.

The question arises whether the complete antigen operative in allergy against
penicillins is formed via an intermediate substance like PNCE [17, 20, 25, 26, 41]

---

[1] The generous gift of semisynthetic penicillins for these experiments by the BAYER-Werke,
Wuppertal-Elberfeld (Prof. E. Auhagen, Dr. Kl. Bauer, Dr. Offe) is gratefully acknowledged.

or some other metabolic degradation product [27] or whether natural and semi-synthetic penicillins can interact with high molecular weight substrates, resulting in the formation of penicilloyl-groups which would subsequently act as antigenic determinants. The latter alternative is the most likely one. Under alkaline conditions the β-lactam ring of PG and other semisynthetic penicillins is easily hydrolysed to form the respective penicilloic acids. Penicilloyl amide derivatives form in vitro with amino acids with free terminal amino groups and also with proteins [2, 19]. We have found that 23 experimental semisynthetic penicillins, synthesized in the laboratories of the BAYER-Werke, Wuppertal-Elberfeld, form the respective penicilloyl derivatives with proteins in vitro at pH 9.0. Since hydrolysis of the β-lactam ring and the formation of penicilloyl derivatives under mild alkaline conditions differs only in extent from the same reactions occuring at pH 7.2 to 7.4 [2, 47] it was concluded, that all these penicillins fullfill the conditions in vitro and probably in vivo to become complete antigens. One can hardly expect to find a nonimmunogenic penicillin among them.

2. Specificity of Antibodies Against Semisynthetic Penicillins

a) *Rabbit antibodies:* All semisynthetic penicillins listed in Table 1, which differ from each other only in the structure of their sidechains stimulated antibody production in the majority of rabbits immunized. It seemed interesting to compare the specificities of the different antisera and to determine the influence of the sidechain structure on the antibody specificity. In a study with a limited number of structurally closely related penicillins [43] it was concluded that the sidechain plays little if any role in the specificity of "antipenicillin" antibodies. These findings were in accord with the known clinical experience that individuals allergic against one penicillin usually show also signs of hypersensitivity against a variety of other penicillins. On the other hand remarkable absence of crossreactivity was noted in some patients hypersensitive to ampicillin. These patients did not show allergic reactions with Oxacillin [49]. Kerp and Kasemir [15] similarly noted an influence of the sidechain structure of penicillins on the elicitability of allergic reactions.

In Table 2 are shown hemagglutination reactions obtained with three different antisera. These antisera are typical for the behaviour of most other "antipenicillin" antisera. The first antiserum was obtained after immunization with 6-APA, a penicillin derivative which has no sidechain at all. This antiserum reacts strongly with its homologous antigen but equally well with determinants of all other penicillins irrespective of the structure of their sidechains. This antiserum is extremely sidechain "unspecific": it recognizes apparently only a structure common to all penicillin antigens. The other extreme is manifest in an antiserum obtained after immunization with oxacillin. This antiserum reacts only with its homologous antigen and not with any of the other penicillin determinants. Here the specificity of the antiserum is strongly if not exclusively determined by the structure of the oxacillin sidechain. An intermediate position with respect to cross reactivity is given by the antiserum against penicillin G. This antiserum does not react at all with 6-APA-determinants. This indicates that the sidechain does indeed play a role in the specificity of the anti-PG antibody. Strong crossreactions are apparent with penicillins which carry a structurally closely related sidechain as exemplified by phenoxymethyl-, phenoxyethyl-penicillin or ampicillin. With growing difference in sidechain structure less and less cross reaction is noticed in the hemagglutination assay with this anti-PG antiserum. Almost no agglutination occurs with erythrocytes coupled with oxacillin. This can be explained by small amounts of sidechain "unspecific" anti-6-APA antibodies in the anti-PG serum, since this cross reaction disappears after absorption of the serum with 6-APA coupled erythrocytes. While anti-"Oxacillin"- and anti-"Dicloxacillin"-sera give no or only very little cross reactions with the PG-antigen strong cross reactions were seen between the two types of sera and their respective antigens.

The reactivity of the anti-6-APA-serum with penicillin coated erythrocytes can be completely absorbed with 6-APA coated erythrocytes and also with any of the other penicillin antigens. However the 6-APA antigen removes only anti-6-

Table 2. *Hemagglutination assay of three rabbit antisera obtained after immunization with 6-APA penicillin G and oxacillin*

| Agglutinogen[a] | Sidechain | Hemagglutination titer | | | Normal-serum |
| | | Antisera | | | |
		anti-6-APA	anti-PG	anti-Oxa.	
E^t·NS	—	O	O	O	O
E^t·NS-6-APA	—	160/320	O	O	O
E^t·NS-PG	Phenylacetyl-	160	160	O	O
E^t·NS-PV	Phenoxymethyl-	160	160	O	O
E^t·NS-Oral.	Phenoxyethyl-	160/320	80	O	O
E^t·NS-Prop.	Phenoxypropyl-	160/320	20	O	O
E^t·NS-Oxa.	5-Methyl-3-phenyl-iso-oxazolyl-	160/320	10	160/320	O

[a] Preparation of agglutinogens is described in the text.

E^t = Sheep erythrocytes treated with tannic acid.

NS = Normal rabbit serum; NS-6-APA, NS-PG, NS-PV etc. = Normal rabbit serum coupled with 6-APA, Penicillin G, Penicillin V etc. E^t·NS-PV therefore means: Tanned sheep erythrocytes coated with rabbit serum proteins previously coupled with Penicillin V.

APA antibodies. It has no effect on antibodies with specificity to any of the other penicillin antigens. This finding indicates that the anti-6-APA antibody is directed against a structure common to all penicillin determinants and that this antibody is much more restricted in its specificity compared to the other antipenicillin antibodies. The specificity of antibodies against PG or semisynthetic penicillins is strongly influenced by the structure of the sidechain of the penicillin used for immunization.

The sidechain can however not be the only factor which determines the antibody specificity. Phenylaceticacid and phenylacetylalanin in 0.01 molar concentration have no inhibitory effect on the hemagglutination reaction of anti-PG antibodies, while penicilloic acid and also intact PG show strong inhibition. The best haptenic inhibition is obtained with penicilloyl amide derivatives as already reported by DeWeck [42, 43] and others [2, 19, 21]. The available data can best be interpreted in the following way: antibodies arising after immunization with penicillins are directed against the penicilloyl derivatives of theses penicillins. The sidechain of the penicillins plays an important role in determining the specificity of these antibodies. Absence of a sidechain (as in 6-APA) or gross structural differences in sidechains (as in PG and Oxacillin) can lead to antibodies with completely different specificities. Penicillins however with structurally closely related sidechains induce antibodies which easily crossreact with related penicillins.

b) *Human antibodies:* In the sera of patients allergic against penicillin antibodies with penicilloyl specificity have been repeatedly demonstrated [1, 7, 9, 14, 21, 23, 24, 29, 35, 38, 39, 40]. In collaboration with Dr. G. Brehm of the Dermatology Department of the University of Mainz and cand. med. H. P. Becker we have also tried to find antibodies with penicilloyl-specificity in the sera of cases with penicillin allergy. Our first attempts in finding specific antibodies using

Table 3. *Complete (A) and incomplete (B) antibodies with penicilloyl specificity in human sera of patients with penicillin allergy*

Sera	Test erythrocytes[a]					
	E-PG		E-Prop.		E-Oxa.	
	A	B	A	B	A	B
42 H. Sch.	+++	+++	O	O	O	O
45 M. G.	O	O	O	+++	O	O
51 R. Z.	O	O	O	O	O	+++
38 G. Kl. A.	O	+++	O	+++	O	O
49 J. H.	+++	+++	O	O	O	+++
39 W. E.	O	+++	O	+++	O	+++
43 A. L.	O	+++	O	+++	O	+++
54 H. R.	+++	+++	+++	+++	+++	+++

[a] Test erythrocytes for the hemagglutination assay were prepared by incubating human bloodgroup 0-rh-negative erythrocytes directly with alkaline solutions of Penicillin G, Propicillin and Oxacillin. Details of the coupling procedure and of the method for the demonstration of complete (A) and incomplete (B) antibodies are given in the text. All sera with penicilloyl specific antibody titers higher than 1:5 are listed as +++.

erythrocytes coupled directly with penicillins were rather disappointing. In only 28.6% of the cases were complete hemagglutinating penicillin specific antibodies demonstrable. However the number of positive sera rose considerably when we applied a modified anti-globulin-test for the demonstration of incomplete antibodies. The technique used will be described below.

Incomplete antibodies could be shown to be present in the serum of 49 out of 84 cases (58.3%) of patients which for anamnestic and clinical reasons were suspected to suffer from penicillin allergy. No complete antibodies with penicilloyl specificity were found in 182 randomly taken human control sera, send to our laboratory for other tests. In only 4 (i.e. 2.1%) control sera were incomplete antibodies with penicilloyl specificity demonstrable in low titers.

With respect to specificity human antibodies specific for penicillin reflect the situation found with rabbit antibodies. As seen in Table 3 some sera contain antibodies specific for the penicilloyl-derivative of one penicillin only. Some sera provide antibodies which cross react with two or three of the penicillins used to prepare the agglutinogen. Some patients produce only incomplete others also complete hemagglutinating antibodies. One patient with high titers of circulating complete as well as incomplete antibodies gave extensive crossreactions with erythrocytes coated with PG, 6-APA-, Propicillin and oxacillin determinants. In this case it was at first not possible to draw any conclusions about the specificity of the antibodies other than that they were penicilloyl-specific. However absorption with various penicillin antigens showed that this antiserum contained a mixture of antibodies with different specificities. Some of these were specific for the 6-APA determinant others showed marked sidechain specificity. The results of this analysis are given in Table 4. It is shown that erythrocytes coated with

Table 4. *Absorption of a polyvalent serum from a patient with penicillin allergy by different penicilloyl-erythrocytes conjugates*

Serum H. R. (54) absorbed with	Test erythrocytes[a]	Antibodies	
		A	B
E	E-PGK	+++	+++
	E-Oxac.	+++	+++
	E-6-APS	+++	+++
E-6-APS	E-PGK	+++	+++
	E-Oxac.	+++	+++
	E-6-APS	O	O
E-Oxac.	E-PGK	+++	+++
	E-Oxac.	O	O
	E-6-APS	O	O
E-PGK	E-PGK	+	O
	E-Oxac.	+++	+++
	E-6-APS	O	O

[a] See footnotes Table 3.

6-APA remove only antibodies specific for the 6-APA determinant from this serum. Antibodies with "sidechain" specificity are unaffected by the absorption with 6-APA coated erythrocytes. Erythrocytes coated with either of the other two penicillins (i.e. Penicillin G and Oxacillin) remove 6-APA specific antibodies and in addition those directed against the penicillin used to prepare the erythrocytes for absorption. It is clearly seen that antibodies directed against Penicillin G do not crossreact with those having Oxacillin specificity and vice versa. These findings about the specificity of penicilloyl specific antibodies in human sera are perfectly in line with the observations described above for rabbit antisera. The antibodies are directed against the penicilloyl structure of a given penicillin, however the sidechain plays an important role in shaping the final specificity of the antibody.

3. Physicochemical Properties of Antibodies with Penicilloyl Specificity

The study of human sera from patients with penicillin allergy showed that these sera often contain complete hemagglutinating and/or incomplete antibodies with penicilloyl specificity. For the demonstration of incomplete antibodies the following technique was used: Semisynthetic penicillins were directly incubated with human rh negative erythrocytes of bloodgroup 0. The coupling conditions were identical with those described above for the coupling of penicillins to rabbit or sheep erythrocytes. Freshly collected erythrocytes of citrated blood samples were used and usually washed three times with 0.01 mol EDTA in isotonic saline before incubation with penicillins. This eliminates traces of fibrinogen on the surface of the erythrocytes which occasionally favor unspecific spontaneous agglutination of the red cells. After the coupling procedure the erythrocytes were washed three times with isotonic saline and incubated with the patients sera for 30 min at 37°. Thereafter the erythrocytes were washed again three times with isotonic buffer and incubated with anti-human-gammaglobulin obtained either from the BEH-RING-Werk, Marburg, or prepared by injecting rabbits with antigen-antibody complexes consisting of Brucella abortus Bang and human antibodies against these organisms.

H-chain specific anti-human-globulin sera were obtained from the BEHRING-Werke, Marburg, against the H-chains of the γM-, γG- and γA-immunoglobulin class. These sera served to determine the immunoglobulin class of penicilloyl specific antibodies in the modified anti-globulin-test as described above. In addition we have determined the heat and mercaptoethanol stability of the antibodies, their sedimentation behaviour in the preparative ultracentrifuge, their elution pattern from sephadex G 200 columns and finally their complement fixing properties. The ability of the antibodies to fix complement was checked in three ways: Firstly it was tested whether the antisera could induce lysis of penicillin coated erythrocytes in the presence of fresh complement. Secondly the promotion of immunadherence by erythrocytes coated with penicilloyl specific antibodies and exposed to complement was determined. The third method consisted of a conventional complement fixation test where the inactivation of a limited amount of complement by erythrocytes coated with penicilloyl specific antibodies is taken as evidence for their complement fixing properties. The last method ought to be the most sensitive, since the disappearance of only one for example the first component of complement should be sufficient to render the test positive. Immunadherence occurs not before the fixation of the third component of complement and involves several steps in the reaction sequence whereas overt lysis of sensitized erythrocytes is only induced after all nine factors of the complement system have exerted their damaging action on the cell membrane.

The results are summarized in Table 5. Sera from patients with penicillin allergy and from rabbits immunized with various penicillins usually contain two types of antibodies with specificities as outlined above. They can be grouped according to their ability to mediate hemagglutination reactions as complete or incomplete antibodies, the latter being only detectable by means of an antiglobulin test.

Complete antibodies sediment in the ultracentrifuge with the 19s globulins and emerge from Sephadex G 200 columns in the first elution peak. These antibodies fix complement, they are heatstable but can be easily destroyed in whole serum or purified fractions by treatment with mercaptoethanol. They belong to the IgM class of immunoglobulins.

Incomplete antibodies proved to be resistant to treatment with mercaptoethanol, they emerged from Sephadex G 200 columns in the second elution peak,
sedimented in the ultracentrifuge with an S20 value of 7s. They belonged to the
IgG class of immunoglobulins as determined with H-chain specific antisera in the
anti-globulin-test. Antisera specific for the H-chains of IgM, IgG and IgA
immunoglobulins were used in this assay.

Table 5. *Physico-chemical properties of humoral anti-"penicillin"-antibodies*

Properties	Antibodies	
	Complete (A)	Incomplete (B)
Heat stability 56°, 30 min	+++	+++
2-mercapto-ethanol resistance (0.1 mol, pH 7.2)	O	+++
Complement fixation[a]		
a) CFR	+++	O
b) immunadherence	+++	O
c) hemolysis	+++	O
S^{20}_W	19 s	7 s
Immunoglobulin class	IgM	IgG

[a] CFR = Complement fixation reaction. For experimental
details see text.

4. Significance of Humoral Penicilloyl Specific Antibodies in Individuals Allergic Against Penicillin

The description presented above for penicilloyl specific IgM and IgG antibodies in the sera of patients allergic against penicillin is essentially in agreement
and complements observations of other investigators [9, 12, 22, 29, 30, 34]. It
seems doubtful whether these antibodies participate in the mediation of allergic
reactions. Absence of correlation between skin sensitivity and the presence of
humoral antibodies has often been noted [1, 10, 30, 39]. These antibodies certainly
indicate, that the animal or the patient has immunologically reacted against
determinants operative in penicillin allergy. Rabbits with high titers of penicilloyl
specific IgG antibodies can even develop severe Arthus reactions in the skin upon
injection of penicilloyl protein conjugates [13, 18, 47]. However the fact that IgM
and IgG antibodies in humans are very often associated with allergic manifestations against penicillin does not prove that these antibodies are actually mediators
of these hypersensitivity reactions.

We have followed the development of penicilloyl specific antibodies in six
luetic patients under treatment with high doses (1 mill. units of PGK/day
i.m.) of penicillin. Three of these patients apparently had low levels of anti-

bodies from earlier treatments with penicillin. But three patients developed penicilloyl specific complete and incomplete antibodies in considerable titers under therapy. Nevertheless none of these 6 patients showed signs of hypersensitivity against the drug upon skin testing and further treatment. This example can serve to illustrate the fact that an immune reaction with the production of IgM and IgG antibodies of penicilloyl specificity does not necessarily lead to an allergic state.

It appears that a special kind of antibody i.e. reagins must be present in the patients tissues in sufficient amounts to provoke signs of allergy after challenge and contact with the homologous antigen. According to the work of Ishizaka [12] immunoglobulins of the IgE class function as reagins. Reagins are not detected by the normal antiglobulin test which usually indicates antibodies of the IgG class. It seems possible to develop an antiglobulin test for the demonstration of reagins by means of IgE specific antisera [8].

5. Concluding Remarks

Our understanding of the mechanism leading to sensitization against penicillins has been greatly clarified by the detection of the penicilloyl group of penicillins as the major antigenic determinant [18, 25, 26, 42]. The penicilloylgroup seems to become attached to proteins by direct interaction of the penicillin molecule with free amino or other reactive groups of proteins. The lability of the β-lactam-ring certainly favors such a reaction. Lability of the β-lactam-ring on the other hand is also prerequisite for the antibiotic activity of the molecule. Penicillins interfere in the mucopeptide synthesis of the bacterial cell wall [36, 48]. Tipper and Strominger [36] have suggested that the antibiotic activity of the drug is due to its ability to form irreversibly a penicilloyl conjugate in the active center of an enzyme, a transpeptidase, which performes the last step in the synthesis of the cell wall mucopeptides by linking their free peptidechains. If this idea proves to be correct, if formation of penicilloyl conjugates is really the basis of the antibiotic activity of the drug, than the hope has to be abandoned that non-immunogenic penicillins will ever be found. For in this case antibiotic activity and immunogenicity would at one crucial point share the same molecular reaction.

Formation of penicilloyl determinants by direct coupling of penicillins to carrier molecules seems to be the way by which the complete antigen is formed in most cases of allergy against penicillin. However it should be kept in mind, that penicillin solutions may from the beginning contain high molecular weight penicilloyl conjugates and penicillin aggregates [4, 33] which by themselves may perhaps serve as sensitizers. Nevertheless for a number of reasons their role as sensitizers seems to be rather doubtful. Purified penicillin solutions appear to be just as mmunogenic as preparations, from which high molecular weight materials have not been removed.

However there is one point, already mentioned by Dr. DeWeck, which should be stressed. Penicillin aggregates and penicilloyl conjugates in penicillin solutions may serve as perfect *elicitors* of allergic reactions. It has been shown by DeWeck [46] that bivalent haptens very effectively elicite hypersensitivity reactions. Until recently it has been difficult to explain why sometimes anaphylactic reactions in individuals allergic against penicillin occur almost instantaneously after the injection of the drug. Native penicillin molecules in solution have to be regarded as monovalent haptens and should rather block than elicit a reaction. Haptenic inhibition of agglutination or precipitation reactions can in fact easily be shown with fresh penicillin solutions [18, 42, 47]. The knowledge however that aggregates occur in penicillin solutions which might serve as multivalent haptenic elicitors of allergic reactions leads us to understand why severe symptoms of hypersensitivity may sometimes develop within seconds after penicillin administration. Penicillin preparations in therapeutic use should be as free as possible of such unwanted substances.

Summary

Ten semisynthetic penicillins tested induced antibody formation in the rabbit. Twenty-three experimental semisynthetic penicillins were found to form penicilloyl derivatives with proteins in vitro. Immunogenicity appears to be an inherent property of natural and semisynthetic penicillins.

The sidechain of penicillins plays an important role in shaping the final specificity of anti-penicillin-antibodies. Absence of a sidechain or gross structural differences in sidechains can lead to antibodies with completely different specificities. However penicillins with structurally closely related penicillins induce cross-reacting antibodies.

In rabbits immunized with semisynthetic penicillins and in men allergic against penicillin antibodies of the IgM and IgG class of immunoglobulins could be demonstrated. The findings are discussed against the background of our knowledge on the pathogenesis of penicillin allergy.

References

1. Van Arsdel, P. P., Jr., A. P. Tobe, and L. J. Pasnik: Association of hemagglutinating antibodies with skin sensitivity in penicillin allergy. J. Allergy 34, 526—534 (1963).
2. Batchelor, F. R., J. M. Dewdney, and D. Gazzard: Penicillin allergy: the formation of the penicilloyl determinant. Nature (Lond.) 206, 362—364 (1965).
3. — —, R. D. Weston, and A. W. Wheeler: The immunogenicity of cephalosporin derivatives and their cross-reaction with penicillin. Immunology 10, 21—33 (1966).
4. — —, J. G. Feinberg, and R. D. Weston: A penicilloylated protein impurity as a source of allergy to benzylpenicillin and 6-aminopenicillanic acid. Lancet 1967, 1175—1177.
5. Brandriss, M. W., J. W. Smith, and H. G. Steinman: Immunologic cross-reactivities of three divers penicillins. Postgrad. med. J. 40, Suppl. 157—160 (1964).
6. Chisholm, D. R., A. R. Englisch, and N. A. MacLean: Immunological response of rabbits to 6-Aminopenicillanic acid. J. Allergy 32, 333—342 (1961).
7. Clayton, E. M., J. Altschuler, and J. R. Bove: Penicillin antibody as a cause of positive direct antiglobulin tests. Amer. J. clin. Path. 44, 648—653 (1965).
8. Coombs, R. R. A.: Detection and significance of membran antigens. Lecture: British council course on Immunology, Cambridge/England, 22. 3. 1968.
9. Fudenberg, H. H., and J. L. German: Certain physical and biological characteristics of penicillin antibody. Blood 15, 683—689 (1960).
10. Harris, J., and J. H. Vaughan: Immunologic reactions to penicillin. J. Allergy 32, 119—127 (1961).
11. Horiuchi, Y., and K. Shibata: Immunochemical studies on the antigenic bindings of benzyl penicillin and five synthetic penicillins with proteins. Int. Arch. Allergy 28, 306—320 (1965).

12. Ishizaka, K., T. Ishizaka, and M. Hornbrook: Physicochemical properties of reaginic antibody. V. Correlation of reaginic activity with γ-E-globulin antibody. J. Immunol. **97**, 840—853 (1966).

13. Josephson, A. S.: The development of antibodies to penicillin in rabbits. J. exp. Med. **111**, 611—620 (1960).

14. —, E. C. Franklin, and Z. Ovary: The characterization of antibodies to penicillin. J. clin. Invest. **41**, 588—593 (1962).

15. Kerp, L., u. H. Kasemir: Untersuchungen zur Antigenspezifität bei Arzneimittelallergien. Beiträge zur Inneren Medizin, pp. 261—269. Stuttgart: Schattauer 1964.

16. Levine, B. B.: Studies on the mechanism of the formation of the penicillin antigen. I. Delayed allergic cross-reactions among penicillin G and its degradation products. J. exp. Med. **112**, 1131—1154 (1960).

17. — Studies on the formation of the penicillin antigen. II. Some reactions of D-benzylpenicillenic acid in aqueous solution at pH 7.5. Arch. Biochem. **93**, 50—55 (1961).

18. —, and Z. Ovary: Studies on the mechanism of formation of penicillin antigen. III. The N-(D-α-benzyl-penicilloyl) group as antigenic determinant responsible for hypersensitivity to penicillin G. J. exp. Med. **114**, 875 (1961).

19. — N-(α-D-penicilloyl) amines as univalent hapten inhibitors of antibody-dependent allergic reactions to penicillin. J. med. pharm. Chem. **5**, 1025—1034 (1962).

20. — Immunochemical mechanisms involved in penicillin hypersensitivity in experimental animals and in human beings. Postgrad. med. J. **40**, Suppl. 146—152 (1964).

21. —, M. I. Fellner, and V. Levytska: Benzylpenicilloyl specific serumantibodies to penicillin in man. I. Development of a sensitive hemagglutination assay method and haptenic specificities of antibodies. J. Immunol. **96**, 707—718 (1966).

22. — — —, E. C. Franklin, and N. Alisberg: Benzylpenicilloyl-specific serum antibodies to penicillin in man. II. Sensitivity of the hemagglutination assay method, molecular classes of the antibodies detected and antibody titers of randomly selected patients. J. Immunol. **96**, 719—726 (1966).

23. —, and A. Redmond: Immunochemical mechanisms of penicillin induced coombs positivity and hemolytic anemia in man. Int. Arch. Allergy **21**, 594—606 (1967).

24. Ley, A. B., J. P. Harris, M. Brinkley, B. Liles, J. A. Jad, and A. Cahan: Circulating antibody directed against penicillin. Science **127**, 1118—1119 (1958).

25. Parker, C. W., J. Shapiro, M. Kern, and H. N. Eisen: Hypersensitivity to penicillenic acid derivatives in human beings with penicillin allergy. J. exp. Med. **115**, 821—838 (1962).

26. —, A. L. DeWeck, M. Kern, and H. N. Eisen: The preparation and some properties of penicillenic acid derivatives relevant to penicillin hypersensitivity. J. exp. Med. **115**, 803—819 (1962).

27. — The immunochemical basis for penicillin allergy. Postgrad. med. J. **40**, Suppl. 141—145 (1964).

28. Peterknecht, W., u. D. Falke: Immun-Adhärenz zum Nachweis virusspezifischer Antigene und Antikörper. I. Ausarbeitung der Methode mit Herpesvirus hominis and serologische Spezifität der Reaktion. Z. med. Mikrobiol. Immunol. **154**, 132—144 (1968).

29. Petz, L. D., and H. H. Fudenberg: Coombs-positive hemolytic anemia caused by penicillin administration. New Engl. J. Med. **274**, 171—177 (1966).

30. Schwartz, R. H., and J. H. Vaughan: Immunologic responsiveness of man to penicillin. J. Amer. med. Ass. **186**, 1151—1157 (1963).

31. Sever, J. L.: Application of a microtechnique to viral serological investigations. J. Immunol. **88**, 320—329 (1962).

32. Stavitsky, A. B.: Micromethods for the study of proteins and antibodies. I. Procedure and general application of hemagglutination and hemagglutination-inhibition reactions with tannic acid and proteintreated red blood cells. J. Immunol. **72**, 360—367 (1954).

33. Stewart, G. T.: Allergenic residues in penicillins. Lancet **1967**, 1177—1183.

34. Swanson, M. A., D. Chanmougan, and R. S. Schwartz: Immunohemolytic anemia due to antipenicillin antibodies. New Engl. J. Med. **274**, 178—181 (1966).

35. Thiel, J. A., Sh. Mitchell, and Ch. W. Parker: The specificity of hemagglutination reactions in human and experimental penicillin hypersensitivity. J. Allergy **35**, 399—424 (1964).

36. Tipper, D. J., and J. L. Strominger: Mechanism of action of penicillins: A proposal based on their structural similarity to acyl-D-alanyl-D-alanine. Proc. nat. Acad. Sci. (Wash.) **54**, 1133—1141 (1965).
37. Walter, A. M., u. L. Heilmeyer: Antibiotika-Fibel, 2. Aufl., pp. 117, 146—149. Stuttgart: Thieme 1965.
38. Watson, K. C., S. M. Joubert, and M. A. E. Bennett: Penicillin as antigen. Nature (Lond.) **183**, 468—469 (1959).
39. — — — Occurence of hemagglutinating antibody to penicillin. Immunology **3**, 1—10 (1960).
40. — Effect of various penicillin compounds on hemagglutination of penicillin-coated erythrocytes. Immunology **5**, 610—620 (1962).
41. De Weck, A. L., and H. N. Eisen: Some immunochemical properties of penicillenic acid. An antigenic determinant derived from penicillin. J. exp. Med. **112**, 1227—1247 (1960).
42. — Studies on penicillin hypersensitivity. I. The specificity of rabbit "Antipenicillin" antibodies. Int. Arch. Allergy **21**, 20—37 (1962).
43. — Studies on penicillin hypersensitivity. II. The role of the side chain in penicillin antigenicity. Int. Arch. Allergy **21**, 38—50 (1962).
44. — Penicillin allergy: its detection by improved hemagglutination technique. Nature (Lond.) **202**, 975—977 (1964).
45. —, and G. Blum: Recent clinical and immunological aspects of penicillin allergy. Int. Arch. Allergy **27**, 221—256 (1965).
46. — Comparison of the antigen's molecular properties required for elicitation of various types of allergic tissue damage. In: Immunopathology pp. 295—303 5th. Internat. Symp. Punta Ala/Italy, 1967. Basel: Schwabe u. Co. Publ. 1968.
47. Wellensiek, H. J., and H. P. Becker: Unpublished observations.
48. Wise, E. M., and J. T. Park: Penicillin: Its basic site of action as an inhibitor of a peptid cross-linking reaction in cell wall mucopeptide synthesis. Proc. nat. Acad. Sci. (Wash.) **54**, 75—81 (1965).
49. Zylka, W.: St. Franziskus Hospitals, Ehrenfeld, Cologne, West-Germany. Personal communication.

Priv.-D z. Dr. H. J. Wellensiek
Institut für Medizinische Mikrobiologie der
Universität Mainz, 65 Mainz, Langenbeckstraße 1

Discussion

DE WECK (Berne): Dr. Wellensiek has drawn attention to a very important point: the immunodominance of so large a determinant as the penicilloyl group and the direct reactivity of the β-lactam ring. We have for example prepared a dinitrophenyl penicillin which — not posessing an acyl side chain — is unable to form penicillanic acid. It does however induce anti-penicilloyl antibodies in the rabbit. — A further remark concerning the question about non-allergenic penicillins: We have attempted to prepare by ultrafiltration within 10 min a very pure penicillin and obtained the purest penicillin we have ever had. When this was tested immediately on highly sensitive patients no difference from commercial penicillin was found. Thus, there is not much hope that a non-allergenic penicillin may be obtained by purification only.

FREIS (Wuppertal): How can one explain the clinical finding of, for example, the different frequencies of skin reactions to penicillin G and ampicillin. In addition, it is always noted that skin reactions are more frequent in certain diseases. According to the studies of Patel [Pediatrics **40**, 910 (1967)] and Brown (Lancet

1967, 1418) as well as those by Pullen (Lancet **1967**, 1176; **1968**, 1090) in Mononucleosa infectiosa, for example, 65 to 100% of the patients show skin reactions.

WELLENSIEK (Mainz): Ampicillin is obviously the most potent allergen among the semi-synthetic penicillins. We do not know, whether Ampicillin functions as a better inducer or a better elicitor of hypersensitivity reactions as compared to other penicillins. In our animal experiments we have not seen essential differences in the immunizing qualities of various penicillins. It may however be worthwhile examining whether ampicillin solutions contain polymers such as Dr. De Weck has mentioned and which have recently been described by Batchelor et al. (Lancet **1967**, 1175). If it turns out, that ampicillin solutions contain polymeric aggregates more often and in greater amounts than other penicillins, the frequent occurrence of anaphylactic reactions following ampicillin therapy could easily be explained.

ROTHER (Freiburg): If complement-binding reactions are involved, the field of anaphylactic reactions has virtually been left. Do tissue lesions, known to depend on complement activity, such as arteriitis or nephritis, also occur in these patients ?

WELLENSIEK (Mainz): No, usually these patients merely have an urticaria. We examined the sera for haemagglutinating antibodies.

WESTPHAL (Freiburg): Is it possible to make penicillins in which the benzyl group is replaced by a long fatty acid ? Such penicillins would have an enormous surface activity and would be fixed on cell borders.

BAUER (Wuppertal): Penicillin K has a long fatty acid radical, but as far as I know, in Dr. Wellensiek's tests it cannot be differentiated from other penicillins.

DE WECK (Berne): There is proof that a conjugation takes place in vivo: using catalysers it is possible to hydrolyse penicillin completely. Once the β-lactam ring has been opened, anti-penicilloyl antibodies can no longer be produced.

WESTPHAL (Freiburg): Has penicillin greater affinity for the bacterium than for the serum proteins ? If one would allow the corresponding bacterial enzymes to compete with the serum protein, primarily a conjugation with the bacterial enzymes would occur.

DE WECK (Berne): We have tested this. There is no doubt that the affinity for the enzyme is stronger than the affinity for the serum or constituents of the serum. It is however possible to create in vitro conditions in which an antibody more easily conjugates with penicillin than with the bacterial enzyme.

WESTPHAL (Freiburg): To me it does not yet seem satisfactorily clarified whether a highly purified protein shows the same affinity. It would be important to know whether patients with a high anti-penicillin titre at the same time have antibodies against other proteins. This is the problem with fungicides: all cause allergy and on closer examination it is found that the antibodies are not only directed against the drug but also against the fungal protein.

21*

FISCHER (Hamburg): Can also in subliminal sensitisation against penicillin, i.e. when no clinical symptoms are present, the penicillin level decrease more rapidly as a result of such antibodies, and a pseudo-resistance be simulated ?

DE WECK (Berne): I don't think that this is possible.

AUHAGEN (Wuppertal): If an allergic urticaria occurs under ampicillin the treatment is often unhesitatingly continued. Normally the allergy disappears while ampicillin is continued. In this case one could say that with the vanishing of the bacteria the real antigen also vanishes.

DE WECK (Berne): A parallel to this is insulin allergy: in generalized urticaria to insulin the patient usually has only very few or barely any insulin binding antibodies in his serum. While the administration of insulin is continued insulin-binding IgG antibodies occur and the rash simultaneously disappears.

WESTPHAL (Freiburg): So one might even say that some antibiotics of the penicillin type, because of their ability to conjugate, are ideal for breaking tolerance. Maybe it is possible to break tolerances with other proteins. So to say one would make a virtue of necessity.

WELLENSIEK (Mainz): We allowed rabbit serum proteins to react with penicillin and purified the conjugates by sephadex filtration. Following the injection of these conjugates into rabbits antibodies possessing penicilloyl specificity appeared. In these experiments each rabbit received penicillin coupled to its own serum proteins. Such penicilloyl conjugates also occur in vivo in penicillin allergics. A few cases of Coomb's positive haemolytic anaemias have been described. In these cases it was possible to break up the erythrocyte-antibody complex and to show that penicilloyl determinants were actually situated on the erythrocytes. At the end of this discussion we should remember, that the penicillins belong to those antibiotics, which show the least side effects. Their high antibiotic potency is unsurpassed and guarantees their outstanding therapeutic value.

BOCK (Tübingen): This concordantia oppositorum gives me the opportunity for a concluding word. For 3 days now in training we have been searching information given by immune competent researchers and — lowering it to the harmless clinical level — have returned to scientific euphoria. We all are happy to have had this opportunity, we have gained very much, and the target of the symposium has been reached: a fruitful discussion between immuno-competent theorists and us clinicians who regrettably often enough feel our incompetence at the bedside. If you ask when we shall have searched it all, I would tell to the Bayer laboratories that a completely uncertain number of such symposia are still needed. Hereby I heartily thank the organisers.

Subject Index